WATER AND ELECTROLYTES IN PEDIATRICS

Physiology, Pathophysiology and Treatment

LAURENCE FINBERG, M.D.

Professor and Chairman
Department of Pediatrics
State University of New York
  Downstate Medical Center
Brooklyn, New York

RICHARD E. KRAVATH, M.D.

Associate Professor
Department of Pediatrics
Montefiore Hospital and Medical Center
Albert Einstein College of Medicine
of Yeshiva University
Bronx, New York

ALAN R. FLEISCHMAN, M.D.

Assistant Professor
Department of Pediatrics
Montefiore Hospital and Medical Center
Albert Einstein College of Medicine
of Yeshiva University
Bronx, New York

With a contribution by PAUL SAENGER, M.D.

1982

W. B. SAUNDERS COMPANY

Philadelphia   London   Toronto   Mexico City   Rio de Janeiro   Sydney   Tokyo

W. B. Saunders Company: West Washington Square
Philadelphia, PA   19105

1 St. Anne's Road
Eastbourne, East Sussex BN21 3UN, England

1 Goldthorne Avenue
Toronto, Ontario M8Z 5T9, Canada

Apartado 26370 – Cedro 512
Mexico 4, D.F., Mexico

Rua Coronel Cabrita, 8
Sao Cristovao Caixa Postal 21176
Rio de Janeiro, Brazil

9 Waltham Street
Artarmon, N.S.W. 2064, Australia

Ichibancho, Central Bldg., 22-1 Ichibancho
Chiyoda-Ku, Tokyo 102, Japan

Library of Congress Cataloging in Publication Data

Finberg, Laurence.

Water and electrolytes in pediatrics.

1. Water-electrolyte imbalances in children.   I. Kravath,
   Richard.   II. Fleischman, Alan.   III. Title.

RJ399.W35F56   618.92'007   81–40736

ISBN 0–7216–3625–X   AACR2

Water and Electrolytes in Pediatrics: ISBN   0-7216-3625-X
Physiology, Pathophysiology and Treatment

Last digit is the print number: 9   8   7   6   5   4   3   2   1

HAROLD E. HARRISON

Premier pediatrician, scientist, teacher, friend

Preface

The course of scientific application to clinical medicine may be said to move along the sequence from basic physical scientist to basic biologic scientist to clinical scientist to bedside clinician. These designations are arbitrary and overlap considerably. No one person in the 1980s will be expert in all these roles or proficient in more than two of them. The electrolyte physiologist–clinician will need to know, in depth, something from each of these areas of knowledge.

The form and balance of this volume reflect the particular mixture we believe to be needed. The varying length and emphasis of the chapters, as well as the extent of documentation, indicate our bias toward the importance of the topics to pediatrics, not necessarily to other branches of medicine. Other books cover information on electrolytes in encyclopedic depth but with different emphases and often with little reference to children.

We attempt in this work to bring together in one volume all subject matter of immediate relevance to water and electrolyte issues in infancy and childhood. Perhaps no other group of concepts and facts has applicability to so many clinical problems—common and uncommon, simple and complex. The literature currently presents such material in texts on general physiology, human physiology, pediatrics, adult electrolyte physiology and therapy, and, finally, in several monographs stressing therapy for children. The effort here combines these perspectives within a pediatric and physiologic historical framework culminating in a clinical, therapeutic section setting forth our biases. We intend to be comprehensive in subjects discussed, although not encyclopedic, in that for the most part only the historically and clinically relevant literature plus some contributions defining known limits will be cited. So many excellent books in renal physiology and kidney disease now exist that we have not treated these subjects in detail here.

The theoretic and pathophysiologic sections are as objective as we could make them, and they are documented with the seminal literature. The clinical section is interpretive and represents the way the authors implement the concepts presented in the other sections. We recognize that others do things a bit differently and probably as well. For simplicity, we have not cited all such approaches, since fundamentally the schemes (the thoughtful ones at least) vary only in nuance and not in substance.

The book is divided into four parts covering, in order, underlying principles, pathophysiology, diagnosis and management of dehydration in general, and the specific disorders encountered in pediatrics. For the student at any stage of career pursuing scholarly knowledge in the field, all parts (plus, indeed, collateral reading) are intended and recommended. For the medical student, the pediatric resident, and for all clinicians caring for children, Part I may well be skimmed, Part II read for refreshment of understanding, and Part III used as a clinical how-to-do-it manual for the treatment of dehydration, particularly that secondary to enteric disease. Specific disorders and techniques are discussed separately in Part IV. They may be referred to individually as the clinical need or the itch of curiosity impels. The appendixes will be of use to the tyro and the history buff. A number of general references are listed at the end of the introduction as well as at the close of some chapters, for course leaders and for those who wish to delve deeper into the science of electrolyte physiology. The clinical expert should find it desirable to have this particular compendium of information in a single volume that is useful as an aid for teaching in courses and seminars.

The authors have worked together over the past 18 years at the Montefiore Hospital and Medical Center and its New York Municipal Hospital affiliate (first Morrisania City Hospital, later the North Central Bronx Hospital). This close association should reduce some of the unevenness characteristic of multi-authored books, perhaps at the expense of a narrower viewpoint. The senior author has edited all the chapters and must take responsibility for any inconsistencies and redundancies.

We wish to express our gratitude to our students for polishing our presentations through the years, and we wish also to thank those who have deciphered handwritings and oral sounds into manuscript form. Mrs. Emmy Brown deserves our particular appreciation. The staff at W. B. Saunders— Al Meier, Mary Cowell, Rebecca Don, and Robert Butler—have been superb in getting the manuscript produced. In a personal note I acknowledge the contribution of my wife, Harriet, for her encouragement, her forebearance, and her indulgence, without which this book would not have happened.

October 1981

Laurence Finberg, M.D.

Contents

Chapter 1
Introduction 1
Laurence Finberg, M.D.

PART I
PHYSICAL, CHEMICAL, AND PHYSIOLOGIC FACTORS
AFFECTING BODY FLUIDS

Chapter 2
Properties of Water, Ions, Solutions, and Cells 5
Laurence Finberg, M.D.

Chapter 3
Composition—Chemical Anatomy 11
Laurence Finberg, M.D.

Chapter 4
Water Metabolism and Regulation 17
Laurence Finberg, M.D.

Chapter 5
Circulatory and Renal Effects on Regulation 23
Richard E. Kravath, M.D.

Chapter 6
Blood Gases, Hydrogen Ion, and pH... 35
Richard E. Kravath, M.D.

Chapter 7
Sodium, Potassium, and Chloride Ions: Metabolism
  and Regulation.. 56
Laurence Finberg, M.D.

Chapter 8
Calcium, Phosphorus, and Magnesium: Metabolism
  and Regulation.. 62
Alan R. Fleischman, M.D.

Chapter 9
Organic Molecules in Extracellular Fluid: Effects
  on Physiology 71
Laurence Finberg, M.D.

PART II
PATHOPHYSIOLOGY AND PATHOLOGY OF FLUID
DISTURBANCES: CLINICAL UNDERSTANDING

Chapter 10
Isotonic and Hyponatremic Dehydration 73
Laurence Finberg, M.D.

Chapter 11
Hypernatremic Dehydration.. 78
Laurence Finberg, M.D.

Chapter 12
Pathophysiology of Hydrogen Ion Disturbance 91
Richard E. Kravath, M.D.

Chapter 13
Pathophysiology of Edema, with a Note on the Mode
of Action of Diuretics.. 108
Laurence Finberg, M.D.

Chapter 14
Pathophysiology of Hyponatremic States 112
Laurence Finberg, M.D.

PART III
CLINICAL IMPLEMENTATION: DIAGNOSIS, ASSESSMENT,
AND TREATMENT OF DEHYDRATION

Chapter 15
Clinical Evaluation of Dehydration... 115
Laurence Finberg, M.D.

Chapter 16
Therapy of Dehydration Resulting from Gastrointestinal
Fluid Loss 121
Laurence Finberg, M.D.

Chapter 17
Therapeutic Management of Hypernatremic Dehydration 129
Laurence Finberg, M.D.

Chapter 18
Interpretations of Laboratory Analyses 136
Laurence Finberg, M.D.

Chapter 19
Solutions and Techniques... 141
Richard E. Kravath, M.D.

PART IV
SPECIFIC DISORDERS OF WATER AND MINERAL
   METABOLISM—RECOGNITION, PREVENTION,
   AND MANAGEMENT

Chapter 20
Diarrheal Disease of Infancy.. 147
   Laurence Finberg, M.D.

Chapter 21
Malnutrition: Marasmus and Kwashiorkor.. 158
   Laurence Finberg, M.D.

Chapter 22
Therapy of Hydration Problems in Renal Disorders............................. 163
   Laurence Finberg, M.D.

Chapter 23
Problems of the Central Nervous System: Anatomic and
   Physiologic Review 167
   Laurence Finberg, M.D.

Chapter 24
Disorders of the Adrenal Gland as Causes of Electrolyte
   Disturbances: Diagnosis and Treatment................................... 171
   Paul Saenger, M.D.

Chapter 25
Heart Failure 186
   Richard E. Kravath, M.D.

Chapter 26
Problems in Liver Failure... 193
   Laurence Finberg, M.D.

Chapter 27
Diabetes Mellitus 195
   Laurence Finberg, M.D.

Chapter 28
Metabolic Disorders Affecting Water and Electrolytes........................ 198
   Laurence Finberg, M.D.

Chapter 29
Electrolyte Problems and Poisonings: Salicylates
   and Phosphates 201
   Laurence Finberg, M.D.

Chapter 30
Asthma 206
   Richard E. Kravath, M.D.

Chapter 31

Cystic Fibrosis 212
  Richard E. Kravath, M.D.

Chapter 32

Sports and Exercise.. 217
  Richard E. Kravath, M.D.

Chapter 33

Special Problems of the Fetus and Neonate..................................... 220
  Alan R. Fleischman, M.D.

Chapter 34

Special Problems of Surgical Patients, Including
  Parenteral Nutrition.. 226
  Alan R. Fleischman, M.D.

Appendix I

Definitional Glossary.. 233
  Laurence Finberg, M.D.

Appendix II

Time Line.. 241
  Laurence Finberg, M.D.

INDEX 245

Chapter 1

INTRODUCTION

Our purpose is to present knowledge bearing on water and mineral metabolism as this subject relates to infants and children. The intersection among physical chemistry, mammalian physiology, and pediatrics is the territory to be covered. Theory and therapy are as related as cause and effect. Knowledge leads not just to implementation but to further knowledge. Thus, consideration of the fundamentals as we now perceive them must precede clinical considerations for the serious student. This concept underlies the organization of what follows. New knowledge as it appears will modify that set forth here, perhaps substantially. Nonetheless, what we now know enables us to accomplish much in clinical settings that was not possible a century ago and that is measurably better than what was possible even a few decades ago.

Clinical disorders of fluid and mineral metabolism, regardless of etiology, are disturbances in physiology. Restoring patients with such disturbances to an optimal state may often be accomplished when it is impossible to combat or even identify etiology. Such correction may be life-saving and life-preserving — sufficient justification, then, for mastery. When etiology is known, specific measures and preventive measures are always in order when feasible. In this exposition, however, we shall pursue the restoration of physiologic homeostasis as the therapeutic goal, recognizing that most of what is perceived as illness is, in fact, disordered physiology or biochemistry.

Three continuing themes influence the subject at hand and the flow of this book: first, the evolutionary processes that set the biologic stage; second, the scientific and clinical histories of our knowledge of water and electrolytes; and, finally, the pe-

diatrician's special province — the study of the influence of growth on electrolyte and water metabolism. Phylogeny will be mentioned, history will be introduced and then recapitulated in an appendix, and growth and development will be introduced in this section and will then permeate the entire text. This last is our principal justification for this book devoted to infants and children.

EVOLUTION AND COMPARATIVE PHYSIOLOGY

The beginnings of life as we know it depend entirely on the presence of water as a solvent. The unique features of this substance will be described in Chapter 2. Suffice it to say here that when life began, approximately two billion years ago, the solvent of the fluid medium of the cell and the cell's surrounding milieu were water. Current understanding of physicogeologic events indicates that the primeval sea was very close in concentration and composition to the extracellular fluid of all living organisms. The modern sea has a similar composition, but its concentrations are roughly fourfold greater, as water separated from the salt by evaporation and returning in rainfall constitutes the fresh water sources of present-day earth.

Probably the inorganic solute profile of both the cell fluid (intracellular) and that sea within us (the extracellular fluid, or ECF) was set from the very beginnings of living things. Single-cell organisms in the sea began the process. Multiple-cell organisms incorporated the sea as ECF. From that point on, over eons, the pattern remained constant as, in addition, specialized

1

cells, tissues, and organs appeared, were modified, and either disappeared or persisted. The evolutionary development of a circulatory system and a complex excretory system had major impact on the method of maintenance of composition of the ECF. Other changes included the adaptations to hyper- and hypo-osmotic watery environments and to terrestrial living. Throughout, the principal relationships of the body fluids were sustained. Experiments on the fluid compartments of various vertebrates show few differences from one species to another, since thermodynamic influences are universal and since ion and water movements are seldom affected by an enzyme change. Interested readers who wish to pursue comparative vertebrate physiology in greater depth are referred to the excellent review by Schmidt-Nielson and Mackay.[1]

HISTORY OF THE DEVELOPMENT OF HUMAN ELECTROLYTE PHYSIOLOGY AND FLUID THERAPY

Four types of historical perspective may be said to bear on the understanding we have achieved to the present. These include the observations of problems in distant times, the development of the physical science underpinnings on which biologic science rests, the contributions of physiologists and clinician-physiologists, and, finally, the innovations and syntheses of the "activist" clinicians, which moved us to our present practices.

The giving of water to quench thirst or to restore dehydrated individuals has both physiologic and intuitive roots. Subhuman species will seek water and drink in response to the thirst produced by fluid loss. The most primitive humans surely recognized the need for fluid when ill, and it seems certain that the ancient physicians, by whatever name, prescribed various fluids for dehydrated patients to drink. The earliest recorded awareness of diarrheal disease is found in the writings of the ancient Greeks, particularly Hippocrates.[2] There are also writings in the Talmud recognizing the effects of diarrheal disease and the wisdom of oral fluid therapy.[3] In more nearly modern times, Benjamin Rush, physician and politician of the American Revolution, contributed a detailed description of an outbreak of an epidemic of diarrheal disease in infants.[4]

The important contributions of chemists and physiologic chemists include the recognition of osmosis by Nollet and later van't Hoff, and the understanding of ionization by Arrhenius and of thermodynamic therapy and principles by J. W. Gibbs, with the subsequent contributions by L. J. Henderson to the understanding of acid-base balance and by Donald Van Slyke to measurement of the substances involved in these phenomena.[*]

Among the physiologic contributions of note, perhaps the earliest is that of a sixteenth century experimentalist, Sanctorius, who demonstrated the existence of insensible water loss.[5] The concept of parenteral fluid therapy for replacement of enteric losses was put forth by O'Shaughnessy in 1831.[6] Carl Schmidt, in 1850,[7] provided extensive analyses of human blood and several other fluids, establishing a broad base for understanding. Nine years later Claude Bernard[8] produced his classic description of the *milieu intérieur.*

In the first part of the twentieth century, pediatricians were particularly productive in advancing in the field of electrolyte physiology and therapy. Howland and Marriot[9] and, almost simultaneously, Schloss[10] described acidosis as a consequence of dehydration. In the second quarter of the century, the leading contributors to the field were James L. Gamble, John P. Peters, and Daniel C. Darrow, two of them pediatricians. Following just the pediatric scientists into the mid–twentieth century, we find Alan Butler, R. E. Cooke, H. E. Harrison, Malcolm Holliday, William Segar, William Wallace, William B. Weil, and Robert Winters. Many others contributed as well. All but one of this last group are still alive (in 1981) and adding to our understanding.

Finally, we have the activists. It is reported that in the seventeenth century the first blood transfusion was given by Denys in France.[11] In 1832, Thomas Latta, a physician in Edinburgh who had read O'Shaughnessy's letter to *The Lancet* of a few months before, attempted replacement therapy in dehydrated victims of cholera.[12] Choosing only those patients who were surely going to die, he saved 8 of 16. Although a few other intrepid physicians followed his lead

---

[*]More information on specific contributions noted in this chapter without citation may be found in Appendix II.

with similar success, the conservative profession of his time denounced this innovation and fluid therapy ceased for another sixty years. It was pediatricians in the early twentieth century who were largely responsible for reviving it. In 1926, a master clinician, Grover Powers,[13] then professor of pediatrics at Yale, acted as a clinical synthesizer of the information thus far gathered. He put forth a comprehensive plan of therapy that formed the basis of therapy for several decades thereafter. The modern approach is a moderate evolution from his plan. In Appendix II of this volume, the historical perspective is set forth in greater detail, with all four types of contributors represented. It should be understood that a number of individuals made more than one kind of contribution. In modern times this is especially true, and the boundaries may now be seen as rather artificial.

INTERRELATIONSHIPS BETWEEN ELECTROLYTE PHYSIOLOGY AND GROWTH AND DEVELOPMENT

The human infant and child differ in many ways from the mature adult. Among these are differences in physiology, which are crucial for the understanding and especially for the management of problems that result from disorders of mineral and water metabolism. These include differences in composition, in metabolic turnover, and in the degree of maturity of the regulating systems.

One can trace differences in chemical anatomy, starting with the viable fetus and proceeding through the newborn infant, the child, and finally the adult. The fetus and newborn infant have an appreciably larger water content than is present later. This is due in part to less fat and in part to the greater proportion of the body mass that is taken up by visceral organs in relation to muscle mass in the fetus and newborn infant.

Muscle tissue accounts for about 60 per cent of the cellular mass of the human after the first months of life. Thus, muscle tissue dominates the calculation for both total water and water in the various body spaces. The differences in the immature organism, however, must be remembered in dealing with newborn infants, especially those born prematurely. At a later age, severe undernutrition may produce a pattern more like that of the fetus and newborn infant than that of the older infant or child.

The skeleton obviously occupies a lesser proportion of the mass of the very young child than of the older child or adult. This, too, has importance in considerations of physiology and therapy. Several constituents of the plasma undergo changes during growth and development. An important example of this is the phosphate concentration, which is very high during the neonatal period, falls gradually during infancy, stabilizes during childhood, and then falls again after puberty. The foregoing are but some of the examples of compositional changes important for clinical assessment and care.

The metabolic turnover of water in particular differs strikingly in the infant from that in the older child and adult. The teaching of this phenomenon was one of the particular contributions of Darrow.[14] In fact, the very high rate of water turnover — about fivefold on a weight basis — for the infant compared to the adult is what makes infants and younger children so vulnerable to illnesses that produce dehydration. This, in turn, is what surely stimulated the very strong interest of pediatricians in this clinical field, particularly in the period from 1910 to 1950.

The third influence of growth and development is found in the differential rates of maturation for the various physiologic regulatory systems of the body. Thus, renal immaturity helps to determine the plasma composition in infants, which is different from that in older children. Similarly, endocrine, gastrointestinal, and pulmonary maturation, separately and together, influence composition, metabolism, and the vulnerability of infants to changes brought by diseases affecting water and mineral balance.

The foregoing form the *raison d'être* for this volume; the matters relating to growth and development recur throughout the chapters that follow.

REFERENCES

1. Schmidt-Nielson BM, Mackay WC: Comparative physiology of electrolyte and water regulation. *In* Maxwell MH, Kleeman CR (eds): Clinical Disorders of Fluid and Electrolyte Metabolism, Chapter 2. McGraw-Hill, New York, 1979.
2. Adams F: The Genuine Works of Hippocrates, Vol I, pp 167, 219; Vol II, p 217. William Wood, New York, 1886. Cited in reference 3.
3. Kramer B, Kanof A: Diarrhea in children. A historical review. J Pediatr 57:769, 1960.

4. Rush B: An inquiry into cause and cure of cholera infantum. *In* Medical Inquiries and Observations, Vol I. Thomas Dobson, Philadelphia, 1794, pp 159–169.

5. Cited by Pratt EL: Presidential address, Society for Pediatric Research, Am J Dis Child 96:419, 1958.

6. O'Shaughnessy WB: Experiments on blood in cholera. Lancet 1:490, 1831–32.

7. Schmidt C: Charakteristik der epidemischen Cholera gegenüber verwandten Transsudationsanomalieen. G. A. Rehyer, Leipzig, 1850.

8. Bernard C: Introduction to the Study of Experimental Medicine (1859), trans HC Greene. Harry Shuman, Inc., New York, 1949.

9. Howland J, Marriot WM: Acidosis occurring with diarrhea. Am J Dis Child 11:309, 1916.

10. Schloss OM, Stetson RE: Occurrence of acidosis with diarrhea. Am J Dis Child 13:218, 1917.

11. Cited in Smith HL: Historical notes on parenteral fluid therapy of diarrhea in infants. J Pediatr 57:611, 1960.

12. Latta T: Letter to Secretary of Central Board of Health, London, Affording View of Rationale and Results of His Practice in Treatment of Cholera and Saline Injections. Lancet 2:274, 1831–32.

13. Powers GF: A comprehensive plan of treatment for the so-called intestinal intoxication of infants. Am J Dis Child 32:232, 1926.

14. Darrow DC: The significance of body size. Am J Dis Child 98:416, 1959.

GENERAL REFERENCES

Andreoli TE, Grantham JJ, Rector FC (eds): Disturbances in Body Fluid Osmolality. American Physiological Society. Williams & Wilkins, Baltimore, 1977.

Comar CL, Bronner F (eds): Mineral Metabolism: An Advanced Treatise, 3 vols. Academic Press, New York, 1960–1969.

Davson H: A textbook of General Physiology, 4th Ed. Williams & Wilkins, Baltimore, 1970.

Dick DAT: Cell Water. Butterworths, Washington, 1966.

Maxwell MH, Kleeman CR (eds): Clinical Disorders of Fluid and Electrolyte Metabolism. McGraw-Hill, New York, 1979.

Strauss MB: Body Water in Man. Little, Brown, Boston, 1957.

Widdowson EM, Dickerson JWT: Chemical composition of the body. In Comar CL, Bronner F (eds): Mineral Metabolism: An Advanced Treatise, Vol II, Part A, p 1. Academic Press, New York, 1964.

Wolf AV: Thirst. Charles C Thomas, Springfield IL, 1958.

Physical, Chemical, and Physiologic Factors Affecting Body Fluids

Chapter 2

PROPERTIES OF WATER, IONS, SOLUTIONS, AND CELLS

The underlying physical sciences on which biology rests have to be understood before any comprehension in depth can be attained by the student. The purpose of this chapter is to review briefly the most important concepts that are used regularly in considering problems of water and electrolytes. We shall assume that the reader has a level of understanding of physical chemistry at least equal to that of the entering medical student. Thus, we will not review in this chapter such concepts as atomic weights, atomic structure, the gas laws, or the principles of mass action. For those who want to refresh their memories of such definitions, Appendix I will be helpful. For those who wish a more detailed analysis, the references at the end of this chapter plus the general references at the end of Chapter 1 will provide deeper insights.

STRUCTURE AND PROPERTIES OF WATER

Water, the universal solvent, is an extraordinary substance, having properties that seemingly make it the unique solvent for living things. L. J. Henderson noted this in his landmark publication. *The Fitness of the Environment*, in 1913.[1] To quote him, "The following properties appear to be extraordinarily, often uniquely, suited to a mechanism which must be complex, durable, and dependent on a constant metabolism: heat capacity, heat conductivity, expansion on cooling near the freezing point, density of ice, heat of fusion, heat of vaporization, vapor tension, freezing point, solvent power, dielectric constant and ionizing power, and surface tension." Henderson wrote this before modern understanding of the structure of water had been achieved; his observations proved prescient.

There are two basic features of the arrangement of the water molecule. The three atoms do not lie in a straight line: two hydrogen atoms are bonded to the oxygen atom so that the O–H bonds are at an angle of 105° to one another. The second feature is that the electrical charge is not evenly distributed. A partial transfer of the electrons in the formation of the molecule leaves the hydrogen atoms with a strong positive charge and the oxygen atom with a strong negative charge. From this structure, in turn, come two important properties. First, the water has a dipole moment and thus tends to orient itself in an electrical field. The four pairs of electrons in water occupy four orbits, which extend tetrahedrally from the oxygen atom. Two pairs are associated with the O–H bonds. The other two pairs are called the "lone pairs." This asymmetry accounts for the dipole moment and is responsible for the electrostatic interaction between water molecules and ions.

Second, water molecules tend to stick together by forming hydrogen bonds. The formation of a hydrogen bond is due to the interaction of the "lone pair" electrons of one water molecule with the protons of a second water molecule. This property leads to the formation of a tetrahedral lattice. This occurs in liquid water as it does in ice, and it gives water some unique properties as a solvent. Thus, in the liquid state, water molecules form a structured lattice into which crystalloid charged ions may displace successive water dipoles and move rapidly.

Another property of the structure of the water molecule is its high dielectric constant (78.5 at 25° C). This means that water reduces the intensity of an external electric field. A reduced electrical field or reduced electrostatic attraction between the pairs of oppositely charged ions (e.g., Na^+ and Cl^-) to $1/78$ of their original field allows the ions to separate sufficiently to move independently. Once the electrostatic attraction is lowered, Brownian and thermal motions of the ions make each behave like an independent molecule.

At any given moment, one of the two protons possessing thermal energy may (and frequently will) leave the water molecule to which it is attached and latch on to a neighboring molecule, producing a hydroxyl (OH^-) ion and a hydroxonium (H_3O^+) ion.

Re-combination of these two ions takes place equally readily.

One liter of water contains 55.5 moles of water, of which on the average only 1 in 555 million *molecules* is dissociated. It takes 10.5 Kcal of energy per mole to remove a water molecule from the pure liquid.[2] Water molecules have an effective radius of less than 0.15 nm and they tumble rapidly. Furthermore, they diffuse rapidly, taking 10 psec to diffuse their own length.

In protein solutions the arrangements are more complex because of the binding of water on the surface of the protein. For some reactions this phenomenon will undoubtedly prove to be important. For the kinds of problems that are of interest to clinicians, the model of cells as leaky containers of a solution of proteins, nucleic acids, and numerous small molecules continues to be useful and (for our purposes) accurate for explaining the effects of disturbances and of therapeutic repair.

Thermodynamics and Chemical Potential

The universal first two laws of thermodynamics govern what happens in solutions. Within major subgroups of living things, such as all vertebrates, among which there is anatomic similarity for the fluid compartment, it is not surprising that there is little species difference in homeostatic mechanisms and responses to disorders. These thermodynamic mechanisms are quite unlike the more complex biochemical changes that depend on the presence of enzymes, enzyme kinetics, and other complex features. This enables the physiologist to do experiments with a variety of species with considerable confidence that the results will be applicable to all.

It is useful, particularly in doing research and in describing the more detailed aspects of salt and water behavior, to speak in rigorous terms of concentrations and gradients that are based on thermodynamic considerations. For this purpose we would like to introduce here the concept of referring to a substance, solvent or solute, in terms of its chemical potential or mole fraction. Chinard stated this with particular clarity:

Consider a system comprising several phases with water a constituent of each phase.

Each phase can be characterized by its pressure P, its temperature T, its volume V, and its chemical composition (expressed in terms of the mole fractions of the several constituents). Equilibrium with respect to water obtains when there is no mass transfer of water among the several phases. Molecular *exchanges* of water take place in and out of each phase at equal rates though the values of P, T, V, and composition may differ for different phases. With these molecular exchanges taking place at equal rates it may be considered that the average energy available per molecule of water is the same in the different phases. At equilibrium with respect to water the chemical potentials of water in all the phases is the same. If equilibrium does not obtain with respect to water, there will be mass transfer of water between the phases provided a pathway is available; molecular exchanges occur at unequal rates between the phases; the chemical potentials of water are not equal. The mass transfer occurs from the phase or phases where the average energy or chemical potential of water is higher to the phase or phases where the chemical potential of water is lower. Experimentally, it is found that mass transfer may occur when there are differences between the phases in the values of one of the variables, P, T, or chemical composition. These variables, therefore, determine the relative values of the chemical potential of water in the several phases.[3]

To amplify a bit further, we will refer to the colligative (or "bound together") properties of a solution, i.e., osmotic pressure, freezing point depression, boiling point elevation, and vapor-pressure depression. All of these relate to the chemical potential of the species of molecule. To make it easier to understand, we will use *molal* and *osmolal* (not *molar* or *osmolar*) concentrations throughout, since this expresses the quantity of solute per kilogram of solvent (water). In practice, in medical problems the differences are usually, although not always, small.

IONS AND EQUILIBRIA

Since the time of Arrhenius it has been understood that salts dissociated into water solutions are called ions. In dilute solutions (such as those under consideration) the dissociation of electrolyte molecules is virtually complete. Ions travel with a shell of hydrating water molecules, details of which are omitted here. A solution will remain, overall, electrically neutral, although there may be polarized regions. For our purposes, however, body fluids seem to be electrically neutral and obey what may be called the law of electroneutrality, even though potential differences are found on boundaries.

When an electrolyte dissolves in water, the ions will substitute for a water molecule in the tetrahedral lattice. This substitution leads to changes in the water lattice. Since the ion is a monopole rather than a dipole, its electrostatic field will interact with the dipole moment of the water molecules and tend to rotate two of the four adjacent water molecules. Carrying this thought further, the aqueous electrolyte solution may be regarded as a liquid crystal of variable composition.[4]

An *equilibrium state* is one in which composition remains constant with nothing entering or leaving the system. *Steady state*, on the other hand, describes a constant composition with concentration maintained by entry of, and simultaneous equivalent egress of, one or more constituents.

Diffusion

Diffusion is the process by which dissolved particles move by molecular energy through solvent along a gradient from higher concentration to lower concentration. In dilute solutions, ions diffuse rapidly through water. Diffusion is easily expressed quantitatively by Fick's law, which relates the water diffusion to concentration and an area of a plane across which the diffusion is occurring. Numerical values of the rate of diffusion of a species of molecules vary with the size and concentration of the molecules and can be expressed by a coefficient of diffusion. The solute moves from regions of high chemical potential to areas of lower chemical potential until, at equilibrium, the chemical potential of the substance is everywhere equal. Later in this chapter, under Permeability and Transport, some special kinds of diffusion will be discussed further.

Membranes

Our current notion is that, structurally, a cell membrane is a lipid bilayer into which globular protein molecules are embedded in single leaflets or which the protein molecules sometimes traverse. Cell membranes have the property of being permeable to some solutes, slightly permeable to others, and relatively impermeable to still others. The semipermeable nature (or selective impermeability) of membranes was discovered long before modern understanding of the chemical composition of membranes was achieved. For our purposes here, the important property is semipermeability, although we will come back to the permeability of membranes in other contexts.

Osmosis

It was discovered long ago that if a semipermeable membrane separating two solutions is impermeable to the solute on one side only, then water moves toward the side containing that solute until hydrostatic pressure counterbalances the movement and produces an equilibrium. This osmotic pressure, one of the colligative properties referred to earlier, represents a hydrostatic pressure difference — the chemical potentials of water in the two compartments having become equal. This may be expressed mathematically by $\pi = CRT$, where π is the osmotic pressure, C the molal concentration of the solute, R the gas constant, and T the absolute temperature. This is sometimes referred to as van't Hoff's law.

Of particular interest in problems of water and mineral metabolism is the fact that when two solutions are separated by a membrane impermeable to an ion, such as protein, on one side only, the opportunity for developing hydrostatic pressure does not exist. What happens instead is an asymmetric distribution of the particles. If we use sodium and chloride ions together with a negatively charged, nondiffusible ion, for example, then the chloride ions on the side without the nondiffusible ion will have a higher concentration than the chloride ions on the side with the nondiffusible ion. The reverse will be true of sodium ions, with the concentration less on the side without the nondiffusible ion.

Mathematically, this relationship at equilibration can be expressed

$$\frac{Cl_1}{Cl_2} = \frac{Na_2}{Na_1}.$$

The degree of difference in a given system can be determined experimentally for the interface between the blood plasma and the interstitial fluid across the capillary membrane. The experimentally determined vari-

ation can be expressed numerically. This number, known as the Donnan factor, is approximately 0.95 for sodium and other cations. This means that if the concentrations of sodium and chloride on the plasma side are known, multiplying the sodium concentration by this factor and dividing the chloride (or other diffusible anion) level by the same factor gives the concentrations on the interstitial fluid side. The foregoing is referred to as the Gibbs-Donnan equilibrium, Donnan having worked out the mathematical implications of Gibbs's thermodynamic laws. For this particular illustration, it should be remembered that the concentrations of sodium and chloride usually expressed by a clinical laboratory are the concentrations in the total volume of serum or plasma and not the chemically active concentrations, which would have to be expressed as molal concentrations in the serum water. Thus, in addition to the calculation for osmosis, a correction for the solid phase of serum must be made by dividing both concentrations by approximately 0.93 or 0.94, depending on the actual protein concentration. It should be noted further that the osmolal concentration of a substance refers to the number of particles of that substance per weight of solvent and is quite independent of any pressure that might develop, since a concentration exists without a semipermeable membrane and a balancing pressure cannot.

If the valence of small crystalloid electrolyte ions is 1, then milliequivalents and milliosmols are identical. If the valence is 2, then the milliequivalent value will be twice the milliosmolar value. Very high molecular weight substances like proteins may have a very high electrical valence but make a minute contribution to the osmolal concentration. For example, the protein content of blood plasma contributes up to -16 mEq but only 1 or 2 mOsm. In mixed solutions, not all electrolyte ions will continue to diffuse freely. Some may become bound either to each other or, especially, to protein molecules. In the event of such binding, the osmolal concentration is accordingly reduced.

PERMEABILITY AND TRANSPORT

As can be gathered from the previous discussion, various solutes are capable of penetrating biologic membranes. Details of this are too complex for presentation here. Suffice it to say that there is variability in the rate of penetration. One particular set of relationships, however, is important to describe in some detail — that is the pressure and osmotic relationships across blood capillaries. Water and electrolytes move freely across the capillary membrane. Protein molecules, although contributing only a tiny portion of the osmolal concentration, are relatively nondiffusible and therefore act to pull water toward the capillary lumen. The hydrostatic pressure at the arterial end of the capillary is about 37 mm Hg. At the venous end of the capillary it falls to 15 mm Hg. Oncotic pressure (as it is called) inherent in plasma protein can be expressed in the same units. It is about 25 mm Hg, which is the height of the column that would be supported if the appropriate experimental apparatus were employed. From the difference between the pressures at either end of the capillary, one can see that water will be pushed out from the arterial end, where hydrostatic exceeds oncotic pressure, to some midpoint of the capillary, and that water molecules will tend to be pulled in from that midpoint to the venous side, where oncotic pressure is greater. This state of affairs was first appreciated and described by Starling[5] (see Fig. 5–1).

Because protein concentrations in plasma may vary, especially in disease, it is sometimes useful to be able to estimate oncotic pressure from the measured concentrations of plasma protein. The following values express this relationship approximately:

albumin   1 g/dl = 5.5 mm Hg
globulin   1 g/dl = 1.4 mm Hg

Transport of ions and other substances in biologic systems occurs in several ways. The simplest type involves two fluids separated by a membrane; diffusion is influenced by the diffusion characteristics of the substance and the permeability characteristics of the membrane. Diffusion in this system is bidirectional until equilibrium is achieved, with equal chemical potentials of solvent and solute on both sides. This is referred to as a passive process, since it takes no input of energy from a living organism. The rate of diffusion is proportional to the concentration gradient over the range of dilute solution concentrations found in biology.

A second type of transport is called *facilitated diffusion*. This occurs when some type of molecule in the membrane has a chemical affinity for the solute. This molecule is called a carrier molecule, and it preferentially binds with and so enables the solute to move to the other side more rapidly than by simple diffusion. This type of transport is also passive and, like simple diffusion, is therefore unable to move solute against a concentration gradient. Since there are a limited number of carrier molecules, the system will show the characteristics of saturation phenomena as the concentration increases — that is, once the binding sites are all taken, the initial, more rapid rate of diffusion (more than simple diffusion) slows in a curvilinear fashion.

Finally, there is *active transport*, which is unlike the previous types in that the substance can be transported against an electrochemical concentration gradient. For charged particles, the electrical as well as the chemical aspect is important. For uncharged particles, we need speak only of the concentration gradient. This type of transport requires energy from the living organism, since work must be done to move solute thermodynamically "uphill," i.e., to a higher chemical potential.

THE MAINTENANCE OF BODY FLUID SPACES

We have already alluded to the difference between concentrations of substances in the plasma and in the fluid that bathes the capillaries (called interstitial fluid). The principal determinants are the concentration of plasma proteins, particularly the smaller ones such as albumin, and the hydrostatic forces of blood pressure and tissue pressure described by Starling.

The boundary between cells and the interstitial fluid is highly asymmetric. In the interstitial fluid, as shown in Figure 2–1, there are predominantly sodium and chloride ions. Inside the cell (using the muscle cell as the example) the solutes are predominantly potassium, magnesium, and phosphate ions along with protein and other organic molecules.

Clearly, this asymmetry has to be maintained by some sort of process. The precise mechanism is still somewhat controversial, and some workers believe that purely physical factors determine the ionic distribution

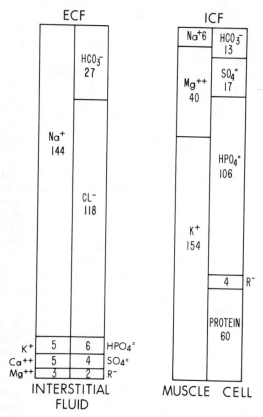

Figure 2–1. Ionic profiles of body fluids: contrast between interstitial fluid and intracellular fluid. The difference between total charges is explained in the text. The concentrations assigned are from a range of normal values.

numbers of water molecules until the cell membrane burst. Thus, the boundary between the interstitial fluid and the cell determines the volume of each in accordance with the amount of sodium that is present. The laws of thermodynamics and the processes of diffusion require that the water concentration, or osmolality, be everywhere equal. The law of electroneutrality requires equal numbers of positive and negative charges on each side. Thus, the asymmetry of the profiles of adjacent body fluid solutes, shown in Figure 2–1, are sustained.

The concept of *coupled transport* has also proved to be of some importance in electrolyte physiology. This occurs when two particles cross a membrane together in enhancement of what either of them will do alone. In particular, sodium couples with organic solutes such as glucose and amino acids in crossing a number of membranes, including the small intestine. Obviously, an anion must also accompany the sodium.

Another type of coupling has been called *solvent drag*, in which water is coupled with solute. This was first described by Anderson and Ussing,[7] who noted that when certain solutes are transported across membranes, there is an accelerated flow of water accompanying the solutes. It is thought that this movement occurs primarily in intercellular spaces.[8]

by binding ions and water to the cell protein.[6] This hypothesis, called the association-induction hypothesis, includes the feature of accepting that the hydration shell of ions determines some of their chemical characteristics in movement through pores and in binding with cell proteins. Most workers, however, believe that the asymmetric composition results from an active transport system. The molecular basis for this is thought to be the enzyme sodium/potassium ATPase, which is found in all cell membranes. The essential purpose of this transport system, which is also sometimes called the "sodium pump," is to move sodium ions from the cell water, actively exchanging sodium ions for potassium ions. This enables the cell to maintain its volume, for otherwise its high nondiffusible molecule content would attract unlimited

REFERENCES

1. Henderson LJ: The Fitness of the Environment. The Macmillan Co., 1913.
2. Kuntz ID, Zipp A: Water in biological systems. New Engl J Med 297:262, 1977.
3. Chinard P: Colligative properties. J Chem Educ 32:377, 1955.
4. Podolsky RJ: The structure of water and electrolyte solutions. Circulation 21:818, 1960.
5. Starling EH: On the absorption of fluids from the connective tissue spaces. J Physiol 19:312, 1896.
6. Ling GN: A Physical Theory of the Living State: The Association-Induction Hypothesis. Blaisdell Publishing Co., New York, 1962.
7. Anderson B, Ussing HH: Solvent drag on nonelectrolytes during osmotic flow through isolated toad skin and its response to ADH. Acta Physiol Scand 39:228, 1957.
8. Ussing HH: Effects of ADH in transport paths in toad skin. In Ussing HH, Thorm NA (eds): Transport Mechanisms in Epithelia (Alfred Benzon Symposium V), p 11. Marksgaard, Copenhagen, 1973.

Chapter 3

COMPOSITION — CHEMICAL ANATOMY

Composition and turnover are the two key elements in understanding body water and mineral balance. In this chapter, the first of these will be considered. After stating our present knowledge, we shall examine the methodologies by which that knowledge has been achieved, indicating gaps and uncertainties as well as working definitions useful for clinical purposes. Each of the body fluids of interest, as well as the interrelationships among them, will then be described. Figure 3–1 illustrates in a diagrammatic way the current concept of the distribution of body water and solids in a fat-free infant, which differs somewhat from that in a fetus, a newborn, or a chemically mature human.

Chemical maturity in terms of body space distribution is reached at a chronologic age of 3 years. From that point through at least middle adult life, there is little change in body water and its distribution as functions of the lean body mass (LBM). Fat deposited in the adipose tissue has little water associated with it and, of course, represents a considerable variable when comparing the weight or mass of one person to another. At maturity, the water content of the human is approximately 70 per cent of the LBM (60 per cent of normal body weight). This figure (70 per cent of LBM) is reasonable for infants after the newborn period as well. The newborn infant has about 5 per cent more water. The fetus has appreciably more, and the young embryo consists of perhaps 95 per cent water. The first physiologic division of body water is into two compartments, with cell walls forming the boundary. Water that is in cells is referred to, with its solute, as

intracellular fluid. In the infant this amounts to about 45 per cent of the LBM. At chemical maturity, it is more like 50 per cent of the LBM. The extracellular water in the infant accounts for about 25 per cent of the

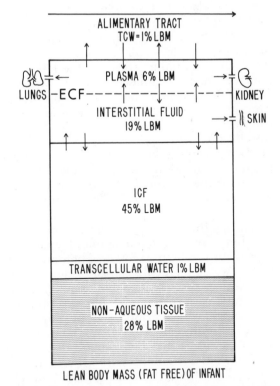

LEAN BODY MASS (FAT FREE) OF INFANT

Figure 3–1. Diagram of body fluids in the infant as a proportion of the lean body mass (LBM), showing the rapid movement of water molecules (arrows) among compartments. Part of the transcellular water (TCW) is in the alimentary tract, part is in the urinary tract, and part comprises inaccessible cartilage and bone water. The cerebrospinal fluid (about 4 ml/kg in infants, 140 ml in adults) is included here in the interstitial fluid. ECF = extracellular fluid; ICF = intracellular fluid.

11

LBM. At chemical maturity, somewhere between 20 and 23 per cent of the LBM may be allocated to the extracellular fluid, depending somewhat on assignment of subcompartments, as will be discussed later.

Within the extracellular fluid there is an extremely important subcompartment —the vascular fluid, or *plasma*. The volume of plasma at all ages is approximately 6 per cent of the LBM. This leaves the other compartment of the extracellular fluid, the interstitial fluid, at about 19 per cent of LBM in infants. Water in the lumen of the gastrointestinal tract and in the urinary tract is considered physiologically outside the body. Fluids in these tracts, along with some others, are sometimes referred to as *transcellular water*. At most, 2 to 2½ per cent of the LBM consists of transcellular water. These concepts will be discussed later in this chapter.

It is easily recognized, of course, that the composition of the animal body represents a steady-state system in which there is continuous intake of water and other substances through the gastrointestinal tract and continuous loss and excretion of water and excretory products through the kidney, skin, and lungs. The mechanisms by which the individual compartments maintain their integrity with respect to volume and content have been touched upon in the previous chapter.

Before proceeding, it is worth calling attention to an additional important characteristic of the various body compartments. With significant exception (e.g., the urinary bladder), water flows freely and quickly among all the various compartments and, therefore, except at the moment of a pathologic disturbance, the chemical potential of all the water molecules is the same. This means that the solute concentration expressed in milliosmols per kilogram (mOsm/kg) will be identical or moving toward identity at all times. The implication of this is that the osmotic distribution space of any solute within the body is always the volume of the entire body water.

The most important example of this concerns sodium and chloride ions. The body's sodium chloride, as we shall see later on, is largely (and necessarily) extracellularly located. If one adds sodium chloride without water to the extracellular fluid, even though the ions added will remain essentially with the extracellular fluid, the addition of the salt will influence all the major body water compartments, because water will move by osmosis to equalize the osmolal concentrations. Thus, if one wishes, for example, to calculate the amount of sodium it takes to raise the extracellular concentration of sodium by 10 mEq/l, one has to determine how much sodium is needed to raise the concentration that much in a volume equal to 70 per cent of the LBM, not in the smaller volume (25 per cent of LBM) that represents the actual sodium distribution. It is clear that this action, if the salt is added with minimal water, will sharply redistribute a significant volume of water from the intracellular fluid to the extracellular fluid. This calculation, of course, presumes an almost instantaneous action, which does not allow for excretion of sodium and water. Conversely, if one adds water without solute to the system, fluids in all the compartments will be diluted. However, because of the particular role played by sodium and chloride, excess water, while retained, will be distributed proportionately, with the largest quantity entering the ICF.

In the discussion that follows, the chemical anatomy of the aqueous portions of the body is described. First, however, some consideration will be given to the ways in which body fluids may be analyzed, since some of these methods must be indirect.

Methodology

There are four types of methodologies applicable to studying the chemical anatomy of the human. Two of these involve whole carcass and tissue analyses as the most direct possible approaches for determining water content. A number of humans of varying ages have been analyzed this way, and the results have been summarized by Widdowson and Dickerson.[1] Because of the general similarity among mammalian species, many more analyses have been carried out on laboratory animals. Most of the results of these analyses may be satisfactorily transferred to humans, at least mature humans. The third technique involves chemical analysis by means of biopsies of muscle tissue, since muscle tissue is the dominant cellular mass of the body. The specimen may be dried to constant weight, giving a total water content, and then a variety of chemical techniques can be applied to analyze the mineral content.[2, 3, 4] The most recent of these studies has been neutron analysis.[5] Finally, many studies have been carried out by injecting a substance and measuring its degree of dilution. Depending on the distribution of the substance, one can then calculate and appropriate space. These methods have been used to approximate total body water, extracellular fluid, and intracellular fluid. Each of these is discussed briefly here. For a more extensive treatment of methodology, the reader is referred to the review by Widdowson and Dickerson.[1]

Total Body Water. As already indicated, total body water (TBW) can be determined by drying a tissue specimen to constant weight or, in a living whole subject, by the dilution technique. Although a variety of agents have been used in dilution studies, probably the most satisfactory is deuterium oxide, D_2O.[6] Tritium may also be used but has the disadvantage, for human work, of being radioactive.

The calculation for the TBW or any other "space," physiologic or not, into which a substance is distributed, is as follows:

$$V = \frac{A - E}{C}$$

where V is the volume into which test substance has diffused at equilibrium; A is the amount of substance administered; E is the amount of substance excreted in urine during equilibration; and C is the concentration of substance in body water (or a portion of it) after equilibration, measured in serum or plasma and corrected to a molal value.

From about the second week of life, total body water remains approximately 70 to 72 per cent of the LBM.[7]

Extracellular Fluid. The extracellular fluid (ECF) has been estimated by a variety of dilution techniques, which include techniques using halides (either stable or radioactive), thiocyanate, thiosulfate, and radioactive sulfate[8] in addition to complex polysaccharides such as inulin.[9] These various substances are distributed somewhat differently, in terms of both distribution space and time of penetration. Inulin and sulfate spaces tend to be somewhat smaller than thiocyanate or bromide spaces. There are several reasons for this. The ECF, in fact, has several subcompartments: One, already referred to, is the plasma. Another is the interstitial fluid, which, for our considerations, includes the lymph and a fairly large volume of water bathing tissues. All the molecules of this fluid are rapidly exchanging with plasma. There is also a slower exchanging fluid in the tendons and the dense connective tissue in cartilage; it is at least partially in a gel state, accounting for the slow exchange and sometimes the accumulation of certain ions. Finally, there is transcellular water, which, although not part of the ECF, exchanges readily with it. The various difficulties of estimating ECF seem more formidable than they actually are, because several of the substances used give values very close to one another and the reasons for the differences are generally known.

The alternative way to estimate ECF is by tissue biopsy and analysis, preferably of muscle tissue.[3, 10] Tissue should be made as free of blood as possible. In the experimental animal this is easily accomplished by exsanguination preceding the biopsy. In the living human, it is desirable to remove as much blood from the biopsy specimen as possible. A simultaneous specimen of plasma is obtained so that the chloride and other substances under investigation can be measured in that fluid as well as in the whole tissue. Since the chloride ion is totally excluded from muscle cell water, at least in the order of magnitude of measurement under consideration, one can use these analyses and calculation to determine the distribution of the water between ECF and intracellular fluid. The water content of both the muscle and plasma can be ascertained by drying to constant weight. Fat is extracted, and the concentration of chloride in plasma and in the remaining muscle tissue can be determined. The concentration of chloride in the interstitial fluid can then be calculated from the plasma concentration by correcting for the water content of the plasma and by the Donnan factor. Since the interstitial fluid chloride represents all the chloride in the muscle and since the concentration of the interstitial fluid is known, the volume can be readily calculated. This volume represents the ECF or, more precisely, the chloride space.[3]

As noted above, there is water in tendon and cartilage that is part of the ECF that exchanges slowly. The amount is relatively small, and for clinical purposes at least it is not very important to take it into account. There are some specialized fluids in the central nervous system, the eye, and the joints that exchange readily with the ECF and that will be discussed below.

Intracellular Fluid. There is no good direct method for estimating the volume of intracellular fluid (ICF); therefore, it is calculated by subtracting the ECF from total body water or total tissue water, as the case may be.

COMPOSITION OF INDIVIDUAL FLUIDS

The composition of the three principal fluids of importance in clinical medicine is shown in Figure 3–2. The diagrams are arranged to stress electroneutrality. Therefore, the anion and cation compartments are identical in height. It should be recognized that electric charge and number of particles may diverge so that the osmolal contribution is not necessarily the same as the concentration expressed in milliequivalents. For univalent ions, the two measurements are the same.

On the other hand, in the *plasma* the large protein molecules contribute anywhere from 10 to 16 negative charges, (mEq) but only 1.5 to 2 mOsm/kg of water. This plasma protein is responsible for the oncotic pressure, since the capillary membrane is relatively impermeable to these molecules, whereas all the other substances shown diffuse readily. There are usually

about 4 to 4.5 gm of albumin in each deciliter of plasma. Each gram of albumin contributes about 5.5 mm Hg of potential oncotic pressure. The globulin content of plasma contributes only about 1.4 mm Hg/gm. When a disorder alters the plasma protein concentration, plasma volume will adjust accordingly. Other factors important in determining the final volume include the arterial blood pressure and the tissue back-pressure produced by the elasticity of the tissues. These two factors are dynamic and adjustable, making possible a wide variety of volumes under varying circumstances. In practical terms, when the albumin concentration is 2.5 gm/dl, there is a balance point at which plasma volume may be lost. Below this level, the loss will be continuous; above it, the compartment will usually be well sustained. The foregoing is a useful if somewhat oversimplified description. Plasma volume may be measured directly by the dilution method described previously, using a dye (Evans Blue, T1824) or a radioactive tag on a protein molecule.[6]

Clinicians customarily deal with electrolyte and other substances as reported from clinical laboratories that have analyzed plasma or, more commonly, serum. The reporting from these laboratories is in milliequivalents per liter (mEq/l), millimoles per liter (mmol/l), or milligrams per deciliter (mg/dl), depending on the substance. The volume referred to is the whole fluid including the solids. As discussed earlier, the chemical and physical activity is accurately reflected in the molal or mol fraction

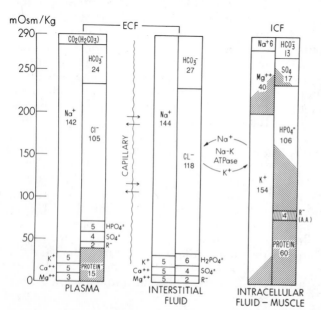

Figure 3–2. Ionic profiles of body fluids: approximate representation of cations and anions of the three principal body fluid compartments. All are electrically neutral and all have the same osmolality despite differences in total charges. The shaded areas represent large molecules or bound ions whose osmolal contribution (mOsm/kg) is quantitatively much less than their electric charge (mEq/kg) but which are of great importance to the distribution of ions because of their impermeability.

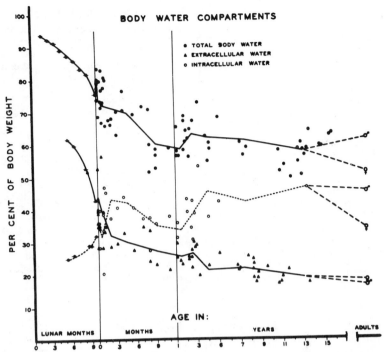

Figure 3–3. Total body water, extracellular water, and intracellular water as percentages of body weight in infants and children, compared to corresponding values for the fetus and adults. (From Friis-Hansen BJ: Body water compartments in children. Pediatrics 28:171, 1961. Copyright © 1961 American Academy of Pediatrics. Used with permission.)

related to a volume of water, which, in fact, is what the analytic instrument measures. The numbers are different but not ordinarily a problem in clinical work, because the whole scale is proportionate. When, for research or for other reasons, highly accurate calculations are required, it is necessary to correct the numerical values, first by measurement of serum (plasma) solids (or water content) and then by calculation, including use of the Donnan factor, discussed in Chapter 2. In the clinical portion of this book, the familiar clinical notation and measurement terminology will be used.

The *interstitial fluid* is essentially protein-free; the concentration of electrolytes in it thus reflects the Gibbs-Donnan effect when compared to that in plasma. A few specialized tissues having modified interstitial fluids should be mentioned. The cerebrospinal fluid (CSF) and the fluids in the eye are not true transudates but rather exhibit the influence of a secretory process. Thus, in the CSF, potassium concentration is lower than in the interstitial fluid and magnesium is higher. Over most concentration ranges, sodium and chloride concentrations, on the other hand, are very close, if not identical, to their interstitial fluid concentrations. Synovial fluid contains considerable hyaluronic acid. This makes it a mucopolysaccharide-protein gel. The water

therein can be properly thought of as part of the interstitial fluid, although the exchange rate is slow and the ionic distribution may vary. The quantity of this fluid is apparently small; it is seldom of clinical significance in electrolyte problems.

The interstitial fluid volume shows change with age from fetal to neonatal life, to infancy, and finally to chemical maturity at the age of approximately 3 years. At birth, perhaps 22 per cent of the LBM is interstitial fluid. By 3 years of age, it is down to roughly 15 per cent of the LBM. There are not enough data on intermediate points to establish whether the change is linear or exponential. There is no difference between the sexes in this respect, and, in general, human muscle tissue is similar to the muscle tissue of most mammals.[4] Data from Friis-Hansen[7, 11] are displayed in Figure 3–3 and Table 3–1.

The profile of the intracellular fluid of muscle shown in Figure 3–2 is characterized by an absence of chloride and a small amount of intracellular sodium. As noted earlier, the mechanism for sustaining this composition and, indeed, cell volume as well is thought to be the active transport of sodium from the cell to the interstitial fluid. The transport process, sometimes referred to as the sodium pump, involves the sodium-potassium–dependent form of the en-

Table 3–1. Distribution of Body Water Between Extracellular and
Intracellular Fluid as a Percentage of Body Weight

Age	Total Water	Extra-cellular Water	Intra-cellular Water	Extracellular Water / Intracellular Water
0–1 day	79	43.9	35.1	1.25
1–10 days	74	39.7	34.3	1.14
1–3 months	72.3	32.2	40.1	0.80
3–6 months	70.1	30.1	40	0.75
6–12 months	60.4	27.4	33	0.83
1–2 years	58.7	25.6	33.1	0.77
2–3 years	63.5	26.7	36.8	0.73
3–5 years	62.2	21.4	40.8	0.52
5–10 years	61.5	22	39.5	0.56
10–16 years	58	18.7	39.3	0.48

Compiled by L Finberg from the data of BJ Friis-Hansen (Acta Paediatr Scand 110(Suppl), 1958), using the volume of distribution of deuterium oxide for total body water and of thiosulfate for extracellular water. Intracellular water is obtained by subtracting the average of extracellular water from total body water. From Maxwell MH, Kleeman CR: Clinical Disorders of Fluid and Electrolyte Metabolism, 3rd Ed. New York, McGraw-Hill, 1979, Chapter 30. Reprinted with permission.

zyme ATPase. This enzyme, fueled by phosphate-bond energy, extrudes sodium, allowing potassium to accumulate in the cell. Sodium extrusion takes water molecules from the cell, preventing excessive cell swelling, which might otherwise occur because of the nondiffusible protein and complex phosphate molecules. The anions within the cell are in part determined by attraction to the protein, so cell content is essentially free of chloride. In other cells of the body — for example, the red cell and the cells of the gastric mucosa — there is a considerable concentration of chloride ion. In terms of mass, however, their total is small, and most cells of the body are generally similar to the muscle cell.

Some work has been done on the electrolyte content of the organelles, particularly the mitochrondria.[12] For example, although the profile in Figure 3–2 shows no calcium content for muscle cell water, the mitochondria are capable of accumulating considerable calcium and phosphorus.[13] It remains true, nonetheless, that there is no millimolar order of magnitude for the concentration of calcium in muscle cell water.

REFERENCES

1. Widdowson EM, Dickerson JWT: Chemical composition of the body. In Comar CL, Bronner F (eds): Mineral Metabolism: An Advanced Treatise, Vol II, Part A, p 1. Academic Press, New York, 1964.
2. Bergstrom J: Muscle electrolytes in man. Scan J Clin Lab Invest 14:1, 1962.
3. Harrison HE, Finberg L, Fleischman E: Disturbances of ionic equilibrium of intracellular and extracellular electrolytes in patients with tuberculosis meningitis. J Clin Invest 31:300, 1952.
4. Elliot DA, Cheek DB: Muscle electrolyte patterns during growth. In Cheek DB (ed): Human Growth. Lea & Febiger, Philadelphia, 1968, p. 260.
5. Dubois J: Water and electrolyte content of human skeletal muscle: variations with age. Rev Eur Etudes Clin Biol 17:595, 1972.
6. Edelman IS, Olney JM, James AH, et al: Body composition studies in the human being by the dilution principle. Science 115:447, 1952.
7. Friis-Hansen BJ: Body water compartments in children. Pediatrics 28:169, 1961.
8. Barratt TM, Wilson M: Extracellular fluid in individual tissues and in whole animals: the distribution of radiosulfate and radiobromide. J Clin Invest 48:56, 1969.
9. Schwartz JL: Measurement of extracellular fluid by means of a constant infusion technique without collection of urine. Am J Phys 160:526, 1950.
10. Flear CTG, Carpenter RG, Florence I: Variability in the water, sodium, potassium and chloride content of human skeletal muscle. J Clin Pathol 18:74, 1965.
11. Friis-Hansen BJ: Changes in body water compartments during growth. Acta Paediatr Scand 110 (Suppl), 1958.
12. Tarr JS, Gamble JL Jr.: Osmotically active space in mitochondria. Am J Phys 211:1187, 1966.
13. Mathews JL, Martin JH: Intracellular transport of calcium and its relationship to homeostasis and mineralization. Am J Med 50:589, 1971.

Chapter 4

WATER METABOLISM REGULATION

Water turnover is the second fundamental consideration in dealing with clinical disorders of hydration. Obviously, daily water replacements exist because there are daily water losses. Losses of water are secondary to heat production. Most of the energy expended by humans eventually becomes heat, which in turn is lost to environment. For homothermic animals such as mammals, heat production in a temperate climate is necessary and must be appropriately balanced by heat loss to maintain a constant body temperature, usually above that of the environment. In normal humans, body temperature is approximately $37°$ C $\pm 1°$ C. The balance between heat production and heat loss is a function of both mass and surface area. An implication of this relationship is the fact that, for each unit of mass, the human infant will have to produce much more heat than the adult to balance the losses, because the infant's surface area–to-mass ratio is about fivefold that of the adult.

Because of the foregoing relationship, it is possible to think of metabolic heat and water loss in terms of either energy expended directly or surface area. At the present time there is no simple way for clinicians to measure either caloric expenditure or surface area. We will here choose to express metabolic water losses in terms of energy expended rather than surface area. It seems to us that this stresses the fundamental relationship. If there is marked obesity or edema, surface area considerations become inaccurate. Furthermore, surface area estimation does not work without qualification in the newborn infant immediately following birth, because of metabolic differences at that time of life. Otherwise, the systems are interchangeable.

The unit of energy that we will use is the Calorie. There has been a recent tendency by specialists in mensuration and terminology to standardize all measurements and, in this case, to substitute the joule; but we will here, at least, retain the more traditional unit, believing that it will be many years, if ever, before such nomenclature change will occur (1 Kcal equals 4.19 Kjoules). The Calorie referred to here is the "large Calorie," or kilocalorie, which equals one thousand of the calories used by physicists. This enables nutritionists and physiologists to use smaller numbers in describing heat units of interest to them. Henceforth in this book when we refer to *calories* (cal), we will always mean the large Calorie, or kilocalorie, even though the unit will not be capitalized.

The source of energy for mammals is, of course, the diet. Only four kinds of substances are utilizable by humans for energy; namely, protein, fat, carbohydrate, and alcohol. Although different species of each of these general categories have slightly different caloric potentials per unit mass, in general it may be said that fat supplies about 9 cal per gram, protein and carbohydrate 4.1 cal per gram, and alcohol about 6 cal per gram. It is important to realize that, in the fasting state, the body draws on its stores of carbohydrates, protein, and fat, in that order, to provide the minimal work and necessary heat of basal metabolism. When the patient is eating, owing to intermediary metabolism some additional obligatory heat, independent of useful energy, is produced immediately following digestion and absorption, which is referred to as the specific dynamic action. Presumably, this develops because of the inefficiency of conservation of energy in metabolizing amino acids. Although the final pathways for energy involve either glucose or fat, protein participates through gluconeogenesis and through ongoing tissue breakdown. This will be referred to again, because consumption and breakdown of protein is always associated with excretory products removable only through urine.

OBLIGATORY WATER LOSSES

The obligatory water losses following the expenditure of energy may be divided into three categories: insensible water loss, urine production, and losses in the stool. All these losses are ongoing at a state of rest. Table 4–1 shows the values for basal caloric expenditure and consequent water loss over the various age ranges including adult life. It is not difficult to remember three or four points and to interpolate between them.

Metabolism has as its major end products carbon dioxide and water. This "water of oxidation" is produced at the rate of 12 ml/100 cal metabolized. In assessing problems of hydration this water must be remembered, particularly when long-term maintenance fluids are being given. As can be seen in the table, metabolic turnover differences extend from birth to postpuberty, unlike the compositional considerations discussed in the previous chapter.

Insensible water loss is water lost by evaporation through the interstices of the skin and by the exhalation of water vapor through the lungs. It is not to be confused with sweating, which is an active process that is not ongoing in most conditions in a temperate atmosphere. The phenomenon of insensible water loss has been known since the sixteenth century, but it was not until the late nineteenth and early twentieth centuries that calorimeter measurements were made by Lusk[1] and Dubois,[2] giving a precise definition of the phenomenon.[1,2] Since that time, though sophistication of instrumentation has increased markedly, the results of experimental determination have remained very close to those of Dubois. Various observers have placed the quantity of water lost at basal conditions of room temperature and humidity between 42 and 48 ml/100 cal metabolized (expended). We shall use the figure 45 ml/100 cal expended in calculations and estimates throughout. At basal conditions, 30 ml (per 100 cal expended) is lost through the skin and 15 ml is lost in the exhaled air. In abnormal states, insensible increases from the skin are proportional to caloric expenditure modified by ambient humidity. Abnormal ventilation, on the other hand, may triple the water loss from the lungs independently of energy expenditure. An increase in body temperature from 1° C over basal conditions increases calories expended by 13 per cent.[2] It should be noted that when body temperature decreases by 1.5° C, heat production (and evaporation loss) increases owing to shivering. Special conditions have to be evaluated in the light of their various physiologic implications and known physical-chemical laws.

Water loss in the urine is also obligatory. The end products of protein breakdown are small nitrogeneous products, chiefly urea. Either the conversion of protein foods or tissue breakdown will cause the associated mineral salts to be added to body fluids. The function of the kidney is to maintain homeostasis by very close regu-

Table 4–1. Basal Caloric Expenditure for Infants and Children*

AGE	WEIGHT (KG)	SURFACE AREA (M²)	CALORIC EXPENDITURE (CAL/KG)
Newborn	2.5–4	0.2–0.23	50
1 week–6 months	3–8	0.2–0.35	65–70
6–12 months	8–12	0.35–0.45	50–60
1–2 years	10–15	0.45–0.55	45–50
2–5 years	15–20	0.6–0.7	45
5–10 years	20–35	0.7–1.1	40–45
10–16 years	35–60	1.5–1.7	25–40
Adult	70	1.75	15–20

*Water expenditure equals 1 ml/cal

lation of the composition of the extracellular fluid. Therefore, the excess concentration over normal for both urea and minerals will be removed in the urine when it is present in the body fluids. Protein breakdown occurs to some extent under almost all conditions so that there is always an endogenous supply of solute requiring excretion.

The mammalian kidney can excrete only liquid urine and that within a fixed range of solute concentrations. For the human being, the range is from approximately 60 to 1400 mOsm/kg. This capacity of the kidney to do the osmotic work of concentration or dilution is important as a protection against disturbances in hydration, although somewhat less for the human than for most other mammals. For the physiologist or clinician, it is useful to do calculations for the repair of dehydration as though the urine to be produced will have approximately the same solute concentration as do the normal body fluids. This gives a factor of safety of over fourfold for the urine volume when the patient has maximal concentrating ability. On the other hand, any water given beyond the patient's absolute need is easily excreted, owing to the kidney's capacity for dilution. In doing calculations we shall assume for the purpose of estimation that the urine formed will have a concentration of from 250 to 300 mOsm/kg. Estimated in this way, obligatory urinary losses will be approximately 50 ml/100 cal expended.

Stool water for elimination occurs even in the fasting state from secretions into the gastrointestinal tract. In health, these losses are small, averaging around 5 ml/100 cal expended. The sum of the three obligatory routes of water loss then equals 100 ml/100 cal expended, or 1 ml/cal expended.

It is important to call attention to the fact that this ongoing water loss related to heat expenditure will occur over all conditions of health and disease. Note that we refer to calories expended rather than calories ingested or absorbed. Excess calories ingested may result in deposition of fat, which does not cause heat loss or water expenditure.

Table 4–1 contains the values determined experimentally for various ages at *basal* conditions. The clinician must also know what to do when the conditions are not basal. Among these conditions are those involving changes in environmental temperature and humidity, changes in body temperature, changes in ventilation volume per minute, and changes in muscular activity. These features increase what we have referred to as the obligatory water loss and in turn are largely dependent on energy expenditure. They are to be distinguished from *abnormal water losses* such as those found in diarrhea, polyuria, sweating, and others. Suffice it to say here that the ordinary patient in a hospital bed, with normal body temperature, rate of ventilation, and physical activity, who has a low energy intake through a diet consisting mainly of carbohydrate, will expend about one and one-half times the basal number of calories.

ABNORMAL WATER LOSSES

In addition to the obligatory water losses, abnormal water losses induced by diseases or unusual environmental conditions should be given some consideration here. These losses are not necessarily related to caloric expenditure. It has already been indicated that an increase in ventilatory rate and depth may triple the rate of water loss in the exhaled vapor. The usual water loss by this route is 15 ml/100 cal expended. It is clear that hyperventilation as induced by disease such as pneumonia or by drug action such as that of toxic levels of salicylate may cause as much as 45 ml/100 cal to be lost.

The amount of water vapor lost is affected by the humidity of the environment in which the patient is placed. Low humidity increases and high humidity decreases water loss. Supersaturated, ambient air at or near body temperature can actually result in the uptake of water through the lungs.

Sweating cools the body by increasing the amount of water evaporated. Under usual circumstances, about 20 ml of sweat is formed per 100 cal of heat production induced by disease or such events as exercise. At an environmental temperature of 34° C, sweat is about 90 ml/100 cal.[3]

The gastrointestinal tract is the site of water ingestion and also, under conditions of disease, a place where abnormal water losses may occur. Certain intestinal disorders — e.g., that induced by the cholera bacillus through its toxin — induce a secretory diarrhea in which the loss of water may be enormous, up to 30 per cent or more of the body weight per day. Vomiting is a symptom that can also lead to considerable water loss, although usually the importance of vomiting lies more in the fact that oral intake is prevented. For hospitalized patients, drainage tubes in the stomach or intestine may remove very considerable volumes of water and electrolytes.

Water losses in the urine can become abnormal from increased solute intake, which induces an osmotic diuresis. Disturbances in antidiuretic hormone (ADH) metabolism may lead to diabetes insipidus with large abnormal losses of water in the urine. There is a congenital disorder in which collecting tubules are unresponsive to ADH and in which large water losses occur. Finally, advanced renal disorders lead to a defect in concentration that removes any margin of safety on the renal control of water loss.

The final type of abnormal water loss from the body spaces is not truly a loss from the body but rather a sequestering of water in some area of the body, owing to tissue injury or a pathophysiologic process involving a single organ tissue. Such accumulations include an edema secondary to burns or mechanical injury; the inflammation that follows surgery, particularly in a hollow cavity such as the abdomen where fluid can accumulate; and fluid accumulation secondary to infection, again particularly in such regions as the peritoneum or pleura. In this connection, it should be pointed out that the transcellular water of the intestinal lumen may also be greatly increased. Such fluid, although weighed with the body on a scale, is, in fact, physiologically outside of the body.

THIRST AND ANTIDIURETIC HORMONE (ADH)

Under conditions of health, water losses, normal and sometimes abnormal, are offset by the intake of water, the process governed by thirst mechanism. Thirst, in turn, is controlled by the central nervous system centers that are sensitive to small changes in body fluid osmolality as well as to other types of stimuli, including changes in blood volume and perhaps to sensations arising from membranes in the mouth. The most important of these is the brain region containing the osmolality sensors. An increase of 1 to 2 per cent in osmolal concentrations causes thirst, and a decrease to normal or below stops the thirst sensation. The volume stimuli, particularly a reduction in the effective plasma volume, becomes important when plasma volume is reduced despite an increase in total body water. Thus, thirst may occur even when the body water is hypo-osmotic.

Coordinated with the thirst mechanism is a hormonal regulator of water metabolism, ADH. This hormone is also known as vasopressin or arginine vasopressin, since it is a peptide hormone consisting of nine amino acids with arginine in the 8 position, as shown below.* The arginine is stressed because in a few mammalian species (e.g., the Suidae, or pig, family) lysine replaces arginine. A number of synthetic compounds have been made by substituting molecules in the 1 or 8 position.

ADH synthesis occurs in the supra-opticohypophyseal tract. It begins in a hypothalmic neuron and extends along an axon terminating in either the median eminence or the posterior lobe of the pituitary. Oxytocin is also produced in this cell system, although, most believe, by a separate set of neurons. Both of these hormones apparently split off from a large precursor protein, which also gives rise to the large binding proteins for the two hormones.

After synthesis, ADH and its binding protein are packaged and stored as granules in the axon. The release of the hormone occurs from the same physiologic stimuli that arouse thirst, hypertonicity, and volume depletion.[4, 5, 6, 7] Other stimuli are also important. Alpha adrenergic compounds (norepinephrine) will lead to ADH release, which in turn will be blocked by alpha blocking agents. Beta adrenergic agents inhibit ADH release. Acetylcholine stimulates it.[6, 7]

After release into the blood, ADH has a short half-life, probably 20 to 25 minutes.[8] It is thought to circulate as a free peptide, with the kidney degrading 60 to 70 per cent and

---

*

$$\underset{1}{\text{Cys-Tyr-Phe-Glu(NH}_2\text{)-Asp(NH}_2\text{)-Cys-Pro-Arg-Gly-NH}_2}\underset{8}{}$$

the liver 20 to 30 per cent, and about 10 per cent appearing in the urine.[6] The principal site of action of ADH is in the collecting tubules and collecting ducts of the kidney. The luminal membrane of these portions of the nephron is nearly impermeable to water. ADH markedly increases the permeability of the luminal membrane to water, leading to reabsorption of water. It also increases the permeability to urea and sodium so that these solutes also have enhanced reabsorption. Our understanding of the mechanism of action has been advanced markedly in the last decade.[4, 5] The hormone binds to specific receptors on the serosal side of the collecting ducts. This leads to activation of adenylate cyclase within the basolateral membrane, which leads to the generation of cyclic adenosine monophosphate (AMP). Precisely what happens next is not yet fully understood. The cyclic AMP may activate an enzyme, which in turn phosphorylates a membrane protein.[9] An alternate hypothesis suggests that the cyclic AMP stimulates formation of microtubules or microfilaments. Whatever the molecular basis, the reaction results in a marked increase in the permeability of the luminal membrane to water and solutes.

ADH acts very rapidly after its release in the circulatory system, implying that no induction of a protein is required for its action. Therefore, concentration or dilution of the urine will bear a close relationship to the level of ADH in the blood. There is no specific normal resting level for ADH. However, in a hydrated individual in a seated position, an expected blood level is 1.0 to 1.5 μU/ml (2.6 to 3.9 picogm/ml).[6] Pain and anxiety cause ADH release. So do many drugs, including morphine and barbiturates. A few other drugs inhibit ADH release. It is probable that some hypothalamic center modulates stimuli arising from three sites: osmol receptors, volume receptors, and so-called higher cortical centers. The volume receptor system is a very important one. Contraction of the intravascular space leads to release of ADH and thus antidiuresis, whereas intravascular expansion results in inhibition of ADH release and thus diuresis. Two receptor sites are sensitive to these volume stimuli: the stretch receptors of the left atrium, which respond to filling changes in that heart chamber; and the carotid sinus receptors, which respond to changes in arterial pressure. The atrial system is probably the more significant. A change of only 1 cm of water pressure will have a significant effect of the circulating ADH level.[10]

From the preceding discussion it should be understood that changes in sodium concentration, a marker of osmolality, and changes in plasma volume represent the two leading stimuli for controlling ADH release. Superimposed on this dual system, however, may be the effects of drugs, pain, and anxiety. Drugs such as morphine, barbiturates, and many anesthetic agents stimulate ADH release and may override the inhibitory effect of a low osmolality or even a low atrial pressure. The same sequence may result from pain or anxiety, which also stimulates ADH release via the cerebral cortical centers.

SUMMARY

The turnover of water has special significance in clinical pediatrics. A higher rate of metabolism per unit mass causes the infant to have a corresponding higher rate of water turnover in comparison with the adult. The obligatory losses are fixed by the need to maintain constant body temperature and by the ways in which homeothermy is achieved. To maintain water homeostasis, there is a marvelously complex system involving thirst and antidiuresis. This system may be overwhelmed by disease, however, most particularly when oral intake of water is reduced or prevented. The details of the regulatory mechanisms need to be understood so that correction of disturbances in physiology will lead to resumption of appropriate homeostatic systems.

REFERENCES

1. Lusk G: Clinical colorimetry, paper 1. A respiration colorimeter for the study of disease. Arch Int Med 15:793, 1915.
2. DuBois EF: The basal metabolism in fever. JAMA 77:352, 1921.
3. Darrow DC, Cooke RE, Segar W: Water and electrolyte metabolism in infants fed cow's milk mixture during heat stress. Pediatrics 14:602, 1954.
4. Hays RM: Antidiuretic hormone. New Engl J Med 295:659, 1976.
5. Schafer JA, Andreoli TE: Action of antidiuretic hormone on water and nonelectrolyte transport processes in mammalian collecting tu-

bules. In Andreoli TE, Grantham JJ, Rector FC (eds): Disturbances in Body Fluid Osmolality. American Physiological Society. Williams & Wilkins, Baltimore, 1977.

6. Friedman AL, Segar WE: Antidiuretic hormone excess. J Pediatr 94:521, 1979.

7. Weitzman R, Kleeman CR: Water metabolism and the neurohypophyseal hormones. In Maxwell MH, Kleeman CR: Clinical Disorders of Fluid and Electrolyte Metabolism, Chapter 12. McGraw-Hill, New York, 1979.

8. Baumann G, Dingman JF: Distribution, blood transport, and degradation of antidiuretic hormone in man. J Clin Invest 57:1109, 1976.

9. Schwartz IL, Shlatz LJ, Kinne-Saffran E: Target cell polarity and membrane phosphorylation in relation to the mechanism of action of antidiuretic hormone. Proc Natl Acad Sci USA 71:2595, 1974.

10. Robertson GL, Shelton RL, Athar S: The osmoregulation of vasopressin. Kidney Int 10:25, 1976.

Chapter 5

CIRCULATORY AND RENAL EFFECTS ON REGULATION

The circulation can be seen as a transportation system between the external environment and the internal environment. Water and salt as well as combustibles, vitamins, and minerals are picked up in the gastrointestinal tract, and oxygen is picked up in the lungs and delivered to cells. Carbon dioxide, metabolic debris, cell by-products, and heat are brought to the organs of excretion by the circulation. These services must be provided continuously throughout the life of the organism. If they are interrupted for more than minutes, death follows.

THE HEART

The heart has high energy requirements, and maintenance of its blood supply is critical to survival of the organism. Cardiac circulation is even more intermittent than that to the rest of the body, since during systole, when blood pressure is highest, no blood flows to the myocardium, with flow only during diastole. Inadequate pressure, flow, or composition of blood in the coronary circulation may quickly result in death of the organism.

Metabolic processes in the heart, which has high oxygen and caloric requirements, eventuate in forceful muscular contraction followed by relaxation. The amount of blood ejected with each systole is the stroke volume, which, when multiplied by the heart rate per minute, gives the minute volume. Cardiac output can be calculated by means of the Fick principle, which is based on the self-evident principle that the amount of something (A) equals its concentration (C) times its volume (V):

$$A = C \times V$$

In other words, the volume equals the amount divided by the concentration:

$$V = \frac{A}{C}$$

The amount of oxygen consumed in a minute divided by the change in concentration of oxygen between venous and arterial blood gives the volume of blood that carried that amount of oxygen, or the cardiac output in liters per minute (see below).*

In the absence of right-to-left or left-to-right shunting, the cardiac output from the left and right sides of the heart is equal.

The blood is ejected into compliant and elastic arteries, which maintain pressure during diastole so that forward blood flow continues. Were the large arteries rigid tubes, systolic pressure would shoot up quite high and diastolic blood pressure would approach zero, as would blood flow to the heart itself. In addition, there would be back-and-forth, or tidal, blood flow to parts of the body that have high tissue pressure or are elevated above the heart.

---

*
$$\text{(V) Cardiac output (l/min)} = \frac{\overset{\text{(A)}}{\text{Oxygen consumption (ml/min)}}}{\underset{\text{(C)}}{\text{Arteriovenous oxygen difference (ml/l of blood)}}}$$

The arterial blood pressure is, therefore, a function of the compliance and elasticity of the blood vessels as well as a function of the stroke volume, the heart rate, and the peripheral resistance.

The flow of liquid in a vessel is expressed by the Poiseuille-Hagan equation:

$$F = (P_A - P_B) \cdot \frac{(\pi)}{8} \cdot \frac{1}{\eta} \cdot \frac{(R^4)}{\ell}$$

where F is the total flow, $(P_A - P_B)$ is the pressure difference between any two points A and B in dynes/cm², η is the viscosity in poises, and R is the radius and ℓ the length of the segment of vessel between A and B. Flow is, therefore, a direct function of the pressure gradient and the fourth power of the radius and is inversely related to the viscosity and the length of the vessel. Increased viscosity of blood can become an important factor in impeding blood flow. When the hematocrit rises over 60, viscosity starts to rise at an increased rate, and as the hematocrit reaches 70 and 80, blood flow can become significantly impaired and produce tissue ischemia. Raising the hematocrit is, therefore, beneficial in increasing oxygen delivery only to the point where increasing viscosity interferes with blood flow to tissue. This probably occurs in most patients at a hematocrit around 60.

Vascular resistance is calculated for the systemic circulation by the equation below.* Resistance to flow occurs mainly in the arterioles, which can change their diameter under neural and humoral control and therefore can regulate blood flow and blood pressure to satisfy local tissue demands. In times of stress, less needed capillary beds can be closed off and flow diverted to more vital areas.

Within a capillary bed, blood flow can be controlled by humoral or neural factors, which can direct flow either into thoroughfare capillaries that act as small, low-resistance arteriovenous shunts, or into true capillaries supplying tissues.[1] This control may be deranged in such diseases as endotoxin shock and hepatic failure and may be the capillary equivalent of the hepatorenal and hepatocerebral syndromes.[2]

Capillaries to such tissues as brain, muscle, and lung are subject to local regulation: a low level of oxygen, a low pH, and a high level of carbon dioxide in the tissues causes dilation and increased blood flow to beds in the brain and muscle, with the opposite effect occurring in the lung, so that blood flow is not directly related to blood pressure. High oxygen and pH and low carbon dioxide have the reverse effect. When acting locally, this allows blood to be distributed to areas where it is needed. But systemic hypoxia and acidemia can result in pulmonary hypertension by increasing pulmonary vascular resistance while tending to produce systemic hypotension by decreasing systemic resistance.

Venous return to the heart is aided by muscular contraction, particularly when the muscles compress veins that contain one-way valves, such as those in the legs, as well as by gravity and respiratory pressure changes in the thorax. It is probably no accident that the heart and lungs are in the same chamber. The lower intrathoracic pressure during normal inspiration, in particular, aids venous return to the heart. This is important, since the heart, unlike most other muscles, has no readily apparent opponent muscle. Since muscles can only actively contract, a contracted muscle must have an opponent to return it to its original stretched position so that it can contract again. Our extremities have flexor and extensor muscle groups to serve this function. Opposition to the heart muscle is provided by the residual kinetic energy generated by the force of contraction of the heart, the elasticity of the blood vessels, and these other forces that return blood to the heart and stretch the atria. The contractions of the atria act in turn as opponents to the contractions of the ventricles by returning them to their stretched positions. If this return of blood to the heart is inadequate, cardiac output drops, because there is less blood to pump and because the force of cardiac contraction is reduced. Inadequate return can be produced by vasodilation with venous pooling, inadequate blood volume (dehydration, blood loss), gravity (rigid standing at attention, "brown-out" in pilots), or increased intrathoracic pressure (excessive airway pressure).

---

* $\dfrac{\text{Systemic resistance}}{\text{(resistance units/m}^2)} = \dfrac{\text{Mean Pressure, Aortic–Right Atrial (mm Hg)}}{\text{System flow (liters/min/m)}}$

Cardiac diseases can decrease cardiac output so that the supply of blood to tissues is inadequate for normal functions and tissue hypoxia results, as in obstructive cardiac lesions and myocardiopathy. If demands for blood flow are excessive, a normal heart may not be able to keep up with the requirements. This can occur with hyperthyroidism, anemia, beriberi, arterial shunts, and septic shock. The state is known as high-output heart failure.

Various causes of heart failure may occur simultaneously and produce additive effects, so that mild anemia in a patient with mild cardiomyopathy may have profound effects. Raising the hematocrit to normal or above normal in such a patient can be very beneficial. In such states, cardiac output is low with respect to tissue needs and can be called "forward failure." In congestive heart failure, the cardiac output may be adequate for tissue needs but venous pressure is elevated, owing to the inability of the heart to pump the volume of blood returning to the heart without the higher venous pressure. This may be due to diseases of the heart itself, as in cardiomyopathy; to increased pumping loads, as in hypertension or obstructions to flow; or to increased blood volume, as in renal failure with excess fluid administration or with hypertransfusion. This can be called "backward failure."

The rise in venous pressure increases the outward movement of water from capillaries by means of Starling forces[3] (see Fig. 5–1), producing an increased interstitial fluid volume with the typical findings of congestive heart failure, such as distended veins, enlarged liver and spleen, and pitting edema. Pulmonary edema may also occur, which increases the work of breathing, requiring greater blood flow and cardiac output, and also impairs gas exchange, impeding cellular respiration further. The response to decreased cardiac output is increased renal sodium and water retention, which increases blood volume and which may make congestion worse.

GASTROINTESTINAL TRACT

Ingested food and water are processed in the gastrointestinal tract and transported by the circulation, first to the liver in the portal circuit, then to the lungs in the pulmonary circuit, and then to all parts of the body by the systemic circulation. The contents of the gastrointestinal tract depend on the availability of food and water in the external environment as well as on hunger, thirst, physical agility, intellectual ability, habit, and social customs.

Following a meal, the circulatory system contains portions of what was ingested, pointing up the problem of trying to analyze a blood specimen of a non-fasting individual. Water, salt, and minerals leave the circulatory system by leaking into interstitial fluid and cells, by sliding down concentration gradients, and by active or facilitated transport.

SUPPLY OF CELLS

The circulatory system, in addition to providing means for transport to the capillaries, provides means for transport through the capillary walls (Fig. 5–1). The pressure head generated by the contraction of the heart counters the inward pull of the plasma proteins on water (oncotic pressure) at the arterial end of the capillary, and water is forced into the tissues. This holds true only for those capillaries that do not have tight cell junctions, thus excluding capillaries going to the brain tissue, the testes, and the eye. The capillaries to these organs are semipermeable with respect to salt as well as to the plasma proteins, so the effective osmotic gradient across them is much greater, with 280 effective milliosmoles per kilogram of water on both sides of the membrane. Capillaries to the rest of the body, however, have loose junctions through which bulk flow of fluid can occur and, in addition, are effectively permeable to salt but semipermeable to plasma protein. The effective osmolality across these capillary membranes is therefore only about 1.5 mOsm per kilogram of water. For every effective milliosmole per kilogram of water, an osmotic pressure of 19.3 mm Hg can be generated.[4]

The capillary pressure provided by the force of the cardiac contractions is in the range of 35 mm Hg. The oncotic pressure of the plasma protein is lower, about 28 mOsm/kg of water, so that the pressure gradient differential can have a major effect on the movement of water through the ordinary capillary wall.

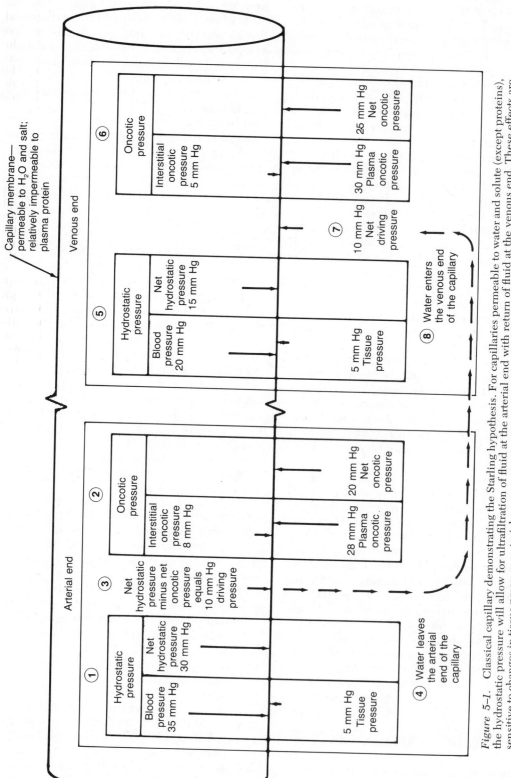

Figure 5–1. Classical capillary demonstrating the Starling hypothesis. For capillaries permeable to water and solute (except proteins), the hydrostatic pressure will allow for ultrafiltration of fluid at the arterial end and with return of fluid at the venous end. These effects are sensitive to changes in tissue pressure, arterial pressure, venous pressure, concentrations of protein in serum and in interstitial fluid, and capillary integrity. Changes in NaCl concentration will have little effect. In vivo the process is bidirectional across the capillary bed; the diagram shows the net effect of these flows.

On the other hand, the blood pressure in capillaries with tight junctions is only a small fraction of the osmotic pressure and will, therefore, have only a minor effect on the movement of fluid through these capillaries, because as water molecules leave the vascular compartment, osmolality rises in the blood in proportion to its fall in the interstitium (Fig. 5–2). For example, if osmolality were to rise to 281 mOsm/kg of water in the plasma and fall to 279 mOsm/kg of water on the outside of the capillary, the pressure gradient would be effectively countered. This change in osmolality would occur when only $1/280$ of the volume of the plasma had crossed the capillary. Thus, bulk movement of fluids may occur in tissues with capillaries with loose junctions but not in those with tight junctions.

A reverse effect will occur after accumulation of edema fluid. As edema increases, tissue pressure builds up. In most tissues this will result in increases in the lymphatic flow and the flow of interstitial fluid back into the capillary, with a decrease in edema according to Starling's hypothesis. The use of elastic bandages and the elevation of a swollen extremity take advantage of this phenomenon. This increase in tissue pressure will have little effect on reabsorption of fluid in the brain, the testes, and the eye, however, since capillaries in these areas are semipermeable to salt. This accounts for the difficulties produced by edema in these tissues, as in Reye syndrome, glaucoma, and mumps. As edema fluid accumulates, tissue pressures in the brain, the eye, or the testes can go up extremely high and can even exceed arterial pressure. This will tend to counter the continuing accumulation of edema fluid, but it is extremely inefficient, since the pressure rise can cause little water movement and tissue death may ensue.

The pulmonary circulation is a low-pressure circulation with a mean pressure of 7 mm Hg in the pulmonary capillaries (Fig. 5–3).[5] The pulmonary interstitium probably has a negative pressure of about 8.3 mm Hg, giving an outward hydrostatic pressure gradient of 15.3 mm Hg from the capillary to the interstitium. The plasma oncotic pressure of 28 mm Hg counters this hydrostatic pressure, but this is reduced by 13 mm Hg, owing to the oncotic pressure of the protein in the interstitial fluid, to a net oncotic pressure of 15 mm Hg. Therefore, there is a mean pressure gradient of 0.3 mm Hg, which favors osmosis of water through the pulmonary capillary, with flow directed toward the lymphatics. Derangements of capillary integrity, alveolar surface tension, protein levels, lymphatic function, and capillary, interstitial, and intrathoracic pressures can upset this balance and produce pulmonary edema.

Most tissues, therefore, have bulk movement of fluid into and out of the interstitium. The leaky capillary wall thus provides easy access for the transport of nutrients and waste products to and from most cells. Organs supplied by capillaries with tight junctions require specialized secretory organs and transport systems to receive adequate fluids and nutrients (in the brain, the choroid plexus; in the eye, the ciliary body) and specialized means for the return of fluid to the circulation (in the brain, the arachnoid granulations; in the eye, the sinus venous sclerae), and these organs do not have lymphatics.

KIDNEY

Since the kidney plays the major role in maintaining salt and water balance, an understanding of renal physiology is important.[6] A large portion of the cardiac output — around 25 per cent — goes to the kidney, where approximately 22 per cent of renal blood flow is filtered in the glomerulus (Fig. 5–4). The glomerular membrane is similar to the usual capillary membrane in that it is permeable to water and salt and relatively impermeable to serum proteins and red blood cells. As filtration proceeds, the concentration of the plasma proteins increases. This process, usually called ultrafiltration, may also be viewed as reverse osmosis. The glomerular filtrate then flows down the renal tubule, where active and passive transport processes add or subtract water and solutes as required by the organism.

The mean blood pressure in the glomerular capillary is about 60 per cent of the mean arterial pressure, or approximately 50 mm Hg. The pressure in the proximal tubule is about 10 mm Hg, leaving a hydrostatic pressure gradient of 40 mm Hg in favor of filtration. There is little pressure drop along the glomerular capillaries, so this gradient tends to persist throughout the

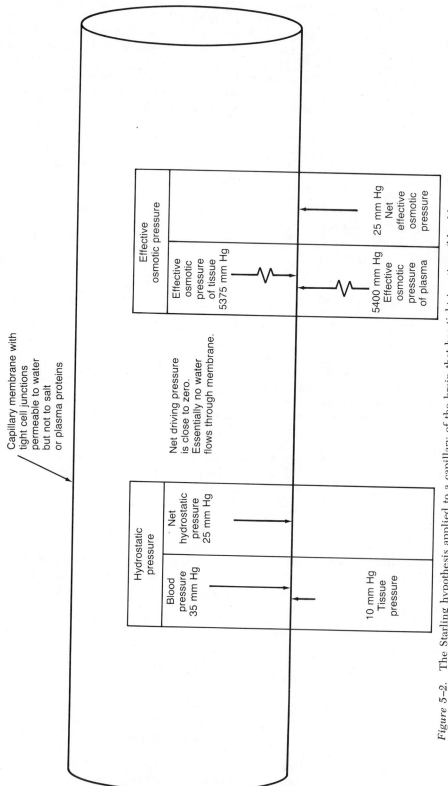

Figure 5–2. The Starling hypothesis applied to a capillary of the brain that has tight junctions (blood-brain barrier). The capillary membrane is permeable to water but not to most solutes. The effective osmotic pressure is therefore very high (approximately 280 mOsm/kg $H_2O \times 19.3$ mm Hg). The hydrostatic pressure is easily balanced by the osmotic pressure. Changes in blood pressure, tissue pressure, or protein concentration will have little effect, but changes in the concentration of NaCl or other nondiffusible solute will cause large water shifts.

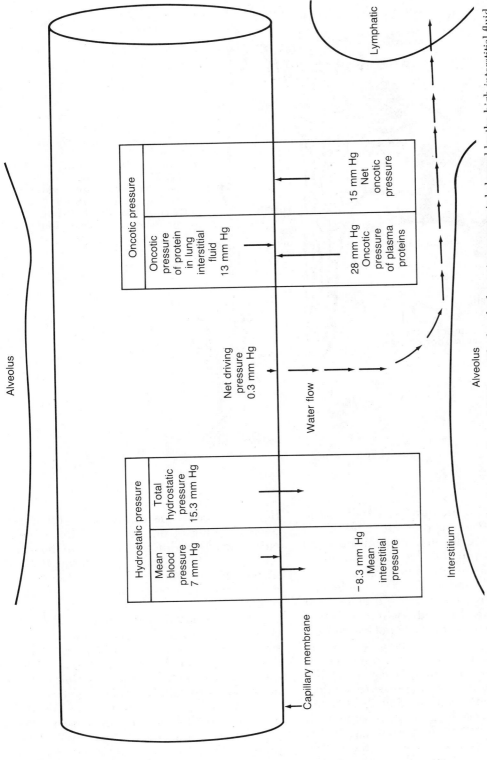

Figure 5–3. The Starling hypothesis applied to a capillary of the lung. The low hydrostatic pressure is balanced by the high interstitial-fluid protein concentration. There is minimal pressure drop along the capillary, since the pressures are low to start with and pulmonary capillaries have low resistance to flow. The lymphatics carry off a small amount of filtered water and protein. The process is otherwise similar to that shown in Figure 5–1.

That portion of the pulmonary capillary wall adjacent to the alveol us is composed of contiguous alveolar and capillary membranes. The alveolar membrane has tight junctions so that this portion of the capillary has characteristics similar to capillaries in the brain, shown in Figure 5–2. (Based on Fishman AP, and Renkin EM (eds): Pulmonary Edema. American Physiological Society/Clinical Physiology Series. Williams & Wilkins, Baltimore, 1979.)

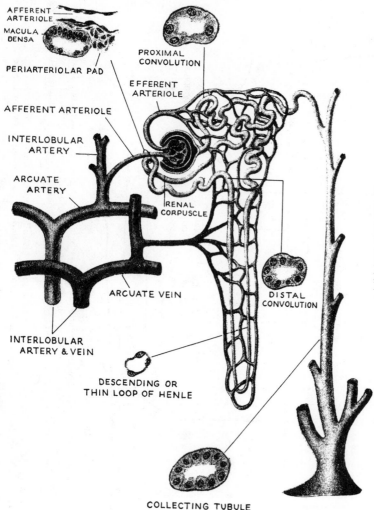

AFFERENT ARTERIOLE
MACULA DENSA
PERIARTERIOLAR PAD
PROXIMAL CONVOLUTION
EFFERENT ARTERIOLE
AFFERENT ARTERIOLE
INTERLOBULAR ARTERY
ARCUATE ARTERY
RENAL CORPUSCLE
ARCUATE VEIN
DISTAL CONVOLUTION
INTERLOBULAR ARTERY & VEIN
DESCENDING OR THIN LOOP OF HENLE
COLLECTING TUBULE

M. LURENG

Figure 5-4. Diagram showing the essential features of a typical nephron in the human kidney. (From *The Kidney* by Homer W. Smith. Copyright © 1951 by Oxford University Press, Inc.; renewed 1979 by Homer Wilson Smith. Reprinted by permission of Oxford University Press, Inc.)

glomerulus. This pressure is partially countered by an oncotic pressure gradient of about 25 mm Hg due to the oncotic pressure of the plasma proteins, leaving a net filtration pressure of about 15 mm Hg.

Particles under 70,000 molecular weight pass freely through the glomerular membrane from the capillary lumen. Therefore, these small particles do not exert effective osmotic pressure, which is why the osmotic gradient is attributable only to the content of protein in the plasma. Thus, the relatively low hydrostatic pressure is effective. Owing to the constant flow through the capillaries, the concentration of protein in the plasma in the glomerular capillaries does not rise enough to counter the hydrostatic pressure substantially. In addition, the constant flow decreases the concentra-

tion of solute at the membrane, with lessened clogging of the pores. Smaller molecules such as inulin, which has a molecular weight of 5000, pass easily through the glomerular membrane and have the same concentration in the filtrate that they have in plasma.

The glomerular membrane may increase in permeability in certain disease states such as nephrotic syndrome, allowing the larger molecules to pass through. The decrease in effective osmolality due to the increased permeability of the membrane to the proteins, which thus reduces oncotic pressure, should cause an increase in glomerular filtration, since the hydrostatic pressure then has even less opposition. In addition, the decrease in concentration of the protein that remains in the plasma decreases oncotic pressure, also serving to increase glomerular filtration, increase further the amount of filtrate, and lead to a decreased blood volume. The decrease in oncotic pressure should also affect capillaries in tissues throughout the body, except the brain, the eyes, and the testes, and produce edema, further reducing blood volume.

The hydrostatic pressure within the glomerular capillary is dependent upon the tone of the afferent and efferent arterioles, and in this way the extent of glomerular filtration can be controlled. The capillaries of the glomerular network, which form by branching of the afferent arteriole as it enters the glomerulus, rejoin to form the efferent arteriole that leaves the glomerulus. This is called an efferent arteriole and not a venule, because it branches again to form another capillary bed that supplies the renal tubules and then joins the renal venous system.

Each of the nephrons (see Fig. 5–4), of which there are approximately 1 million per kidney, consists of a glomerulus, a proximal convoluted tubule, a loop of Henle, and a distal convoluted tubule. The glomerular filtrate travels down the tubule. In the proximal tubule, two thirds of the filtered water and sodium chloride are reabsorbed along with bicarbonate, glucose, potassium, phosphate, protein, and amino acids. H^+ and NH_4^+, penicillin, p-aminohippurate, and radiographic contrast materials are secreted. The solute transport is generally by active mechanisms, and water always moves passively along osmotic gradients through membranes of varying permeability. Although vasopressin and aldosterone have no effect on water and salt reabsorption in the proximal tubule, the unknown "third factor," which possibly influences salt and water balance, has its effect here. Expansion of extracellular fluid volume results in decreased reabsorption of salt and water in the proximal tubule.

In the juxtamedullary nephrons, the thin segment of the loop of Henle dips down into the medulla toward the papilla of the kidney, through areas of increasing hypertonicity with an osmolality up to 1300 mOsm/kg of water. The thin segment then makes a hairpin turn and ascends to form the thick segment of the loop of Henle. The postglomerular capillaries follow the course of the loop of Henle. The proximity of the descending and ascending portions of the loop, owing to the hairpin turn, allows it to function as a countercurrent multiplier, and the capillaries serve as countercurrent exchangers. This preserves the hyperosmolality of the renal medulla and allows for leveraged sodium chloride reabsorption against a concentration gradient. Approximately 25 per cent of the filtered sodium chloride and 5 per cent of the filtered water are reabsorbed in the loop of Henle.

A detailed discussion of the countercurrent multiplier and exchanger mechanism with all the supporting evidence is beyond the scope of this work. It may be found in texts and articles on renal physiology and nephrology.[6, 7, 8] The maintenance of the countercurrent multiplier/exchanger depends upon the architecture just described and upon the different permeabilities of the nephron segments to sodium and chloride ions, urea, and water. These are shown in Table 5–1.

Active (energy-driven) removal of salt in the thick ascending limb, which is impermeable to urea and water, leaves urea in an increasingly hypotonic tubular fluid. Driven by hydrostatic pressure, this fluid moves along the nephron to the distal tubule, which is impermeable to urea but permeable to water controlled by ADH.

Table 5–1. Permeability of Nephron Segments

SEGMENT	NA^+ AND Cl^- IONS	UREA	WATER
Descending loop of Henle	Impermeable	Impermeable	Permeable
Thin ascending loop	Very permeable, passive	Permeable	Impermeable
Thick ascending loop	Active Cl^- transport	Impermeable	Impermeable
Distal tubule and cortical collecting duct	Na^+-K^+, Na^+-H^+ exchange	Impermeable	Permeable with ADH
Medullary collecting duct	Permeable	Permeable only at duct junctions of inner medulla	Permeable with ADH

Water under antidiuretic conditions diffuses out, and salt also moves out (by active transport), leaving a highly concentrated urea solution to enter the outer collecting ducts. This region of the nephron is also impermeable to urea. The junctions of the collecting ducts are, however, permeable to urea (Table 5–1).[7] Thus, as the luminal fluid moves down the collecting ducts to the inner medulla, urea molecules diffuse down a concentration gradient into the interstitium. This, in turn, draws water from both the collecting ducts and the adjacent descending limbs of the loop of Henle. In the descending limb, which is impermeable to salt, this results in increased salt concentration while the neighboring interstitium is being diluted. As the fluid turns the bend, it enters a region impermeable to water but permeable to salt. Salt then diffuses down its concentration gradient to the interstitium. Still more water molecules are then drawn from the adjacent collecting ducts, thus diluting the urea. In this manner, the urea gradient (collecting ducts → interstitium) is recreated. Urea diffusion to interstitium is renewed and water is pulled from descending limbs, re-establishing the salt gradient. The water is partially carried away by the ascending vasa recta as the water moves rapidly down its own concentration gradient.

The osmolality of the interstitium in the inner medulla is the sum of salt and urea; passive diffusion of urea from collecting ducts and passive diffusion of salt from the thin ascending limb are made possible by the energy of active transport of chloride (salt) from the thick ascending limb in the outer medulla. The active transport (and different permeabilities) creates a high urea concentration, which establishes the solute gradient movements described previously, and salt and urea gradients "recreate" each other at specific points in medullary portions of the nephron. This cycle has been designated a "bootstrap" model in which urea and salt gradients re-establish each other in an escalating fashion.[7]

In the course of these events, urea molecules undergo medullary recycling and urea is "trapped" in the medulla.[8] Therefore, the presence of adequate urea in urine is necessary for a maximal medullary gradient in the human.

In the distal convoluted tubule, the dilute urine (100–200 mOsm/kg of water) is also further modified, as needed, by excretion of NH_4^+, H^+, and K^+. The distal convoluted tubule then releases its contents to the collecting duct, which passes alongside the loops of Henle through the hypertonic medulla to open into the renal pelvis. In the well-hydrated individual, little happens to the urine in the collecting duct, and therefore a dilute urine is excreted. In a poorly hydrated person, antidiuretic hormone is excreted by the posterior pituitary, which makes the collecting duct permeable to water, starting the sequence described previously. As it passes through a hypertonic medium, water diffuses out of the collecting duct down the osmotic gradient, providing a small volume of concentrated urine. The maximal adult human concentration of urine is about 1300 mOsm/kg of water. In newborn infants it is about 600 mOsm/kg of water, and by 1 year of age it approximates the adult level.

BLOOD

Hyperosmolality, while protecting plasma volume during dehydration, also has an interesting effect on red cell volume.[9] The red cells respond like other cells in the body by losing water during hyperosmolality, and this water serves to increase blood volume at the same time the hematocrit is decreasing owing to water loss from the cell. This is reflected in a drop in hemoglobin, an even greater drop in hematocrit, and a rise in mean corpuscular hemoglobin concentration (MCHC) as the hemoglobin remaining in the red cell becomes more concentrated as water is withdrawn (Fig. 5–5). Thus, hypertonic dehydration may produce an apparent anemia, which may be corrected as the hypertonicity is corrected.

The opposite phenomenon occurs with hypotonic dehydration, in which the red cells swell as plasma water enters them. Because there is less plasma and the red blood cells are larger, hematocrit increases to a greater extent than hemoglobin, and the MCHC decreases. In this way a mild degree of anemia may be obscured, but as the hyponatremia and dehydration are corrected, the anemia becomes apparent.

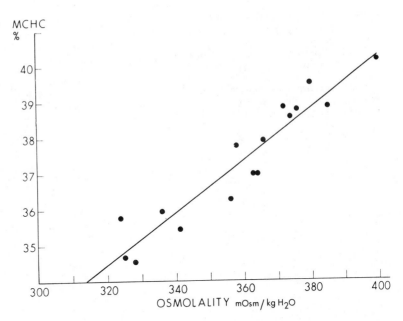

Figure 5–5. Correlation of mean corpuscular hemoglobin concentration (MCHC) with osmolality for one cat. (From Kravath RE, Aharon AS, Abal G, and Finberg L: Clinically significant physiologic changes from rapidly administered hypertonic solutions: acute osmol poisoning. Pediatrics 46:267, 1970. Copyright © 1970 American Academy of Pediatrics. Used with permission.)

Hyponatremia also exaggerates the effects on the circulation of the fluid loss in dehydration, since excess extracellular fluid is lost to the intracellular space. The treatment of disturbances of osmolality should, therefore, take into consideration their effects on blood volume and on the circulatory system.

SUMMARY

The integrity of the circulatory system is dependent on adequate cardiac activity, sufficient volume, composition, and fluidity of the blood, and intact vasculature. Derangements of any of these have profound effects on the entire organism. If the derangements are mild, temporary, or local, the organism may survive; otherwise, the organism dies. When functioning, the circulatory system enables water and salt balance to be maintained, but it requires reasonably normal levels of water and salt to function adequately; thus, a vicious cycle can be easily set up, so that derangement of circulation may adversely affect salt and water balance, which, in turn, may make circulation worse. Fortunately for the therapist, this cycle also works in reverse, so that improvement in water balance may improve circulation, which, in turn, may improve salt and water balance.

Dehydration will usually cause a decrease in blood volume and impair circulatory efficiency, which will impair cerebral, motor, gastrointestinal, and renal functions and will rapidly make matters worse unless corrected. An occasional exception is hypertonic dehydration, in which the rising extracellular osmolality pulls water from cells, tending to preserve extracellular volume. More frequently, however, this form of dehydration is accompanied by decreased blood volume.

Disease processes affecting the circulatory system will have important effects on homeostasis and on responses to stress. Severe heart disease will produce increased blood volume, increased venous pressure, edema, and engorgement of the lungs, kidney, liver, spleen, and other organs, as well as decreased blood flow, which further impairs their function. Diuretic agents cause electrolyte as well as water depletion and may lead to metabolic alkalosis and other abnormalities. Metabolism is increased in heart disease and heart failure, and increased circulatory demands increase the burden on the circulatory system.

Patients with diseases of the circulatory system who have derangements of salt and water balance require precise management that avoids further stress, as well as attention to the treatment of the underlying disease.

REFERENCES

1. Zweifach BW: Functional Behavior of the Microcirculation. Charles C Thomas, Springfield, IL, 1961.

2. Kravath RE, Scarpelli EM, Bernstein J: Hepatogenic cyanosis: arteriovenous shunts in chronic active hepatitis. J Pediatr 78:238, 1971.
3. Starling EH: On the absorption of fluids from the connective tissue spaces. J Physiol 19:312, 1896.
4. Wolf AV: Aqueous Solutions and Body Fluids. Harper & Row, New York, 1966.
5. Fishman AP, Renkin EM: Pulmonary Edema. American Physiological Society. Williams & Wilkins, Baltimore, 1979.
6. Leaf A, Cotran R: Renal Pathophysiology. Oxford University Press, New York, 1976.
7. Britton KE, Carson ER, Coge PE: A "bootstrap" model of the renal medulla. Postgrad Med J 52:279, 1976.
8. Jamison RL, Maffly RH: The urinary concentrating mechanism. New Engl J Med 295:1059, 1976.
9. Kravath RE, Aharon A, Abal G, Finberg L: Clinically significant physiologic changes from rapidly administered hypertonic solutions: acute osmol poisoning. Pediatrics 46:267, 1970.

Chapter 6

BLOOD GASES, HYDROGEN ION, AND pH

Two gases, oxygen (O_2) and carbon dioxide (CO_2), play a vital biologic role, and an understanding of these gases is essential to an understanding of acid-base metabolism.

Our understanding of the biologic role of these gases is a surprisingly recent development, even when compared with the historical development of concepts of water and electrolyte metabolism. In fact, the word *gas* was not invented until the seventeenth century, when a Belgian physician, J. B. Van Helmont, coined it to fill the need caused by the new idea that different types of air existed. He had discovered that a kind of air (i.e., the gas carbon dioxide) was formed when limestone was treated with acid. It did not support life and was heavier than the usual kind of air. It was not until 1774 that Joseph Priestley announced the discovery of a gas that supported combustion even better than air and could also support life.

BASIC CONCEPTS

In order to understand some recent developments in our understanding of the role of gases in physiology, pathophysiology, and therapy, it helps to understand some basic terminology and concepts.[1-11]

Partial Pressure of Oxygen, Nitrogen, and Water in Air

As you know from daily weather reports, the usual barometric pressure at sea level is 760 mm, or 30 inches, of mercury. The barometric pressure varies inversely with the water vapor content of the air, since water vapor, with a molecular weight of 18, is lighter than O_2 or N_2, with molecular weights of 32 and 28 respectively. (Since 22.4 liters of an ideal gas at standard conditions contains one mole, the density of an ideal gas is directly proportional to its molecular weight.) Dry air is, therefore, heavier than moist air and consists of approximately 21 per cent oxygen and 78 per cent nitrogen (N_2). When air is fully saturated with water vapor, its water content will vary directly with the temperature (which is why a cold front is frequently accompanied by rain). At a body temperature of 37°C, fully saturated air is about 6.2 per cent water vapor, with a partial pressure (P) of 47 mm Hg. (6.2% $\times$ 760 mm Hg = 47 mm Hg). The partial pressure of a gas is proportional to its fractional concentration, or percentage composition in a mixture. The partial pressure of a pure gas is the same as the barometric pressure. The rest of this warm, fully saturated air — or 93.8 per cent of the total, with a partial pressure of 713 mm Hg (93.8% $\times$ 760 mm Hg = 713 mm Hg) — contains 21 per cent oxygen, with a partial pressure (PO_2) of 150 mm Hg. The remainder is mainly nitrogen, with a partial pressure (PN_2) of 563 mm Hg.

Relatively dry room air, when inhaled, becomes warmed to body temperature and fully saturated with water vapor in the upper airway. This takes place mainly in the nose, which is optimally designed for this purpose. If the nose is bypassed, this process takes place with less efficiency in the lower airway, with the problem of drying of secretions. As the air is warmed and humidified, its volume expands slightly, decreas-

35

ing the concentration of both nitrogen and oxygen. Thus, for air at 37°C that is fully saturated with water vapor, 47 mm Hg of the total 760 mm Hg pressure will be contributed by the water vapor.

Partial Pressure of Oxygen, Nitrogen, Carbon Dioxide, and Water in the Lung

In the lung some oxygen is removed from the inhaled air and carbon dioxide is added. The respiratory quotient (R) is the ratio between the amount of CO_2 added and the amount of O_2 removed, or CO_2/O_2. When the amount of CO_2 added and the amount of O_2 removed are equal, R equals 1 and the total volume of the gas does not change. If the amount of CO_2 added is less than the amount of O_2 removed, R is less than 1 and the total volume of the gas decreases; consequently, the proportion of nitrogen in it increases slightly and the proportion of oxygen decreases. This change is expressed by the alveolar air equation, which is used for calculating ideal alveolar oxygen tension:

$$P_A O_2 = P_I O_2 - \frac{P_A CO_2}{R}$$

where $P_A O_2$ is the alveolar partial pressure of oxygen, $P_I O_2$ is the partial pressure of inhaled oxygen, and $P_A CO_2$ is the alveolar partial pressure of carbon dioxide.

Since the usual $P_A CO_2$ is 40 mm Hg, at an R of 1 there would be a decrease of 40 mm Hg in the $P_A O_2$. Thus, although the partial pressure of inhaled oxygen is about 150 mm Hg, it drops to about 110 mm Hg in the alveolus. At other respiratory quotients, the $P_A O_2$ can be calculated from the alveolar air equation or from nomograms such as that shown in Figure 6–1. Estimation of the alveolar PO_2 may be useful in assessing pulmonary function by comparing it with the concurrently measured arterial PO_2.

Oxygen and Carbon Dioxide in the Blood

Oxygen diffuses from the alveolus into the blood in the pulmonary capillary, and carbon dioxide diffuses the opposite way. Diffusion is the ability of a substance to pass from a point of higher pressure to one of lower pressure. In the gas phase, the rate of diffusion is inversely proportional to the square root of the molecular weight of the gas and directly proportional to the pressure difference and the temperature. But when gases are dissolved in liquids, the rate of diffusion is modified by the degree of solubility of the gas in the liquid. Although CO_2 is denser than O_2 and diffuses more slowly than O_2 in the gas phase, it is more soluble in solution than oxygen. Since CO_2 is far more soluble than O_2 and only slightly more dense, it diffuses 20 times more rapidly in liquids. This is why diseases impairing diffusion do not cause a significant rise in PCO_2. Before CO_2 will be significantly affected, the patient will die of hypoxia. Since oxygen diffuses so much more slowly, it will be the limiting factor.

In an adult, the alveolar surface available for diffusion is estimated to be 50 to 90 m² , with a capillary area of about 140 m² and a total capillary length of 970 to 1540 miles (1550 to 2460 km). The thickness of the membrane separating blood and air is of the order of 0.2 to 0.6 micron, and the time spent by a particle of blood in the alveolus is estimated at 0.75 sec at rest and 0.34 sec during exercise.

Inhaled atmospheric air contains 0.04 per cent CO_2, a small amount. The CO_2 output in a resting individual on a normal diet is about 190 ml/min and O_2 consumption is about 240 ml/min, giving a respiratory quotient, CO_2/O_2, of 0.8.

Carbon dioxide diffuses from cells in the body tissues into the capillaries, where it is transported in the blood in several ways. A small amount is carried in the plasma as dissolved CO_2. A very small portion of this forms carbonic acid (H_2CO_3), which dissociates to form H^+ and HCO_3^-. The H^+ is buffered in the plasma. Dissolved CO_2 in plasma also reacts with the amino group of plasma proteins to form carbamino compounds. Most of the CO_2 passes into the erythrocytes, where some remains as dissolved CO_2. Some combines with $-NH_2$ groups of hemoglobin to form carbamino compounds:

$$R-NH_2 + CO_2 \rightleftarrows R-NHCOO^- + H^+$$

with H^+ buffered by other parts of the hemoglobin molecule. This reaction is facilitated by the simultaneous loss of oxygen to the tissues, since the reduced hemoglobin has an increased affinity for H^+:

$$HbO_2 + H^+ \rightleftarrows HHb + O_2.$$

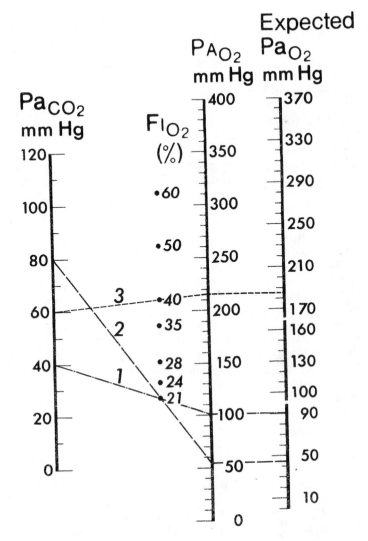

Figure 6–1. Alveolar air equation nomogram. Note that it assumes a respiratory quotient of 0.8 and makes use of the value of arterial PCO_2, not alveolar PCO_2. (Prepared for the American Lung Association by Dudley F. Rochester, M.D. Copyright © 1976 American Thoracic Society — Medical Section of the American Lung Association. Used with permission.)

Solution of alveolar air equation, assuming sea level and R=0.8. To determine alveolar oxygen tension, locate Pa_{CO_2} to the left, and FI_{O_2} in the middle. Join the points with a ruler, and read PA_{O_2} at the right. At the far right are approximate values of Pa_{O_2}, assuming normal values for the (A-a) O_2 gradient. If the observed Pa_{O_2} is lower than the Pa_{O_2} on the far right scale, the (A-a) O_2 gradient is increased. The dash and dot lines illustrate sample calculations:

Example	Pa_{CO_2}	FI_{O_2}	PA_{O_2}	Expected Pa_{O_2}
I	40	21%	102	92
II	80	21%	54	44
III	60	40%	216	186

Most of the CO_2 combines rapidly with water, owing to the presence of carbonic anhydrase in the red cells, to form carbonic acid, most of which rapidly dissociates to hydrogen ion (H^+) and bicarbonate (HCO_3^-). The H^+ is buffered by hemoglobin and other buffers.

$$CO_2 + H_2O \underset{\text{carbonic anhydrase}}{\rightleftharpoons} H_2CO_3 \rightleftharpoons H^+ + HCO_3^-$$

HCO_3^- diffuses from the red blood cell into the plasma, and Cl^- shifts into the cell to maintain electrical neutrality. Although the plasma actually transports more than 60 per cent of the CO_2 added to the blood in the tissues, the chemical reactions within the cell supply most of the HCO_3^- in the plasma.

In the lung, the conversion of H^+ and HCO_3^- to CO_2 and H_2O is aided by the carbonic anhydrase present in lung tissue.[12] All the above processes are reversed as the CO_2 diffuses from the liquid to the gas phase down a pressure gradient, from a partial pressure of carbon dioxide (PCO_2) of 46 mm Hg in the pulmonary arterial blood to one of 40 mm Hg in the alveolus. Since the concentration of free H^+ in the blood is so minute, the vast amount of it comes from the nonbicarbonate buffers, which act as sinks for it. The PCO_2 and the CO_2 content have an almost linear indirect relationship with alveolar ventilation. Doubling alveolar ventilation halves PCO_2 and CO_2 content, and halving alveolar ventilation doubles PCO_2 and CO_2 content. In blood in the physiologic range, for every millimeter of mercury of PCO_2, 0.03 mmol/l of carbonic acid plus carbon dioxide will dissolve in the solution:

$$PCO_2 \times 0.03 \text{ mmol/l} = CO_2 + H_2CO_3 \text{ (in mmol/l)}$$

Mixed venous blood usually has a PCO_2 only about 6 mm Hg higher than that of arterial blood. Since carbon dioxide diffuses faster than oxygen, it requires a lower pressure head.

The blood in the pulmonary vein is usually virtually fully equilibrated with alveolar air, so that the oxygen and carbon dioxide pressure difference between alveolus and pulmonary vein is, therefore, very slight. Normally, about 2 per cent of the cardiac output bypasses the alveoli by way of the bronchial venous drainage and thebasian veins. Therefore, the partial pressure of oxygen in the arterial blood (P_aO_2) is lowered to around 90 to 100 mm Hg by this venoarterial admixture. Oxygen is carried in the blood by physical solution and in reversible combination with hemoglobin. The peculiar relationship between the degree of this combination with oxygen and the partial pressure of oxygen is apparent from the shape of the oxyhemoglobin dissociation curve (Fig. 6–2). At a PO_2 of 90 mm Hg the hemoglobin saturation with oxygen is about 97 per cent. Each gram of hemoglobin when fully saturated can combine with 1.39 ml of oxygen. With a hemoglobin level of 15 gm/100 ml, 100 ml of blood can contain 15×1.39, or 20.8, ml of oxygen when the hemoglobin is fully saturated with oxygen. If it were 97 per cent saturated, it would have 97 per cent of that value, or 20.2 ml/100 ml.

In addition to the oxygen that is combined with the hemoglobin, about 0.003 ml of oxygen physically dissolves in 100 ml of blood for every millimeter of mercury of PO_2. Therefore, at a PO_2 of 100 mm Hg, 100 ml of blood would contain 0.3 ml of dissolved oxygen. In a person breathing room air, the total oxygen contained in 100 ml of blood at a PO_2 of 100 mm Hg would then be $20.2 + 0.3$, or 20.5, ml of oxygen. By breathing 100 per cent oxygen, a person with normal lungs could raise the arterial PO_2 to over 600 mm Hg. This would fully saturate the hemoglobin, adding 0.6 ml of oxygen per 100 ml. of blood, and 500×0.003, or 1.5, ml. of dissolved oxygen would also be added. This would equal the oxygen-carrying capacity of about 1.5 gm of hemoglobin and would be equivalent in oxygen-carrying capacity to a transfusion of whole blood of about 10 ml/kg. This can be accomplished without waiting for blood typing and cross-matching. At 3 atmospheres pressure ($760 \text{ mm Hg} \times 3 = 2280 \text{ mm Hg}$) with oxygen breathing, the PO_2 of arterial blood may go up to 2100 mm Hg. The dissolved oxygen would then be 2100×0.003, or 6.3 ml/100 ml of blood. Since the usual arteriovenous oxygen difference at rest is about 5 ml/100 ml of blood, the hemoglobin of venous blood could remain fully saturated and respiration could take place without the functioning of hemoglobin.

Diseases of the heart and lungs that produce increased venoarterial admixture, hypoventilation, imbalance of ventilation and perfusion of the alveoli, or barriers to diffusion will produce a fall in PO_2 of arterial blood, which may be partially or completely reversed by breathing oxygen. Unfortunately, oxygen toxicity limits the application of these principles to relatively short durations or relatively low partial pressures of oxygen. Although it is the high arterial PO_2 going to the eye that is thought to cause retrolental fibroplasia, it is possible for pulmonary oxygen toxicity to occur even with low arterial PO_2, since high alveolar PO_2 can be toxic to the lung.

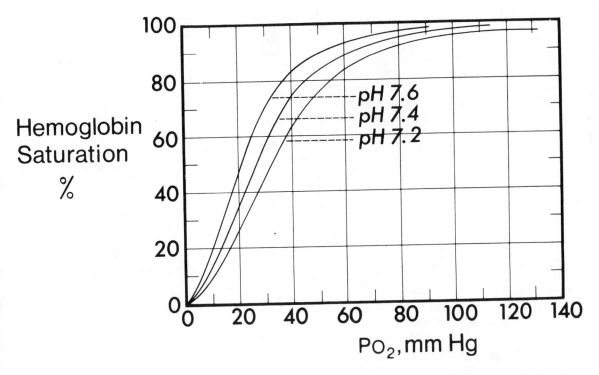

This graph plots oxyhemoglobin saturation as a function of blood oxygen tension at three pH values. Intermediate pH values may be extrapolated.

• To find saturation from P_{O_2} locate P_{O_2}, move vertically to the correct curve, then move horizontally to the saturation axis.
• To find P_{O_2} when saturation is known, reverse these steps.

Figure 6–2. Oxyhemoglobin dissociation curve. (From the American Lung Association. Copyright © 1976 American Thoracic Society — Medical Section of the American Lung Association. Used with permission.)

Owing to the shape of the oxyhemoglobin dissociation curve (Figure 6–2), there is a large margin of alveolar O_2 that can be tolerated with very little drop in O_2 content or saturation, whereas small changes in tissue P_{O_2} can markedly change the amount of O_2 delivered. A lower pH causes a shift of the oxyhemoglobin dissociation curve to the right. This shifting of the curve to the right does not much affect the oxygen saturation at the usual P_{O_2} in the alveolus, but it will affect the delivery of O_2 to the tissues. At the same P_{O_2}, blood with a lower pH will deliver more oxygen to the tissues. Decreasing pH and increasing P_{CO_2} have the same effect in increasing the unloading of oxygen from hemoglobin, which is known as the Bohr effect:

$$HbO_2 + H^+ \rightleftarrows HHb + O_2$$

In this way the local effects of increased metabolic activity at the tissue level can have a direct effect on the availability of O_2.

Cyanosis is usually apparent at an oxygen saturation of 75 to 85 per cent or when there is about 5 gm of reduced hemoglobin in the capillaries. Cyanosis is not a reliable sign of hypoxia, since poor lighting, dark skin pigmentation, and anemia may negate its usefulness as a sign. Rapid infusions of bicarbonate, by raising pH and increasing the affinity of hemoglobin for oxygen and by increasing plasma volume and lowering hemoglobin concentration, may eliminate cyanosis without correcting hypoxia. Cyanosis will also not be observed in a patient who is hypoventilating in oxygen. The P_{CO_2} can then rise to extremely high levels without cyanosis becoming apparent, pointing out the need for arterial P_{O_2} measurements in such patients.

The red blood cells of the newborn infant have a greater affinity for oxygen, shifting the oxyhemoglobin dissociation curve to the left. Thus, cyanosis will not be apparent until the P_{O_2} is close to 40 mm Hg, so it is not a good sign for hypoxia in the newborn infant.

The difference between the affinities of adult and fetal blood for oxygen relates to the greater effect of erythrocyte 2,3-diphosphoglycerate (2,3-DPG) levels on adult hemoglobin. The higher the levels of 2,3-DPG in the red blood cells, the less affinity adult hemoglobin has for oxygen and the more the oxyhemoglobin dissociation curve shifts to the right.[13-16] This increases unloading of oxygen to tissues. Although levels of 2,3-DPG are similar in adult and fetal red blood cells, fetal hemoglobin interacts with 2,3-DPG to a lesser extent and therefore has a higher oxygen affinity. Hypoxia brings about increased levels of 2,3-DPG, which increases oxygen delivery to tissues and serves as an adaptation to the hypoxia.

Animal life requires mitochondrial function, and mitochondria require adequate amounts of oxygen at adequate pressure. If the PO_2 is normal in arterial blood but the amount of oxygen supplied is inadequate, as in severe anemia or circulatory failure, tissue hypoxia results. If the oxygen affinity of hemoglobin is increased, as with hemoglobin-H, then even though adequate amounts of oxygen may be present in the blood, the partial pressure will not be high enough to deliver adequate amounts of oxygen to the mitochondria.

Hypoxia causes a shift from aerobic metabolism toward anaerobic metabolism. Instead of carbohydrate being metabolized to carbon dioxide and water with production of 38 moles of ATP, lactic acid is formed with production of only 2 moles of ATP, depriving cells of their major energy source and further increasing catabolism and production of acids. The production of organic acids increases hydrogen ion concentration, which may further impair cellular function. Hypoxia may quickly cause severe metabolic acidosis and permanent damage. Ameliorating to some extent the adverse effects of the resulting acidemia is the shift of the oxyhemoglobin dissociation curve to the right by the Bohr effect, which will aid in the unloading of oxygen at the tissues, although chronic acidosis will tend to shift the curve back to the left again through its effect on erythrocyte 2,3-DPG levels. Tissue hypoxia is a very common cause of metabolic acidosis and accompanies severe ventilatory or circulatory failure.

The development of metabolic acidosis is, therefore, a good index of tissue hypoxia and should be used in assessing the adequacy of tissue oxygenation.

Hypercapnia. In ventilatory failure CO_2 excretion falters and PCO_2 rises, virtually by definition. The concentration of carbon dioxide in plasma is almost directly proportional to the partial pressure of carbon dioxide, giving an almost linear graphic relationship, unlike the sigmoid curve of oxygen. This is because there is no equivalence of hemoglobin in CO_2 transport. As CO_2 accumulates and PCO_2 rises, there is increased formation of H_2CO_3, which dissociates to form H^+ and HCO_3^-. This can easily be seen by application of the law of mass action to the equilibrium reaction:

$$CO_2 + H_2O \underset{}{\overset{\substack{\text{carbonic}\\ \text{anhydrase}}}{\rightleftharpoons}} H_2CO_3 \rightleftharpoons H^+ + HCO_3^-$$

A rise in CO_2 causes a shift to the right, with an increase in H^+ and HCO_3^-.

Law of Mass Action. The mathematical relationship between these reactants is expressed in the Henderson-Hasselbalch equation:[17]

$$pH = pK + \log \frac{[HCO_3^-]}{[H_2CO_3]}$$

where $[HCO_3^-]$ is the concentration of bicarbonate and $[H_2CO_3]$ is the concentration of carbonic acid.

Although this equation has been used to estimate the effect of disturbances of acid-base balance, it is simpler and generally adequate to apply the law of mass action to the equilibrium reaction for qualitative assessment and, for actual calculations, to use a graphic solution of the Henderson-Hasselbalch equation, such as the Siggaard-Andersen alignment nomogram (see Fig. 6–4).[18] For example, hyperventilation causes a fall in carbon dioxide and a shift to the left of the equilibrium reaction, producing decreases in HCO_3^- and H^+ concentrations. It is easy to see the effects of buffering, compensation, and correction on the equilibrium reaction.

pH

Water dissociates slightly into H^+ and hydroxyl ion (OH^-):

Table 6–1. Acids, Bases, and Neutral Ions

ACIDS	BASES	ELECTROLYTES
H_2CO_3	HCO_3^-	K^+
NH_4	Acetate$^-$	Na^+
R-COOH (organic acids)	NH_3	Ca^{2+}
$H_2PO_4^-$ (in blood)	Lactate$^-$	Mg^{2+}
H_2SO_4	Protein$^-$	Cl^-
HCl	Hemoglobin$^-$	NaCl
	$HPO_4^{2-} =$ (in urine)	KCl
	OH^-	
	THAM	

$$H_2O \rightleftarrows H^+ + OH^-$$

In pure water at 25°C, the velocity of the reactions is such that the concentration of the ions is 1/10,000,000 or 10^{-7} mole per liter.

$$-\log [H^+] = 7$$
$$\text{or pH} = 7$$

Therefore, by definition, a rise in the hydrogen ion concentration and a fall in pH are synonymous. In biologic systems the pH must be maintained in a narrow range. This requires active measures, since metabolic and environmental factors are constantly stressing the mechanisms that maintain stable pH levels. The extreme of range compatible with enzymatic function and, indeed, life in the higher species lies between 7.0 and 7.8 pH. A substance that when added to body fluid will cause a rise in the H^+ concentration is defined as an acid, and something that lowers H^+ concentration is a base (Table 6–1). (See Appendix II for rigorous definitions.)

The substances in column 3 of Table 6–1 are completely ionized in the pH range of body fluids and thus are unable to affect the pH directly. Some of these ions, particularly Na^+, K^+, and Cl^-, may — by active exchange with H^+ and HCO_3^- or by altering metabolic processes as a result of deficit or excess — lead indirectly to changes in pH. They should not be considered acids or bases, however, any more than lead in the form of a bullet should be considered an acid simply because it causes an acidosis in a person who has been shot in the kidney. Acid-base balance should be assessed primarily by attention to pH, acids, bases, and buffer systems.

CLINICAL MEASUREMENTS

An understanding of blood gases and pH is enhanced markedly by knowledge of the principles underlying their clinical measurement. It is not necessary to understand all the technical details involved, however, and they will not be presented here.

pH and Hydrogen Ion Concentration

The commonly used instrument for measuring pH[19] incorporates a glass electrode, which is composed of a glass membrane permeable to hydrogen ions but not to the other anions or cations in solution.

If there is a difference in the concentration of hydrogen ions across this membrane, the hydrogen ions tend to move across the membrane from the side of higher concentration to the side of lower concentration. Since the other particles in solution cannot penetrate the glass membrane, a potential difference will develop across the membrane proportional to the differences in concentration of the hydrogen ion. This potential difference can be measured easily. If known concentrations of hydrogen ions are placed on one side of the glass membrane with a standard solution on the other side, and if the potential differences are measured, the electrode can be calibrated. One can then measure the potential difference created by an unknown solution and thus determine its H^+ concentration. Although the chemical activity of hydrogen ions and not their actual concentration is being meas-

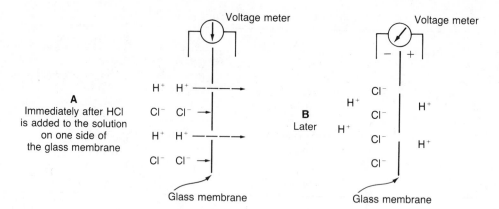

ured, the two values are equivalent in dilute solutions of H$^+$, such as blood. This extremely valuable measure can be made in seconds on microsamples of blood or other fluids. The samples require no preliminary preparation or processing and the procedure can give very reliable results even with technically unsophisticated users of the equipment.

The normal pH of human arterial blood is 7.4. This is the same as a concentration of H$^+$ of $10^{-7.4}$ Eq/l, or 0.00004 mEq/l, or 40 nEq (nanoequivalents)/l. An abnormally low pH of the blood is called acidemia, and occasionally a pH as low as 6.8 may occur, but it will not last very long, since it is not compatible with life for more than minutes to hours. A pH as high as 7.7 occasionally occurs. A high pH in the blood is called alkalemia. The normal pH of 7.4 of the arterial blood has no generally accepted term, although *eupHemia* has been suggested. The pH of venous blood will be affected by the metabolic work of the tissues drained, but in an extremity at rest will generally be around 0.04 pH unit lower than that of arterial blood.

Relationship Between pH and Hydrogen Ion Concentration. pH is the negative logarithm of the H$^+$ concentration measured in equivalents per liter (Eq/l). This relationship, although straightforward mathematically, is a little difficult to use in the field, owing to the difficult arithmetic involved in the conversion. This has lead to a variety of suggestions for simplifying the conversion.[20]

One suggestion is that, since the relationship between pH and [H$^+$] (hydrogen ion concentration) is almost linear in the range of pH from 7.1 to 7.5, a change of 0.01

pH unit will change [H$^+$] 1 nEq/l. At the normal arterial pH of 7.4, H$^+$ concentration equals 40 nEq/l. A fall in pH from 7.4 to 7.2 will increase H$^+$ concentration from 40 to 60 nEq/l.

Another suggestion is to multiply the normal hydrogen ion concentration of 40 nEq/l by 1.25 sequentially for each 0.1 unit decrement in pH and by 0.8 for each 0.1 unit increment in pH. Thus, for a pH of 7.2, which is 0.2 unit below 7.4:

$$40 \times 1.25 = 50$$
$$50 \times 1.25 = 62.5$$

Therefore, the estimated hydrogen ion concentration is 62.5 nEq/l. For a pH of 7.7, which is up 0.3 pH units more than 7.4:

$$40 \times 0.8 = 32$$
$$32 \times 0.8 = 25.6$$
$$25.6 \times 0.8 = 20.5$$

The estimated hydrogen ion concentration, then, is 20.5 nEq/l.

Another method estimates the change in H$^+$ concentration by recognizing that the antilogarithm of 0.3 is 2, so that for every 0.3 unit increase or decrease in pH, there is, respectively, a halving or doubling of H$^+$ concentration. Thus, as pH falls from 7.4 to 7.1, H$^+$ concentration increases from 40 to 80 nEq/l.

A simple and precise method is to use an electronic calculator that does logarithms and antilogarithms. Keep in mind in these calculations that the concentrations must be expressed in equivalents per liter (Eq/l), not in milliequivalents or nanoequivalents per liter (mEq/l or nEq/l). Thus, if the concentration of H$^+$ is 20 nEq/l, or 0.00002 mEq/l, it is 0.00000002 Eq/l. If you enter 0.00000002 into the calculator and then press "log," you get −7.69897. Similarly, with 0.00000004 entered, the result is −7.39794, and with 0.00000008 entered, you get −7.09691, and so on.

If you know the pH and want to calculate the H$^+$ concentration, follow the calculator directions for antilogarithms. On the Texas Instruments Model TI-308 calculator, for example, given a pH of 7.4 and the desire to find the concentration of H$^+$, you enter 7.4; press "+/−", which makes it −7.4; and then press "inv", then "log"; and you get 3.9811 × 10^{-8}, or 0.000000039811, or 39.8 nEq/l. When you enter 6.9, you get 0.00000013, or 130 nEq/l. An electronic calculator makes these interconversions extremely quick and easy. As a matter of fact, an electronic calculator turns solutions of the Henderson-Hasselbalch equation itself into a snap.

Partial Pressure of Carbon Dioxide

The electrode for the measurement of PCO$_2$ utilizes the special glass membrane that is used for hydrogen ion measurement (Fig. 6–3).[21] The glass membrane is covered at a slight distance by another membrane that is permeable to carbon dioxide, so that a small chamber is created whose walls are formed by the glass membrane permeable to H$^+$ on one side and the membrane permeable to CO$_2$ on the other. A solution that contains water and carbonic anhydrase is enclosed in this chamber. If carbon dioxide is placed on the outside of the CO$_2$-permeable membrane, it will diffuse across the membrane into the aqueous solution containing carbonic anhydrase. As noted previously, the carbon dioxide will combine with water in the presence of carbonic anhydrase to form carbonic acid, most of which will immediately dissociate into bicarbonate and hydrogen ion.

$$CO_2 + H_2O \overset{\text{carbonic}}{\underset{\text{anhydrase}}{\rightleftharpoons}} H_2CO_3 \rightleftharpoons H^+ + HCO_3^-$$

The hydrogen ions produced in the reaction will tend to penetrate the glass membrane by sliding down the concentration gradient, whereas the bicarbonate will be excluded, producing a potential difference across the glass membrane proportional to the concentration of carbon dioxide. Known concentrations of carbon dioxide are placed on one side of the CO$_2$-permeable membrane to calibrate the system, and then unknown concentrations can be easily measured.

It should be noted that the pH and PCO$_2$ electrodes are not measuring the amounts of hydrogen ion or carbon dioxide contained in the sample but are directly measuring their chemical activity or concentration, so measurement of the volume of the sample need not be made.

A normal PCO$_2$ of arterial blood is 40 mm Hg. A low PCO$_2$ (e.g., 20 mm Hg) is

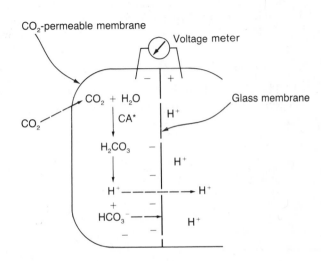

Figure 6–3. Carbon dioxide (CO$_2$) electrode.

*Carbonic anhydrase

called respiratory alkalosis, and a high PCO_2 (e.g., 80 mm Hg) is respiratory acidosis. The PCO_2, as previously discussed, is directly proportional to alveolar ventilation and is therefore of great value in assessing the respiratory system. A normal PCO_2 of 40 mm Hg and a normal pH of 7.4 in arterial blood is rarely seen in normal children, since they almost always are agitated by the procedure and cry or otherwise hyperventilate, tending to give a lower PCO_2 and a higher pH than what one might otherwise expect.

Partial Pressure of Oxygen

The PO_2 electrode does not depend on permeability through a glass membrane but instead depends on flow of electrons from a silver–silver chloride anode to oxygen at the cathode.[21, 22] This electric current is proportional to the PO_2 at the cathode. Calibration is performed with samples of known PO_2.

Normal PO_2 in arterial blood during breathing of room air is 80 to 100 mm Hg. The PO_2 electrode and the ones for pH and PCO_2 require only tiny samples of blood, which need only heparinizing and no further treatment, do not require weighing or measuring of volume, and involve only seconds to minutes to give very accurate and extremely useful results.

The oxygen saturation can be determined colorimetrically, since blood that is fully oxygenated is bright red and blood that is unsaturated with oxygen is darker. The relationship of PO_2 to oxygen saturation is not linear, but the curve has a peculiar shape, which is graphically represented in the oxyhemoglobin dissociation curve (see Fig. 6–2).

Total Carbon Dioxide

The standard method for measuring the oxygen content of blood is the Van Slyke method, which determines the amount of oxygen in a specific volume of a sample.[23] This requires precise measurement of volume and meticulous technique and is therefore rarely done in clinical laboratories.

The Van Slyke method with modifications is still commonly used for measurements of CO_2 in serum.[23] This entails precise measurement of the volume of a sample of serum, the addition of a strong acid to convert the bicarbonate to CO_2, and the application of suction so that the CO_2 is removed as a gas from the serum:

$$H^+ + HCO_3^- \rightarrow H_2CO_3 \rightarrow H_2O + CO_2 \uparrow$$

After oxygen is removed from the specimen, the remaining carbon dioxide is measured and reported in millimoles per liter of serum (mmol/l). Normal total CO_2 in children is 22 to 24 mmol/l. This total CO_2, which is traditionally reported along with the sodium, potassium and chloride as serum "electrolytes," should not be confused with PCO_2 or with bicarbonate. The PCO_2 is reported in millimeters of mercury (mm Hg), torr, or kilopascals, is a function of the chemical activity of the gas (the partial pressure), and is usually determined on whole blood. The total CO_2 includes all CO_2 in the serum, as well as the bicarbonate and the carbonic acid that were present in the specimen and were converted to carbon dioxide. Increased PCO_2 and increased HCO_3^- will, therefore, cause total CO_2 to be increased, and decreased PCO_2 and decreased HCO_3^- will cause it to be decreased. These effects on total CO_2 can be easily visualized by applying the law of mass action to the equilibrium reaction for carbonic acid. The principle of Le Chatelier states that if the conditions of a system that is initially at equilibrium are changed, the equilibrium will shift in a direction that will tend to restore the original conditions. This is also known as the law of mass action.

At anode:
4 Ag$^+$ + 4 Cl$^-$ $\longrightarrow$ 4 AgCl + 4 e

At cathode:
O_2 + 2 H$_2$O + 4 e$^-$ $\longrightarrow$ 4 OH$^-$

High total carbon dioxide due to increase in PCO_2:

$$CO_2 + H_2O \xrightleftharpoons[\text{carbonic anhydrase}]{} H_2CO_3 \rightleftarrows H^+ + HCO_3^-$$

An increase in PCO_2 raises the concentration of the reactants on the left side of the equation, causing a shift to the right. Therefore, carbon dioxide, carbonic acid, and bicarbonate are all elevated and contribute to an increase in total carbon dioxide.

High total carbon dioxide due to decrease in hydrogen ion concentration:

$$CO_2 + H_2O \xrightleftharpoons[\text{carbonic anhydrase}]{} H_2CO_3 \rightleftarrows H^+ + HCO_3^-$$

A decrease in hydrogen ion concentration will shift the equilibrium to the right, increasing the bicarbonate and decreasing carbon dioxide and carbonic acid. As new carbon dioxide is formed in metabolism, its level will return toward previous levels and may even exceed them. This produces an increase in total carbon dioxide.

High total carbon dioxide due to increase in bicarbonate:

$$CO_2 + H_2O \xrightleftharpoons[\text{carbonic anhydrase}]{} H_2CO_3 \rightleftarrows H^+ + HCO_3^-$$

An increase in bicarbonate will shift the equilibrium to the left, increasing carbonic acid and carbon dioxide, which will contribute to an increase in total carbon dioxide. The shift to the left will also, obviously, decrease hydrogen ion concentration.

Low total carbon dioxide due to decrease in PCO_2:

$$CO_2 + H_2O \xrightleftharpoons[\text{carbonic anhydrase}]{} H_2CO_3 \rightleftarrows H^+ + HCO_3^-$$

A decrease in PCO_2 causes the equilibrium reaction to shift to the left, lowering hydrogen ion concentration as well as carbon dioxide, carbonic acid, and bicarbonate, producing a decrease in the total carbon dioxide.

Low total carbon dioxide due to increase in hydrogen ion concentration:

$$CO_2 + H_2O \xrightleftharpoons[\text{carbonic anhydrase}]{} H_2CO_3 \rightleftarrows H^+ + HCO_3^-$$

The increased hydrogen ion concentration will shift the reaction to the left, decreasing bicarbonate and temporarily increasing carbon dioxide and carbonic acid. As ventilation continues, the increased carbon dioxide will be excreted and carbon dioxide and carbonic acid will return toward or below previous levels. The decrease in bicarbonate will be reflected in a decrease in total carbon dioxide.

Low total carbon dioxide due to decrease in bicarbonate:

$$CO_2 + H_2O \xrightleftharpoons[\text{carbonic anhydrase}]{} H_2CO_3 \rightleftarrows H^+ + HCO_3^-$$

As bicarbonate is lost, the equilibrium reaction shifts to the right, raising the hydrogen ion concentration. In addition to the lower bicarbonate, the carbonic acid and carbon dioxide will decrease temporarily and then return toward normal levels as more carbon dioxide is produced. The lowering of bicarbonate will be reflected in a lower total carbon dioxide.

This variety of influences on total CO_2 makes its significance difficult to evaluate unless one takes into consideration the clinical status of the patient, the pH, and the PCO_2. Potential confusion makes the total CO_2 less clinically useful unless derangements are profound, since respiratory changes only affect total CO_2 to a limited extent. Therefore, total CO_2 below 16 or over 45 mmol/l can be presumed to be due to nonrespiratory changes. For less extreme deviations, total CO_2 may not be very helpful.

Base Excess

The PCO_2 gives an accurate reflection of the respiratory component of the acid-base balance. For example, a PCO_2 of 80 mm Hg indicates respiratory acidosis, and one of 15 mm Hg indicates respiratory alkalosis. A simple equivalent to indicate the metabolic (nonrespiratory) component of a pH disturbance would be useful, since respiratory problems entail one type of therapy and metabolic problems usually entail something quite different. It has already been demonstrated that the total CO_2 cannot fill the bill.

The effect of respiratory abnormalities on the pH in a blood sample can be eliminated by bringing the PCO_2 from its initial level to the normal level of 40 mm Hg. By then titrating the blood with standard acid or base to a pH of 7.4, the metabolic component of the disturbance can be measured.

Ponder, for example, a patient with an arterial PCO_2 of 80 mm Hg and a pH of 6.9. It is immediately evident that there is an elevation in the respiratory component of acid-base equilibrium, because the PCO_2 is elevated. Is there a metabolic component of the disturbance affecting the pH as well, and if so, how much? To eliminate the effect of the elevated PCO_2 (the respiratory component) on the pH, the blood can be equilibrated with gas with a PCO_2 of 40 mm Hg. With a lowering of the PCO_2 of the blood to 40 mm Hg, the hydrogen ion concentration should fall and the pH should rise, as indicated by the law of mass action.

Suppose the pH rises from 6.9 to 7.1. We know that a metabolic component to the disturbance must also be present, since the pH would otherwise have risen to 7.4 when the PCO_2 was brought to normal. To determine how much of a metabolic component there is, the blood can be titrated to a normal pH of 7.4 with strong base. If it requires 16 mEq/l of sodium hydroxide (NaOH) to bring the pH of the blood specimen from 7.1 to 7.4, there is a base deficit of 16 mEq/l, or a base excess of −16 mEq/l. This concept of base excess is helpful in understanding acid-base problems and in deciding on therapy, since base excess can be used as an index of the metabolic component of the disturbance. It reflects the changes in the concentrations of H^+ and HCO_3^- and other buffers.[7, 24]

It is not necessary to equilibrate blood and then titrate it in the laboratory each time the base excess must be determined, since it can be calculated by means of a number of appropriate nomograms as long as the hemoglobin concentration and any two of these values — PCO_2, pH, and total carbon dioxide — are known (see Fig. 6–4).

Bicarbonate

It is sometimes forgotten that bicarbonate concentration is not actually measured in clinical laboratories but is a derived value (as is base excess) that is calculated by using the Henderson-Hasselbalch equation or by subtracting the values for dissolved CO_2 and H_2CO_3 from the value for the total CO_2. Thus, the value for bicarbonate is dependent on the validity of certain assumptions, such as the constancy of pK and the solubility of CO_2. The calculation of HCO_3^- values can be made directly from the Henderson-Hasselbalch equation if two out of three of these values — total CO_2, pH, and PCO_2 — are known by means of one of a number of nomograms, by computer program, or by calculator.

Since HCO_3^- values approximate total CO_2 values so closely, they are frequently used interchangeably in clinical practice. This is probably reasonable in most circumstances where great precision is not required, but if the total CO_2 (in mmol/l) and the PCO_2 (in mm Hg) are known, it is very easy to calculate the bicarbonate concentration, since the solubility factor for CO_2 in blood is 0.03 and the total CO_2 is known to be made up mostly of HCO_3^-, a small amount of dissolved CO_2, and a minute amount of H_2CO_3. If the PCO_2 is multiplied by the solubility factor, the product represents the dissolved CO_2 and H_2CO_3. For example, if in a sample of blood the PCO_2 is 40 mm Hg, then dissolved CO_2 and H_2CO_3 are 40×0.03, or 1.2 mmol/l. If the total CO_2 is 26 mmol/l, then the HCO_3^- in that sample of blood is $26 - 1.2$, or 24.8 mmol/l. Since the concentration of H_2CO_3 in the total CO_2 is 0.01 per cent of the concentration of bicarbonate, 0.2 per cent of the concentration of dissolved CO_2, and 0.0095 per cent of the total CO_2, it can be safely ignored.

$$[HCO_3^-] = \text{total } CO_2 - (PCO_2 \times 0.03)$$

SIGGAARD-ANDERSEN ALIGNMENT NOMOGRAM

Figure 6–4 shows the Siggaard-Andersen alignment nomogram. The four

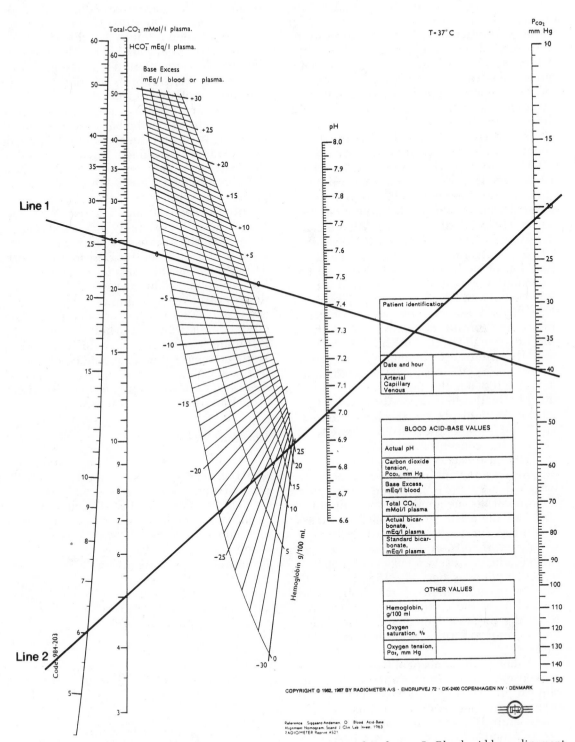

Figure 6–4. Siggaard-Andersen alignment nomogram. (From Siggaard-Andersen O: Blood acid-base alignment nomogram. Scand Clin Lab Invest 15:211, 1963. Radiometer reprint AS21. Copyright © 1962, 1967 by Radiometer A/S. Used with permission.)

straight lines of the nomogram present a graphic solution to the Henderson-Hasselbalch equation. A straight line drawn through any two points on the figures gives the solution for the equation at the points where the drawn line intersects the nomogram lines. Take, for example, a bicarbonate of 24.5 mmol/l (mEq/l on the nomogram scale) and a PCO_2 of 40 mm Hg. A straight line drawn between these points on the PCO_2 and HCO_3^- scales (Line 1) intersects the pH scale at 7.4, indicating that for a HCO_3^- value of 24.5 mmol/l and a PCO_2 of 40 mm Hg, the pH is 7.4 according to the Henderson-Hasselbalch equation. A straight line drawn on the nomogram between HCO_3^- 5 mEq/l and pH 7.0 indicates a PCO_2 of 21 mm Hg (Line 2). Notice that these straight lines intersect a grid shaped like a machete blade and labeled Base Excess and Hemoglobin. At the point where the Hemoglobin line intersects the drawn line, the base excess can be read. For example, Line 2 on the nomogram, drawn from pH 7.0 through HCO_3^- 5 mEq/l and PCO_2 21 mm Hg, intersects Hemoglobin 15 gm at Base Excess −27 mEq/l. At a hemoglobin of 5 gm/100 ml, the base excess is −24.2 mEq/l. On the line drawn between PCO_2 40 mm Hg and pH 7.4, the base excess is zero and is not affected by changes in hemoglobin concentration.

The base excess is very useful in simplifying assessment of problems of acid-base balance, since by intent it gives a measure of the metabolic component of the acid-base disturbance. A normal base excess is 0 mEq/l for adults and −2 mEq/l to −4 mEq/l for infants. A base excess of −20 mEq/l indicates a severe excess of metabolic acids, whereas one of +15 mEq/l indicates a severe deficit of metabolic acids regardless of the clinical status of the patient, the pH, the Henderson-Hasselbalch equation, or any rules of thumb or golden rules.

Although the concept of base excess has proved to be very useful in understanding clinical problems of acid-base metabolism, it should be remembered that this value is based entirely on measurements made on whole blood. Extrapolation may easily be made to interstitial fluid and, less easily, to intracellular fluid. The role of intracellular buffers and bone in total body buffering may prove to be extremely important, but the clinical significance is still relatively

unknown.[25, 26] For most purposes we can assume that the base excess does reflect the acid-base state of the body as a whole, but we should keep in mind that this is only an assumption. Additionally, the Henderson-Hasselbalch equation itself assumes that the pK and the solubility are not variables, but this is not always true.

Another problem, although a minor one, with the use of the base excess is that it does not, to be precise, give only an index of the metabolic component, owing to the flux of bicarbonate between blood and interstitial fluid in acute respiratory changes in PCO_2. The base excess will fall about 2 mEq/l for each 20 mm Hg rise in PCO_2. When the PCO_2 suddenly increases from 40 to 80 mm Hg, the base excess will be expected to drop from 0 mEq/l to −4 mEq/l. This should not be considered a change in the metabolic component. This effect, although of physiologic interest, is relatively small and need not be considered in most clinical circumstances, when deviations in PCO_2 are less severe. Why this distinction between the respiratory and metabolic components is important in diagnosis and in therapy will become obvious in the sections on pathophysiology and disease states.

Carbonic Acid

Carbonic acid is of special importance to pH balance since it is in equilibrium with the alveolar CO_2, which is "volatile."

The Henderson-Hasselbalch equation is derived from the equilibrium reactions of carbonic acid in the following way.

From the law of mass action,

$$H_2CO_3 \rightleftarrows H^+ + HCO_3^-$$

becomes

$$K = \frac{\{H^+\}\,\{HCO_3^-\}}{\{H_2CO_3\}}$$

or

$$\{H^+\} = \frac{K\{H_2CO_3\}}{\{HCO_3^-\}}$$

In logarithmic form,

$$-\log\{H^+\} = -\log K - \log\frac{\{H_2CO_3\}}{\{HCO_3^-\}}$$

or

$$pH = pK + \log \frac{\{HCO_3^-\}}{\{H_2CO_3\}}$$

This relationship is of limited practical usefulness, since only the pH is measured and the bicarbonate and carbonic acid activity and the pK are not.

In order to make some use of this sorry state of affairs, a term representing the approximate pK is introduced, the pK'; instead of the activity of HCO_3^-, the concentration of HCO_3^- is used, and instead of H_2CO_3 concentration, the PCO_2 times a solubility factor (0.03) is introduced. (This can be done because the concentration of H_2CO_3 is proportional to the dissolved CO_2, which is proportional to the PCO_2 times a solubility factor.) Thus, we end up with

$$pH = pK' + \log \frac{[HCO_3^-]}{PCO_2 \times 0.03}$$

where pK' is assumed to be a constant equal to 6.1. Actual measurements have shown it to be surprisingly variable for a constant, depending on ionic concentration, temperature, and pH and ranging from 5.8 to 6.429.[27-31] The solubility factor for CO_2 is somewhat variable with temperature also, a factor taken into account by laboratories conducting measurements of total CO_2.[32]

The relationship between pK', temperature, and pH can be described by the following equation:[29]

$$pK' = -4.7416 + \frac{1840.141}{T} + 0.15906(T)$$

$$-\log \left(1 + \frac{0.020682}{10^{-pH+7}}\right)$$

Under most, if not all, clinical conditions, the variability is negligible, but for extreme precision, this term should replace pK' in the Henderson-Hasselbalch equation.

This equation has been responsible for discouraging generations of physicians from appreciating and understanding problems of acid-base balance. It is a classic example of the emperor's new clothes, for everyone pretends to understand it but few do. For most of us, it is difficult if not totally impossible to figure out the effect of a primary acid-base disturbance with its compensatory effects and, perhaps, a superimposed lesser disturbance while simultaneously balancing an equation containing two negative logarithms, two "constants," and a ratio.

It is far better to go back to the equilibrium reaction from which the Henderson-Hasselbalch equation is derived in order to see the qualitative effects of a disturbance, and then to use a nomogram, such as the Siggaard-Andersen alignment nomogram, or an electronic calculator to make the actual calculations on the rare occasions when this is necessary, rather than referring directly to the Henderson-Hasselbalch equation for this purpose (see Chapter 12).

For human blood at pH 7.4, PCO_2 40 mm Hg, and HCO_3^- 24 mmol/l, the following numerical relationships exist, as calculated from the Henderson-Hasselbalch equation:

$$CO_2 + H_2O \rightleftarrows H_2CO_3 \rightleftarrows HCO_3^- + H^+$$
$$30,000 \qquad\qquad 60 \qquad 600,000 \quad 1$$

For every H^+ ion there are 600,000 HCO_3^- ions, 30,000 CO_2 molecules, and 60 H_2CO_3 molecules. Do not bother figuring out the constants in the reaction and the mathematical relationship, since the result is simply the Henderson-Hasselbalch equation again.

One may wonder what happens to electroneutrality as the equilibrium shifts from left to right and from right to left; the plus signs and minus signs do not seem to add up properly. The nonbicarbonate buffers have been omitted from the equilibrium reaction for simplicity. As H^+ concentration changes, buffer reactions take place with exchange of H^+ for other cations:

$$Na\text{-}Buffer + H^+ \rightarrow H\text{-}Buffer + Na^+$$

It is necessary to visualize Na^+ and all the other cations swimming around in the same soup.

Familiarity with the measurements of pH, PO_2, PCO_2, total CO_2, and base excess is essential in understanding the biological effects of disease and in managing sick patients. It is, therefore, important to feel pleasantly enthusiastic toward their use. This attitude can be acquired with a modicum of effort and with continued use of these measurements.

TERMINOLOGY

Acidemia and Alkalemia

The pH of arterial blood is currently the definitive index of the acid-base balance. An abnormally low pH, indicating an excess of acid in the arterial blood, is called acidemia. An abnormally high pH, indicating too little acid (or too much base) in the blood, is called alkalemia.

Acidosis and Alkalosis: Compensation and Correction

A PCO_2 greater than 40 mm Hg in the arterial blood represents respiratory acidosis regardless of the pH or the HCO_3^- value. A low PCO_2 represents respiratory alkalosis. The ending -osis should be taken to mean a tendency in the direction specified in the stem of the word. In the same way, an elevated arterial base excess may be called metabolic alkalosis and a base deficit, or negative base excess, may be called metabolic acidosis, regardless of the actual pH, HCO_3^- or PCO_2.

If the respiratory or metabolic acidosis or alkalosis is the initiating disturbance, it should be called primary — e.g., primary respiratory acidosis in a patient with lung disease who is hypoventilating and has a high PCO_2. If the disturbance has gone on for a while and physiologic mechanisms that modify it from the opposite side of the carbonic acid equilibrium have come into play, these modifications can be called compensatory. For example, if the PCO_2 has been elevated for several days (1), the kidney may compensate for the low pH by retaining HCO_3^- (2), which is called metabolic compensation or compensatory metabolic alkalosis (see diagram below). When the lung disease has been treated and the PCO_2 returns to normal, it is said that the primary disturbance has been corrected (3). An acute disturbance is one in which maximal compensation has not yet developed; a chronic disturbance is one in which compensation has already occurred, as illustrated by the following values:

1. Normal arterial blood: pH 7.4, PCO_2 40 mm Hg, base excess 0 mEq/l.
2. Acute respiratory acidosis with acidemia: pH 7.2, PCO_2 80 mm Hg, base excess −4 mEq/l.
3. Chronic respiratory acidosis with acidemia and compensatory metabolic alkalosis: pH 7.34, PCO_2 80 mm Hg, base excess +12 mEq/l.

It is relatively common to see patients with "pure" acute respiratory acidosis and respiratory alkalosis, owing to the need for an interval of several hours or days before significant metabolic compensation can occur. If blood is drawn early in the disturbance, compensation may not yet be evident. On the other hand, it is uncommon to see the effects of "pure" metabolic acidosis or alkalosis, since respiratory compensation can take place in seconds to minutes owing to the rapid diffusion of CO_2. A metabolic acidosis, through its stimulatory effects on the respiratory center, almost immediately causes an increase in ventilation and very rapid compensatory lowering of PCO_2. Values for representative arterial blood gases of chronic compensated metabolic acidosis are pH 7.29, PCO_2 18 mm Hg, and base excess −16 mEq/l.

Compensation for a metabolic acidosis occurs through respiratory adjustments to increase alveolar ventilation and lower PCO_2, affecting the opposite side of the equilibrium reaction from the primary disturbance. Correction of the disturbance takes place on the same side of the equilibrium reaction as the primary disturbance and in metabolic acidosis occurs, for example, by excretion of hydrogen ions, retention of bicarbonate, addition of other bases, and metabolic removal of H^+ by its combination with lactate or pyruvate as they enter the citric acid cycle.

In the same way, correction of a respira-

$$CO_2 + H_2O \rightleftharpoons H_2CO_3 \rightleftharpoons H^+ + HCO_3^-$$

(1) ———————————————————————→

(3) ←——————————————————— (2)

(1) increased CO_2: Primary respiratory acidosis
(2) increased HCO_3^-: Compensatory metabolic alkalosis
(3) decreased CO_2: Correction of the disturbance

tory abnormality takes place by adjustment of alveolar ventilation to return PCO_2 to normal. If chronic respiratory acidosis is corrected quickly, the residual compensatory metabolic alkalosis may subsequently take several days for correction.

Buffering

While metabolic compensation may take days and respiratory compensation minutes, buffering takes place with the speed of a rapid chemical reaction. Buffering acts to decrease the impact of changes in the amount of acids or bases in solution by minimizing their effect on hydrogen ion concentration.

A weak acid in solution along with its salts is a buffer system, since addition of strong acid or base results in less change in H^+ concentration than would occur in pure water. "Strong" acids are completely dissociated in biologic solutions, releasing H^+ and the anion:

$$HCl \rightarrow H^+ + Cl^-$$

$$H_2SO_4 \rightarrow H^+ + HSO_4^-$$

$$H_3PO_4 \rightarrow H^+ + H_2PO_4^-$$

"Weak" acids form an equilibrium between the H^+ and the anion in biologic solutions:

$$H_2PO_4^- \leftrightarrows H^+ + HPO_4^{2-}$$

$$R-COOH \leftrightarrows H^+ + R-COO^-$$

$$H_2CO_3 \leftrightarrows H^+ + HCO_3^-$$

$$NH_4^+ \rightleftarrows H^+ + NH_3$$

$$H-protein \rightleftarrows H^+ + protein^-$$

In biologic solutions, sodium or potassium ions are always present to form salts. If hydrogen ions are added to or taken from a solution containing these salts and weak acids and bases, the equilibrium will shift by the law of mass action, or Le Chatelier's principle, so as to decrease the change in H^+ concentration that might otherwise have been expected. The major buffers in blood are hemoglobin, which provides 35 per cent of the total buffer capacity, and bicarbonate, which provides over 50 per cent. The weak carbonic acid plays a central role in physiologic buffering:

$$H_2CO_3 \rightleftarrows H^+ + HCO_3^-$$

In addition to acting like any of the other buffers to lessen changes in pH, carbonic acid converts quickly and reversibly to CO_2 and H_2O in the presence of carbonic anhydrase. There are large reservoirs of carbon dioxide in the body; it is constantly produced by all the cells and is continuously excreted in the lungs, providing a virtually inexhaustible supply of H_2CO_3, unlike the other buffer acids. Since large amounts of CO_2 can be quickly retained or excreted by the lungs, the amount of CO_2 in the body can be quickly increased or reduced. The lungs, by precisely regulating the excretion of CO_2, influence the left side of the equilibrium reaction, and the kidneys, by controlling the excretion of H^+ and HCO_3^-, influence the right side of the equilibrium reaction and thus can control the concentration of H^+.

A teleologic question that may arise is, since a buffer is more effective near its pK, why is the pK of bicarbonate 6.1 rather than 7.4, at which, theoretically, it would be more effective? Or, if chemistry seems more immutable than biology, one might ask, since bicarbonate is the major buffer, why isn't the normal human arterial pH around 6.1? H_2CO_3 dissociates in blood at a pH of 7.4 to such an extent that there is 20 times more HCO_3^- than CO_2. This 20-fold greater concentration of HCO_3^- allows for greater control of pH by respiration. Since H_2CO_3 is in equilibrium with carbon dioxide, which is a volatile gas, small changes in CO_2 concentration produce large changes in H^+ concentration, permitting very great leverage over the effect it would have if it were acting near the pK of bicarbonate.

If the normal human arterial pH were 6.1, at a PCO_2 of 40 mm Hg the HCO_3^- concentration would be 1.2 mEq/l. This would decrease the effectiveness of bicarbonate as a buffer, since its concentration would be lower. In order to have 24.5 mEq/l of HCO_3^- at a pH of 6.1, the PCO_2 would have to be 817 mm Hg, which is 57 mm Hg higher than the barometric pressure at sea level on earth. Perhaps theoretical inhabitants of a planet like Jupiter would have a PCO_2 in this range. Human beings with this PCO_2 on earth would be very effervescent.

There are other characteristics of this system that are very interesting. If you add an amount of acid, such as lactic acid, to the system, buffering will occur as the equilibrium shifts and as H_2CO_3 and then CO_2 and

H_2O are produced. If the patient is apneic, the PCO_2 will rise, countering further shifts in the equilibrium and decreasing the efficiency of the buffer system. This represents a "closed" system. If the patient does not become apneic but continues to have the same alveolar ventilation, the PCO_2 will rise transiently and then fall toward the initial level, since the alveolar air will contain an increased amount of CO_2, which will then be excreted at a greater rate. The CO_2 produced by the shift in the equilibrium induced by the increase in hydrogen ions will thus be excreted via the lung, and the shifted hydrogen ions will end up in new molecules of water.

This represents an "open system" in which the newly produced CO_2 does not stay in the system to decrease its efficiency but is removed instead. One can see this effect in a patient on a respirator with a fixed rate and tidal volume; thus, a patient with a fixed level of alveolar ventilation can be considered an "open" carbonic acid buffer system.

In intact human beings this does not happen, and the intact human being should not be considered an open system. In the normal human being the increased hydrogen ion concentration from the lactic acid is sensed by receptors and respiration is immediately increased, lowering CO_2 below the initial level, thus shifting the equilibrium to the left and lowering H^+ concentration to an extent far greater than would a mere open system. This part of the buffer system is called respiratory compensation. Thus, the carbonic acid buffer system in the intact human organism is not merely an *open* system but a *yawning* system.

Similar schemes can be outlined for metabolic alkalosis, respiratory acidosis, and respiratory alkalosis, and further discussion of these will be found in Chapter 12.

The bicarbonate–carbonic acid–carbon dioxide equilibrium system is also of interest because certain specialized cells of the body that contain carbonic anhydrase can convert CO_2 and H_2O to H^+ and HCO_3^- and can secrete the H^+ and retain the HCO_3^-. This occurs in the kidney and the stomach. In the stomach this serves a digestive purpose, and in the kidney it plays a vital role in the excretion of H^+ and retention of HCO_3^-.

Another important characteristic of this system is that, owing to the fact that carbon dioxide is so readily soluble and highly diffusible, it is available when needed at all body sites. It is a truly marvelous system.

Dilution Acidosis and Contraction Alkalosis. The effects of changes in extracellular volume on acid-base balance can be easily visualized by reference to the equilibrium reaction. If extracellular volume is rapidly expanded or contracted, the concentration of the blood buffers will be increased or decreased proportionately but the level of PCO_2, although initially deviating in the same direction, will quickly return toward normal levels:

Contraction alkalosis

$$\longleftarrow$$
$$H_2O + CO_2 \rightleftarrows H_2CO_3 \rightleftarrows H^+ + HCO_3^-$$
$$\longrightarrow$$

Dilution acidosis

A decrease in the concentration of HCO_3^- will result in a shift of the equilibrium to the right, regardless of the cause of the decrease, with an increase in H^+ concentration or a decrease in pH. The opposite occurs when there is a contraction of extracellular volume increasing the concentration of bicarbonate. This has been reported as a major factor in the alkalosis of pyloric stenosis, but its full clinical significance remains to be determined.[33]

THE CONTROL OF HYDROGEN ION LEVELS

During normal metabolism, the body cells release into the extracellular fluid a number of compounds that are capable of acting as acids. The most important are:

1. Organic acids, which result from incomplete degradation of fats, carbohydrates, and amino acids.

2. Dihydrogen phosphate, which forms

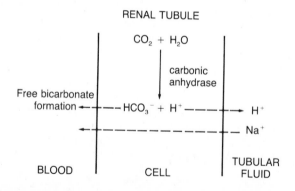

RENAL TUBULE

$CO_2 + H_2O$

carbonic anhydrase

Free bicarbonate formation ← $HCO_3^- + H^+$ ⟶ H^+

⟶ Na^+

BLOOD   CELL   TUBULAR FLUID

when ATP is split to ADP during energy-primed reactions.

3. Carbon dioxide, which is produced by the complete oxidation of carbohydrates, fats, and proteins and which reacts with water to produce carbonic acid, bicarbonate and hydrogen ion.

4. Inorganic acids produced in the metabolism of protein, e.g., H_2SO_4.

In general, metabolism in infants produces an average of 2 to 3 mEq of H^+ per kilogram of body weight per day, so that an increase in H^+ concentration is always likely if the ion if not continuously removed from the body. Four mechanisms prevent such an increase from occurring:

1. *The buffering capacity of the blood and cells.* The various buffers, such as protein, hemoglobin, and bicarbonate, take up hydrogen ion:

$$HCO_3^- + H^+ \rightarrow CO_2 + H_2O$$

$$Protein^- + H^+ \rightarrow Protein-H$$

The H^+ concentration, and therefore the pH, may change little, but the buffer capacity is reduced. The ability of the buffers to prevent an increase in H^+ concentration is limited by their concentrations.

2. *Metabolism.* Anabolic processes in the fat depots, liver, and muscle may remove the organic acids from the blood and incorporate them in tissue protein, fat, and carbohydrate. When lactic or pyruvic acid is involved, H^+ is taken up as the acid is catabolized.

3. *Respiratory Factors.* The modulation of PCO_2 by the respiratory system is the most important minute-by-minute regulator of the blood pH and also the most important system for excreting H^+, since the lung normally excretes about 200 times as much acid in the form of CO_2 as does the kidney. Respiration is very sensitive to changes in PCO_2 and H^+.[34]

4. *Renal Mechanisms.* While the respiratory system can regulate H^+ concentration only by modulating the body content of carbonic acid, the kidney can adjust levels of other acids as well.[35]

An important role of glomerular filtration is the provision of Na^+ and K^+ for exchange for H^+ by the tubular cells as well as of the buffers that lower the H^+ concentration in the urine and so decrease the gradient of H^+ concentration and decrease the work of the tubular cells.

The tubules are concerned with the actual excretion of H^+. The following main mechanisms are involved (Fig. 6–5):

1. Action of carbonic anhydrase in forming H^+ and bicarbonate. The H^+ is excreted into the tubular lumen and the bicarbonate diffuses into the blood. The concentration of H^+ in the tubular urine can be increased more than 1000 times its concentration in the glomerular filtrate, to a pH of 4.0.

2. Energy-primed exchange of H^+ for Na^+ and K^+.

3. The conversion of the bicarbonate in the glomerular filtrate to CO_2 and H_2O upon the addition of H^+. By this means the HCO_3^- content of acid urine can be brought virtually to zero.

4. Formation of ammonia (NH_3) in distal tubular cells, which acts as a buffer to form ammonium (NH_4^+) on combination with H^+ and which then can be excreted in place of Na^+ or K^+. Ammonia formation increases with acidosis but requires several

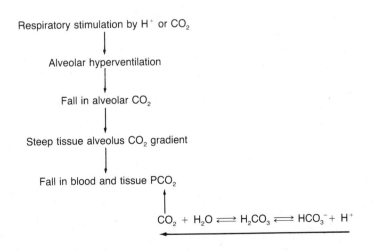

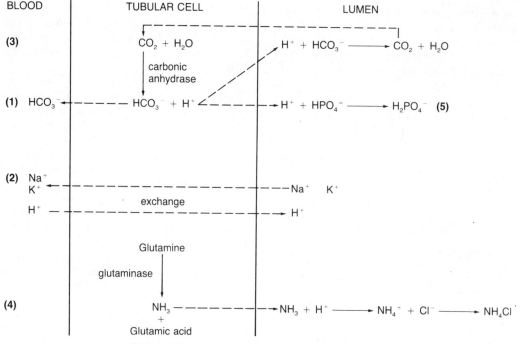

Figure 6–5.   Renal regulation of acid-base balance.

days for a full response. Increased H^+ in the urine decreases the proportion of NH_4^+ returning to the circulation and increases the amount excreted in the urine. The ammonium is generally excreted with chloride or, in the absence of chloride, with bicarbonate.

5. At the usual range of urinary pH, HPO_4^{2-} acts as a buffer, combining with H^+ to form $H_2PO_4^-$, which is excreted in the urine. Other buffers in the glomerular filtrate, such as acetoacetate, creatinine, and urate, work in the same way.

REFERENCES

The first 11 citations are general references containing background concepts, which will aid those wishing to pursue blood gas physiology in greater depth.

1. Gamble JL: Chemical Anatomy, Physiology, and Pathology of Extracellular Fluid, Harvard University Press, Cambridge, MA, 1947.
2. Darrow DC: A Guide To Learning Fluid Therapy. Charles C Thomas, Springfield, IL, 1964.
3. Goldberger E: A Primer of Water, Electrolyte and Acid-Base Syndromes. Lea & Febiger, Philadelphia, 1965.
4. Davenport HW: The ABC of Acid-Base Chemistry. University of Chicago Press, Chicago, 1974.
5. Plum F, Posner JB: The Diagnosis of Stupor and Coma. F. A. Davis Co., Philadelphia, 1972.
6. Comroe JH, Forster RE, Dubois AB, Briscoe WA, Carlsen E: The Lung — Clinical Physiology and Pulmonary Function Tests. Year Book Medical Publishers, Inc., Chicago, 1962.
7. Winters RW, Engel K, Dell RB: Acid-Base Physiology in Medicine. The London Company of Cleveland, Westlake, OH, 1967.
8. Weil WB Jr., Bailie MD: Fluid and Electrolyte Metabolism in Infants and Children: A Unified Approach. Grune & Stratton, New York, 1977.
9. Slonim NB, Chapin JL: Respiratory Physiology. C. V. Mosby Co., St. Louis, 1967.
10. Carroll HJ, Oh MS: Water, Electrolyte and Acid Base Metabolism. J. B. Lippincott Co., Philadelphia, 1978.
11. Statland H: Fluid and Electrolytes in Practice. J. B. Lippincott Co., Philadelphia, 1963.
12. Effros RM, Chang RSY, Silverman P: Acceleration of plasma bicarbonate conversion to carbon dioxide by pulmonary carbonic anhydrase. Science 199:427, 1978.
13. Benesch R, Benesch RE: Intracellular organic phosphates as regulators of oxygen release by haemoglobin. Nature 221:618, 1969.
14. Bauer C, Ludwig M, Ludwig I, Bartels H: Factors governing the oxygen affinity of human adult and foetal blood. Respir Physiol 7:271, 1969.
15. Bromberg PA: Cellular cyanosis and the shifting sigmoid: the blood oxygen dissociation curve. Am J Med Sci 260:1, 1970.
16. Brewer GJ, Eaton JW: Erythrocyte Metabolism: interaction with oxygen transport. Science 171:1205, 1971.
17. Hasselbalch KA: Die Berechnung der Wasserstoffzahl des Blutes aus der freien und gebundenen Kohlensäure desselben und die Sauerstoffbin-

dung des Blutes als Funktion der Wasserstoff-zahl. Biochem Z 78:112, 1916.

18. Siggaard-Andersen O. Blood acid-base alignment nomogram. Scand J Clin Lab Invest 15:211, 1963.

19. Astrup P, Schrøder S: Apparatus for anaerobic determination of the pH of blood at 38° centigrade. Scand J Clin Lab Invest 8:30, 1956.

20. Narins RG, Emmett M: Simple and mixed acid-base disorders: a practical approach. Medicine 59:161, 1980.

21. Severinghaus JW, Bradley AF: Electrodes for blood PO_2 and PCO_2 determination. J Appl Physiol 13:515, 1958.

22. Operator's Manual 113-01 UM Blood pH/Pco_2/Po_2 Analyzer. Instrumentation Laboratory, Inc., Lexington, MA, January 1974, pp. 3, 17.

23. Van Slyke DD, Neill JM: The determination of gases in blood and other solutions by vacuum extraction and manometric measurement. J Biol Chem 61:523, 1924.

24. Rooth G, Thalme B: Validity of buffer base and base excess in perinatal acid-base studies. Am J Obstet Gynecol 108:282, 1970.

25. Lai YL, Attebery BA, Brown EB Jr: Intracellular adjustments of skeletal muscle, heart, and brain to prolonged hypercapnia. Respir Physiol 19:115, 1973.

26. Poyart CF, Fréminet A, and Bursaux E: The exchange of bone CO_2 in vivo. Respir Physiol 25:101, 1975.

27. Trenchard D, Noble MIM, Guz A: Serum carbonic acid pK'_1 abnormalities in patients with acid-base disturbances. Clin Sci 32:189, 1967.

28. Natelson S, Nobel D: Effect of the variation of pK' of the Henderson-Hasselbalch equation on values obtained for total CO_2 calculated from Pco_2 and pH values. Clin Chem 23:767, 1977.

29. Rispens P, Dellebarre CW, Eleveld D, Helder W, Zijlstra WG: The apparent first dissociation constant of carbonic acid in plasma between 16 and 42.5°. Clin Chim Acta 22:627, 1968.

30. Sinclair MJ, Hart RA, Pope HM, Campbell EJM: The use of the Henderson-Hasselbalch equation in routine medical practice. Clin Chim Acta 19:63, 1968.

31. Wills MR, Laite PA: Apparent change in the pK'_1 of carbonic acid in plasma in response to acute metabolic acidosis in normal subjects. Clin Chim Acta 35:514, 1971.

32. Bartels H, Wrbitzky R: Bestimmung des CO_2-absorptionskoeffizienten zwischen 15 und 38°C im wasser und plasma. Pfluegers Arch Ges Physiol 271:162, 1960.

33. Kildeberg P, Engel K: Metabolic alkalosis in infants: role of water depletion and changes in composition of stool. Acta Paediat Scand 60:637, 1971.

34. Sørensen SC: The chemical control of ventilation. Acta Physiol Scand, 361(Suppl):1, 1971.

35. Simpson DP: Control of hydrogen ion homeostasis and renal acidosis. Medicine 50:503, 1971.

Chapter 7

SODIUM, POTASSIUM, AND CHLORIDE IONS: METABOLISM AND REGULATION

SODIUM

Sodium (Na) is sixth in abundance among the elements of the earth's crust, constituting about 2.8 per cent of the crust's weight. Sodium has a single stable isotope with an atomic weight of 22.991 and five artificially produced radioisotopes with half-lives varying from 0.23 second to 3 years. ^{22}Na and ^{24}Na are useful for tracer experiments.[1] The sodium atom has a radius of 5.6 angstroms (0.56 nm); although the metallic atom is smaller than potassium, the hydrated ion is larger. As already indicated, sodium as a cation (Na$^+$) functions in the body primarily as a determiner of body fluid osmolality and volume.

Body Content

The total content of sodium in the body has been found to be between 80 and 96 mEq/kg of fat-free weight with a progressive, gradual decrease from fetal to adult life. In adults, about two thirds of the sodium is exchangeable when isotopes are infused and from 30 to 50 per cent of body sodium is in the skeleton; a much lower proportion is found in infants and children. Probably 90 per cent of the skeletal sodium of adults is not in the bone water portion.[1] In cartilage, some sodium is bound to chondroitin sulfate.

A small amount of sodium is found in cell water, varying among the different tissues and cells (see references 1 and 2 for details). Variation also occurs in connection with changes in pH.[3] Although, in this book, the lean body mass is frequently considered to be constant, it is important to point out that this is an oversimplification, justifiable for most clinical situations but not applicable to all circumstances. Changes resulting from disease, physiologic disturbances, and, perhaps most important, maturation affect the lean body mass and its sodium content.[4] An average concentration of sodium in the intracellular water of human muscle ranges from 5 to 8 mEq/l. A small amount of bound sodium may be found in the sarcolemma.

Requirements and Intake

The requirement for sodium under normal conditions, excluding growth, is very low, so efficient are the physiologic mechanisms for conservation. As little as 0.1 mEq/100 cal expended is needed. On the other hand, the tolerance and excretory capacity for sodium by the healthy individual is sufficiently great to permit as much as 10 mEq/100 cal to be taken in, a difference of 2 in order of magnitude. For practical reasons, in clinical settings the midpoint of the exponential range, 2 to 3 mEq/100 cal, is used, as it is by the authors here (with exceptions noted) and by most investigators. Growth for human infants requires approximately 95 to 115 mEq of sodium per kilogram of weight gain. Since these values have been obtained from balance studies, they are probably on the high side; the errors of the metabolic balance technique tend to exaggerate retention.

The human diet varies markedly in its sodium content. A breast-fed infant gets about 1 mEq/kg/day and grows well. Older children and adults consume up to 10 mEq/kg/day or more, according to various studies.[5] In some human adults and in certain strains of rats, high sodium intake seems to precipitate or cause hypertension. This association is not apparent in the majority of human adults, however, or in other strains of rats. Its significance in young children is less well understood, but prudence would dictate that intake in great excess of need be avoided.

Excretion: Turnover and Regulation

Urine is the main route of excretion for sodium, and small amounts are also lost in stool, sweat, tears, and other bodily discharges. A small amount is also lost via the skin in the absence of sweating. The physiology of sweating, while important, is beyond the scope of this work; a recent review may be consulted as an introduction.[6] Sodium, appearing as it does in all body fluids and secretions, has extremely active metabolism. The biologic half-life of a sodium tracer is approximately 11 days.[7, 8]

Since the effect of sodium salt intake is to expand the extracellular fluid (ECF), it follows that excretion of sodium depends upon the sensing of changes in the volume of ECF (or a portion thereof). Thirst and antidiuretic hormone (ADH) secretion are the important modulators. These mechanisms are triggered by baroreceptors in the left atrium and in arteries (see Chapter 2). There may be baroreceptors in the kidney that also play a role.[9]

Renal Excretion. The principal pathway for excretion clearly involves renal function, and net excretion is the difference between the sodium filtered and that reabsorbed. In the adult, 180 l of glomerular filtrate is formed daily, containing about 25,000 mEq of sodium. Usually, 99.5 per cent is absorbed, leaving 125 mEq for excretion. Adjusting either the glomerular filtration rate (GFR) or the tubular reabsorption rate results in striking changes. A twofold increase in GFR without a change in reabsorption will produce a tenfold increase in sodium excretion. Although this makes glomerular filtration the more potent excretory mechanism, both processes are subject to regulation, making for a safer homeostatic system. Intrarenal blood-flow adjustments, hormonal influences, and segmental differences within the nephron all contribute to regulation.

There are several components to consider in reviewing renal hemodynamics, including peritubular capillary forces, medullary blood flow, and redistribution of intrarenal blood flow. The peritubular forces constitute the familiar hydrostatic pressure–Starling force balance. A fall in capillary pressure or a rise in hydrostatic pressure will decrease uptake from the interstitium, which will decrease the net transport of sodium in the proximal tubule even though active transport is unchanged.[10] It has been postulated that an increase in medullary blood flow dissipates hypertonicity of the medulla and thus depresses sodium absorption in the ascending limb of Henle's loop.[11] Finally, juxtamedullary nephrons may have a greater capacity to reabsorb sodium than superficial ones. If so, redistribution to deeper nephrons would result in sodium retention. This has been disputed,[12] although the possibility remains under some circumstances.

The hormonal influences on the kidney affecting sodium excretion include those of ADH, aldosterone, and "natriuretic hormone." ADH is discussed in detail elsewhere in this work, as are the general effects of aldosterone. The possibility of the existence of a natriuretic hormone stems from the work of deWardener.[13] The postulated substance is an inhibitor of sodium transport that appears in plasma from an as yet unknown site either when volume is expanded[14] or when nephrons are temporarily lost, causing transient sodium retention.[15] An inhibitor of sodium transport in the toad bladder is found in dialysates of plasma from animals after volume expansion.[16] The chemical nature of the substance has not been identified, and there is controversy over its significance.[17]

As filtered sodium passes along the nephron, reabsorption occurs at four discrete sites. The proximal tubule reabsorbs 50 to 75 per cent of the filtered load. The reabsorption is isotonic and occurs largely because of active transport with organic anions. Starling forces also affect sodium and water movement at this level. The descending limb of Henle's loop is virtually impermeable to sodium.[18] In the thin ascending limb there appears to be passive reabsorption of sodium salts, whereas in the thick ascending limb there is active outward transport of chloride ion, with sodium (and potassium) passively moving from the lumen along the electrochemical gradient thus created.[19, 20] In the distal tubule, net sodium reabsorption occurs and is associated with an electric potential difference increasing progressively along the segment.[21] This active transport system involves a cation exchange, with potassium and hydrogen entering the lumen as sodium leaves. Finally, the collecting ducts in both the cortical and medullary portions actively transport sodium outward.[10] The cortical contribution appears greater and is probably mediated by mineralocorticoids.[22] Here again, potassium is exchanged for sodium.

The renin-angiotensin-aldosterone system appears to regulate sodium balance, fluid volume, and possibly blood pressure in the following fashion: The kidney, when its perfusion diminishes, releases renin. Renin, in turn, induces liberation of angiotensin II, which stimulates aldosterone secretion. Angiotensin and aldosterone act to raise arterial pressure and promote sodium retention.[23]

Role of the Skeleton

As indicated, some of the body sodium is lodged in the skeleton and does not mobilize readily. However, under conditions of either marked depletion of sodium or acidemia, the skeleton will release some sodium. In this way, the skeleton participates in buffering the hydrogen ion and in providing a reservoir of buffering capacity, albeit a small one.

Before concluding this section on sodium metabolism, it seems advisable to remind pediatricians that, in the infant, the mechanisms for sodium homeostasis are still developing. Probably toward the end of the first year of life, in well-nourished infants, at least, the systems approach maturity.

POTASSIUM

Like sodium, potassium (K) is abundant in the earth's crust (2.59%). The average atomic weight of the natural isotopes is 39.098. The major isotope is ^{39}K, and small amounts of ^{40}K and ^{41}K occur. ^{40}K is radioactive, with an extremely long half-life (1.3

billion years) which makes it useful in measurement studies. The atomic radius is 1.33 angstroms (0.13 nm) and the hydrated cation radius is 3.8 angstroms (0.38 nm), smaller than the hydrated sodium ion.

Body Content

The potassium content of the body is 50 to 55 mEq/kg of weight in the well-nourished (non-obese) person with an average proportion of muscle tissue. Ninety-five per cent of the potassium is in intracellular fluid, which in turn is found mostly in muscle. The average concentration of potassium in intracellular fluid (ICF) is 150 mEq/l of water, but the range is wide between various tissues and even in muscle under changing conditions. A varying small proportion seems to be bound to protein and is, therefore, osmotically inactive. The ratio K/N (mEq of potassium/gm of nitrogen) in muscle tissue in healthy individuals ranges from 2.6 to 3.0. The ratio is useful as a marker of normal proportions.

Requirements and Intake

The daily requirement of potassium (determined largely by the obligatory losses) is about 2 mEq/100 cal expended. Since all animal and vegetable matter contains potassium, sources are abundant. The average dietary intake for animals is about 1.5 mEq/kg, but some species ingest 10 times this amount. Absorption occurs readily from the small intestine.

Excretion: Turnover and Regulation

About 90 per cent of excreted potassium is in the urine. Small, if any, amounts are excreted in the sweat and stool, although either of these may become important sites of loss in pathologic states. Renal excretion is efficient, so increased intake is followed by increased excretion, with even more excreted than is filtered by the glomerulus. Renal conservation is not very good; only when deficits are extreme does it occur to any significant extent. This in contrast to sodium conservation. Most of the potassium in the glomerular filtrate is absorbed in the proximal tubule, probably by passive mechanisms.[24] Toward the end of the proximal tubule and in the descending loop of Henle, potassium is secreted in part with actively transported organic anion and in part down an electrochemical gradient.[25] In the thick portion of Henle's loop, potassium along with sodium passively accompanies chloride ion as it is actively reabsorbed.

In the distal tubule, potassium is added to the urine in exchange for sodium, an active transport mechanism mediated by aldosterone, which will also stimulate potassium excretion independent of sodium exchange.[26] Aldosterone thus plays a critical role in the renal excretion of potassium.

Control of Plasma Potassium

Unlike sodium levels, potassium levels in the plasma are low (3.5 to 5.5 mEq/l). A change of 2 mEq/l in either direction is a large proportionate change that may have profound physiologic and clinical effects. Diet and renal excretion (thus, aldosterone as well) are the main determinants of the potassium level. Both hypokalemia and hyperkalemia affect myocardial conduction pathways as well as other muscle activity. Altered levels of potassium are reflected in changes in the electrocardiogram. T-wave changes, low in hypokalemia and high in hyperkalemia, are characteristic.

Physiologic factors influencing renal potassium excretion are changes in sodium excretion, changes in acid-base balance, and adrenal steroids. Delivery of sodium to the lumen of the distal tubule is necessary for orderly potassium excretion in exchange for sodium reabsorption by the kidney. The exact nature of the mineralocorticoid effect on potassium excretion has not, however, been established.[27]

Thus, aldosterone, because of its kaliuretic action, plays an important role in the regulation of plasma potassium levels. Changes in serum potassium concentrations have, in turn, profound effects on aldosterone secretion. Increases in serum potassium concentration will stimulate the secretion rate of aldosterone.[28] Even changes within the physiologic range in serum potassium concentration (0.1 to 0.5 mEq/l) prompt an adrenal response in the form of increased aldosterone secretion.

Renin, too, appears to play a role in potassium homeostasis. Recent studies indicate that hyperkalemia, in addition to stimulating aldosterone, directly inhibits renal renin secretion, and that hypokalemia, which retards aldosterone secretion, also

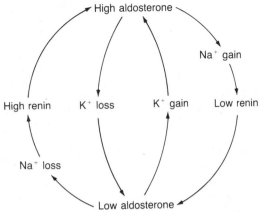

Figure 7–1. Double-cycle feedback system affecting sodium and potassium homeostasis.[23]

stimulates renin secretion. This double-cycle feedback for simultaneous effects of aldosterone and renin on sodium and potassium homeostasis is shown in Figure 7–1.

The glucoregulatory hormones also play a role in this system.[29] The mechanism of action seems to be that insulin stimulates efflux of sodium from cells by stimulating the Mg-dependent Na-K-ATPase. Potassium enters the cell as sodium leaves.[30] If potassium is infused intravenously, insulin and glucagon secretion is stimulated, helping to move potassium into cells.[31] Some potassium is also deposited with glycogen when glucose and insulin are administered together.

This review of potassium in physiology is far from complete. The interested reader is referred to the literature.[32, 33]

CHLORIDE

Chloride ion (Cl^-) is derived from chlorine, a gas and an element that accounts for only 0.031 per cent of the earth's crust. The average atomic weight is 35.453 for two natural isotopes, ^{35}Cl and ^{37}Cl. There are seven radioactive isotopes that may be prepared. The content of chloride in the body has been measured at about 34 to 38 mEq/kg.[34] Chloride is the principal anion of the ECF. It has a very low concentration (<1 mEq/l) in muscle cell water, but nearly 16 per cent of body chloride does appear in a number of cells of mesenchymal origin — in particular, blood and connective tissue cells.[2, 35] The daily turnover of chloride ion is high, about 1.2 to 3.6 mEq/kg of body weight. As with sodium, however, the requirement may be very low (0.1 mEq/100 cal), since renal conservation is excellent.

In ECF, because one cation (sodium) is electrically balanced, for the most part, by two anions (chloride and bicarbonate) and because bicarbonate is independently regulated by changes in carbon dioxide and hydrogen ions, producing an electrical reciprocal relationship between chloride and bicarbonate, it has long been easier and therefore customary to think of extracellular ion changes in terms of sodium. Also, because the earlier studies on active transport seemed to involve cations rather than anions, chloride ion was perceived as passive and "mendicant." More recent data make it clear that the chloride ion has unique importance in body fluid composition and metabolism.

We have already touched on the role of chloride in renal regulation[18, 19] and will later describe its role in intestinal secretion (see Chapter 10). Active chloride (passive sodium and potassium) transport in the ascending loop of Henle, which is followed further downstream in the nephron by a sodium-potassium-hydrogen exchange mechanism, has physiologic and clinical implications that arise whenever there is a deficiency of chloride ion relative to sodium. When there is a lower-than-normal chloride concentration in the filtrate reaching the thick ascending portion of Henle's loop, less sodium will, necessarily, follow the smaller number of chloride ions to the interstitium. This allows more sodium ions to reach the distal tubule. Under these conditions, more than the usual number of sodium ions will be reabsorbed at this locus, and since each reabsorbed sodium ion is exchanged for a hydrogen or potassium ion, these ions will be lost in excess. The result will be, in time, hypokalemia and alkalosis to accompany the hypochloremia. A recent review[36] has delineated these consequences of a dietary chloride deficiency. In later sections several disease states involving chloride deficiency will be discussed.

REFERENCES

1. Forbes GB: Sodium. *In* Comar CL, Bronner F (eds): Mineral Metabolism, Vol 2B. Academic Press, New York, 1962.

2. Manery JF: Water and electrolyte metabolism. Physiol Rev 34:334, 1954.

3. Cooke RE, Coughlin FR Jr, Segar WE: Muscle composition in respiratory acidosis. J Clin Invest 31:1006, 1952.

4. Wedgwood RJ: Inconstancy of the lean body mass. Ann NY Acad Sci 110:141, 1963.

5. Dahl LK: Salt intake and salt need. N Engl J Med 258:1152, and 1205, 1958.

6. Knochel JP: Clinical physiology of heat exposure. *In* Maxwell MH, Kleeman CR (eds): Clinical Disorders of Fluid and Electrolyte Metabolism. McGraw-Hill, New York, 1979.

7. Veall N, Fisher HJ, Browne JCM, Bradley JES: An improved method for clinical studies of total exchangeable sodium. Lancet 1:419, 1955.

8. Miller H, Munro DS, Wilson GM: The human use of ^{24}Na. Clin Sci 12:97, 1957.

9. Tobian LA, Tomboulian A, Janecek J: Effect of high profusion pressure on the granulation of juxtaglomerular cells in an isolated kidney. J Clin Invest 38:605, 1959.

10. Reinich HJ, Stern JH: Regulation of sodium balance. *In* Maxwell MH, Kleeman CR (eds): Clinical Disorders of Fluid and Electrolyte Metabolism. McGraw-Hill, New York, 1979.

11. Early LE, Friedler RM: Observations on the mechanisms of decreased tubular reabsorption of sodium and water during saline loading. J Clin Invest 43:1928, 1964.

12. Lemure NH, Lipschitz MD, Stein JH: Heterogenicity of nephron function. Ann Rev Phys 39:159, 1977.

13. DeWardener HE, Mills IH, Clapham WF, Hayter CJ: Studies on the efferent mechanism of sodium diuresis which follows the administration of intravenous saline in the dog. Clin Sci 21:249, 1961.

14. Buckalew VM, Diamond KA: Effect of vasopressin on sodium excretion and plasma antinatriuretic activity in the dog. Am J Phys 231:28, 1976.

15. Webber H, Lin KY, Bricker NS: Effect of sodium intake on single nephron glomerular filtration rate and sodium reabsorption in experimental uremia. Kidney Int 8:14, 1975.

16. Buckalew VM, Martinez HJ, Green WE: The effect of dialysates and ultrafiltrates of plasma of saline-loaded dogs on toad bladder sodium transport. J Clin Invest 49:926, 1970.

17. Osgood RW, Lemeire NH, Gorkin MI, Stein JH: Effect of aortic clamping on proximal reabsorption and sodium excretion in the rat. Am J Phys 1:92, 1977.

18. Kokko JP: Sodium chloride and water transport in the descending limb of Henle. J Clin Invest 49:1838, 1970.

19. Burg MD, Green N: Function of the thick ascending limb of Henle's loop. Am J Phys 224:659, 1973.

20. Rocha AS, Kokko JP: Sodium chloride and water transport in the medullary thick ascending limb of Henle: evidence for active chloride transport. J Clin Invest 52:612, 1973.

21. Wright F: Increasing magnitude of electrical potential along the renal distal tubule. Am J Phys 220:624, 1971.

22. Gross JB, Kokko JP: Effects of aldosterone and potassium-sparing diuretics on electrical po-

tential differences across the distal nephron. J. Clin Invest 59:82, 1977.

23. Laragh JH, Sealey JE: The renin-angiotensin-aldosterone hormonal system and regulation of sodium, potassium and blood pressure homeostasis. *In* Orloff J, Berliner RW (section eds): Handbook of Physiology, Section 8: Renal Physiology, p. 831. American Physiological Society. Williams & Wilkins, Baltimore, 1973.

24. Malvin RL, Wilde WS, Sullivan LP: Localization of nephron transport by stop flow analysis. Am J Phys 194:135, 1958.

25. Grantham J, Qualizza PB, Erwin RL: Fluid secretion in proximal straight tubules in vitro: role of PAH. Am J Physiol 226:191, 1974.

26. Barger AC, Berlin RD, Tulenko JF: Infusion of aldosterone, 9-α-fluorohydrocortisone and antidiuretic hormone into the renal artery of normal and adrenalectomized, unanesthetized dogs: effect on electrolyte and water excretion. Endocrinology 62:804, 1958.

27. Hierholzer KM, Wiederholt H, Holzgreve G, et al.: Micropuncture study of renal transtubular concentration gradients of sodium and potassium in adrenalectomized rats. Arch Gen Physiol 285:193, 1965.

28. Himathongkam T, Dluhy RG, Williams HG: Potassium-aldosterone-renin interrelationships. J Clin Endocrinol Metab 41:153, 1975.

29. Knochel JP: Role of glucoregulatory hormones in potassium homeostasis. Kidney Int 11:443, 1977.

30. Gavryck WA, Moore RD, Thompson RC: Effect of insulin on membrane-bound Na-K-ATPase extracted from frog skeletal muscle. J Physiol 252:43, 1975.

31. Santensonio F, Falooma GR, Knochel JP, Anger RH: Evidence for a role of endogenous insulin and glucagon in the regulation of potassium homeostasis. J Lab Clin Med 81:809, 1973.

32. Kernan RP: Cell. K. Butterworth, Washington DC, 1965.

33. Schultze RG, Nissenson AR: Potassium: physiology and pathophysiology. *In* Maxwell MH, Kleeman CR (eds.): Clinical Disorders of Fluid and Electrolyte Metabolism. McGraw-Hill, New York, 1979.

34. Forbes GB, Lewis AM: Total sodium, potassium and chloride in adult man. J Clin Invest 35:596, 1956.

35. Cotlove E, Hogben CAM: Chloride. *In* Comar CL, Bronner F (eds): Mineral Metabolism, Vol. 2B Academic Press, New York, 1962.

36. Simopoulis AP, Bartter FC: The metabolic consequences of chloride deficiency. Nutr Rev 38:201, 1980.

Chapter 8

CALCIUM, PHOSPHORUS, AND MAGNESIUM: METABOLISM AND REGULATION

CALCIUM

Calcium is a divalent metal; its atomic number is 20 and its atomic weight is 40.08. There are six natural isotopes and one artificially produced isotope (^{45}Ca) that is used experimentally. Calcium is the fifth most abundant element in the earth's crust and in human body composition.

The calcium ion plays a major role in many fundamental biologic processes. It not only is essential for the formation of adequate osteoid in the process of skeletal mineralization, but also has a major role in intra- and intercellular processes. Many enzymes, such as amylase and lipase, and thromboplastin require calcium specifically for activation. Extracellular calcium concentration affects the release of several hormones not directly regulating calcium homeostasis, such as insulin and glucagon. Intracellular concentrations of calcium affect the excitability of neural tissue in the central nervous system and the conduction system of the heart. Intracellular calcium also triggers the mechanical events of muscle contractility. The functions of many cell membranes and organelles are regulated by the concentration of calcium in their environment. Many vesicles in intracellular organelles or at synapses release their contents upon stimulation by calcium. The importance of calcium as an integral factor in electrical conduction at membranes, muscle contraction, enzyme activity, and skeletal mineralization requires that the control of its concentration in the serum be carefully regulated in order to maintain the concentration of ionized calcium within extremely narrow limits.

The total calcium level in the plasma consists of three fractions: ionized calcium, protein-bound calcium, and calcium bound to diffusible molecules such as citrate and phosphate. Ionized calcium in plasma is the physiologically active fraction of the total calcium; in the normal child, the ionized calcium level is approximately half the total calcium level. Ionized calcium is responsible for the actions of calcium in regulating hormone synthesis and secretion, electrical and mechanical activity, and enzyme activity, and it is the fraction of calcium that is available to cross the placenta from mother to fetus. Ionized calcium exists in equilibrium with protein-bound calcium. This equilibrium is pH-dependent, so when the pH of plasma decreases, there is a decrease in the binding of calcium to protein and a resultant increase in the ionized calcium level. Correction of acidemia, i.e., increasing the pH, can result in an increase in the protein-bound calcium and a decrease in the ionized calcium in plasma with no change in total calcium concentration. The ionized calcium level is maintained between 4.0 and 5.0 mg/dl by multiple regulatory mechanisms.[1]

The amount of ionized calcium in the extracellular fluid is less than 1 per cent of the total calcium in the body, and about 1 per cent is in mitochondria; the other 98 per cent is in the skeleton and teeth. Thus, in order to maintain ionized calcium levels in serum within a narrow range, a complex regulatory mechanism is necessary.

The ultimate extracellular ionized calcium concentration depends on calcium intake in the diet, absorption from the gastrointestinal tract, extraction from the extracellular space into bone mineral, resorption of bone mineral, glomerular filtration of calcium into the nephron, and tubular reabsorption of calcium into the extracellular space. We will discuss each of these aspects of calcium metabolism with reference to the regulation and maintenance of extracellular ionized calcium level.

Calcium intake can vary greatly, depending upon the calcium content of the food ingested. Besides the calcium in milk and dairy products and in bone-containing foods such as sardines, there is little calcium in the average daily diet. Control of absorption of calcium from the gastrointestinal tract is the major regulatory mechanism for prevention of hypercalcemia. Unlimited calcium absorption from the gastrointestinal tract would require that either bone accretion or renal excretion of calcium be the regulatory mechanism to maintain extracellular calcium in a narrow range. However, the amount of calcium accretion in bone is limited even in times of rapid growth, and increasing urinary concentrations of calcium in hypercalcemia might result in the formation of insoluble calcium-phosphate, bicarbonate, or other complexes that can damage renal parenchyma.

There is wide variability in the percentage of ingested calcium that is absorbed by the gastrointestinal tract. This absorption is affected by insoluble calcium salts formed in the gut when large amounts of phosphate, phytate, and other anions are present and interfere with absorption. Calcium is absorbed primarily in the duodenum and upper jejunum. In addition to the calcium ingested in the diet, calcium is added to the intestinal contents by various intestinal secretions. This results in a secretory and reabsorption cycle. However, the most important determinant of the rate of absorption of calcium from the gut is the level of the hormone 1,25-dihydroxyvitamin D or calcitriol.

Calcitriol, the hormonal form of the vitamin, is bound by proteins in the cytoplasm of the intestinal cells and is transported into the nucleus. After the hormone reaches the nucleus, increased production of messenger RNA occurs and a specific calcium-binding protein will be found in the mucosa. This calcium-binding protein appears to increase the rate of transfer of calcium from the intestinal lumen into the mucosal cell and to assist in the transport of the calcium from the mucosal cell into the interstitial fluid and finally into the serum. Even with high intestinal concentrations of calcium, in the absence of calcitriol there is little movement of calcium into the mucosal cell. This mechanism, then, controls the absorption rate of calcium and prevents excessive absorption of calcium in response to high dietary intake. It also can increase the percentage of the total ingested calcium that is absorbed in response to low plasma levels of ionized calcium, even when the quantities of ingested calcium are low.

The movement of calcium out of the extracellular fluid into bone and the reabsorption of calcium from bone into the extracellular fluid compartment is determined by osteoblastic and osteoclastic activity regulated by calcitonin and parathyroid hormone. Plasma inorganic phosphorus levels also have a major regulatory role in the mineralization and resorption of bone. Inadequate levels of inorganic phosphorus in the extracellular fluid hinder the mineralization of osteoid and the movement of calcium from the extracellular fluid compartment into bone. Excessive levels of inorganic phosphorus in the plasma result in increased dissolution of bone and movement of calcium into the extracellular fluid. Movement of calcium ions into the intracellular space, glomerular filtration in the kidney, and bone accretion and dissolution creates a dynamic cycle, with the entire extracellular pool of calcium turning over 40 to 50 times each 24 hours.

Calcium is filtered by the renal glomeruli to the extent that more than 10 times the amount of calcium present in the extracellular fluid is filtered during a 24-hour period. However, renal tubular conservation of calcium accounts for almost 100 per cent of the amount filtered by the glomeruli. Renal tubular reabsorption of calcium can be increased in response to hypocalcemia by endogenous parathyroid hormone. Calcium excretion in the urine is increased by diuresis in general and by potent diuretics, such as furosemide, in particular. Parathyroid hormone levels increased to pathologic concentrations, acidosis, adrenal steroids, and hypophosphatemia can also increase calcium excretion in the urine by decreasing renal tubular reabsorption.

REGULATORY HORMONES

Further discussion of calcium homeostasis requires a thorough understanding of the three regulatory hormones for serum calcium level: parathyroid hormone, calcitriol and calcitonin.

Parathyroid Hormone

Parathyroid hormone (PTH) is a polypeptide consisting of 84 amino acids in a single chain, with a molecular weight of approximately 9500. The biologic activity of the hormone resides in the amino terminal portion of the molecule; carboxy terminal fragments are devoid of any biologic activity. PTH is synthesized from a larger prohormone, proparathyroid hormone, which contains additional amino acids at the amino terminus.[2] PTH is secreted by the parathyroid gland in response to a decreased level of ionized calcium in the plasma. Although this is the major stimulus to the secretion of the hormone, magnesium deficiency may result in inhibition of hormone synthesis and release even when the ionized calcium level in the plasma is low.[3] Increased concentration of phosphate alone does not stimulate PTH secretion but may have an effect through a decrease in the ionized calcium or magnesium level in the serum.

Bone and kidney are the major organs on which PTH acts. In both organ systems PTH activates an adenyl cyclase to form cyclic adenosine monophosphate (cyclic AMP) from adenosine triphosphate (ATP). The activation of cyclic AMP in bone cells results in increased metabolic activity of osteocytes and osteoclasts. Release of lysosomal enzymes results in the solubilizing of bone mineral and the release of calcium and phosphate ions into the extracellular fluid.[4] This action of PTH requires the presence of adequate amounts of calcitriol.[5]

In the kidneys PTH increases cyclic AMP concentration with a resultant inhibition of tubular reabsorption of phosphate and increased phosphate loss in the urine. PTH also has a separate action on renal cells to increase 1α-hydroxylation of 25-hydroxyvitamin D to calcitriol. This hormonal form of vitamin D works to increase intestinal absorption of calcium and phosphate. This indirect mechanism is the means by which PTH affects intestinal absorption of calcium and phosphorus.

PTH concentrations increase in maternal serum during pregnancy in response to a decrease in the plasma ionized calcium level.[6] PTH does not, however, cross the placenta.[7] There is an active placental pump of calcium from mother to fetus, which results in relative fetal hypercalcemia by the end of pregnancy. This fetal hypercalcemia is associated with low or undetectable levels of PTH in the fetus.[8]

Calcitriol

Vitamin D, in actuality a prohormone, is taken into the body in the diet or is synthesized from 7-dehydrocholesterol by ultraviolet irradiation of the skin. Vitamin D, or cholecalciferol, is biologically inactive and must be metabolized to more active forms. The first step in this metabolic conversion is the hydroxylation in the liver at the 25 position of the molecule to 25-hydroxyvitamin D.[9] 25-Hydroxyvitamin D is a physiologically active metabolite of vitamin D, having potency in both the intestines and the bone. However, the hormonal and most potent form of vitamin D, calcitriol, is formed in the kidney by the $1\text{-}\alpha$-hydroxylation of 25-hydroxyvitamin D.[10] This synthesis of 1,25-dihydroxyvitamin D (calcitriol) is controlled primarily by the level of PTH in the kidney.[11] Since the serum level of ionized calcium controls the secretion of PTH, it indirectly controls the formation of calcitriol.

Decrease in extracellular phosphate concentration also results in an increase in calcitriol formation. High levels of calcitriol in the plasma may result in decreased secretion of PTH from the gland, thus completing multiple feedback loops of PTH and calcitriol interaction.[12]

Adaptation to low calcium intake results in increased efficiency of intestinal calcium absorption through an increase in calcitriol concentration. Because the half-life of calcitriol is short,[13] the plasma and tissue levels of the hormone allow fine regulation of the calcium absorption in the gastrointestinal tract.

Calcitriol increases not only calcium absorption in the gastrointestinal tract but also phosphate absorption. Thus, the decrease in synthesis of calcitriol by increased plasma concentration of phosphate helps regulate serum phosphate levels within a broad range.

Recent advances in radioimmunoassays enable measurement of serum levels of vitamin D metabolites. The correlation of serum levels of 25-hydroxyvitamin D in mothers and their fetuses suggests that 25-hydroxyvitamin D crosses the placenta.[14] However, recent reports of fetal plasma levels of calcitriol reveal that term fetuses have calcitriol concentrations in plasma substantially lower than normal adult values as compared with maternal levels, which are significantly greater than normal.[15, 16] This finding suggests a mechanism other than simple passive transport of the hormone across the placenta, as well as a decrease in fetal renal hydroxylation to form calcitriol. Normal levels of calcitriol in plasma vary diurnally and with age.[17] Further understanding of the regulatory mechanism for the synthesis and degradation of this hormone will clarify multiple metabolic abnormalities in calcium homeostasis.

Calcitonin

Calcitonin is a 32–amino acid polypeptide that is secreted by the parafollicular cells of the thyroid gland.[18] The major stimulus for calcitonin secretion is an increased concentration of ionized calcium in the plasma. The primary action of calcitonin is to inhibit bone resorption by affecting osteocytes and osteoclasts. This results in increased bone accretion. This mechanism is not an inactivation or inhibition of PTH metabolism at bone but is a direct action on specific bone cells.[19] It is postulated that there are specific and distinct receptor sites for calcitonin and PTH in the osteocytes. Calcitonin inhibits dissolution of bone and causes a reduction in the number of osteoclasts formed. In adults, the physiologic importance of calcitonin is somewhat obscure. Thyroidectomized adults show little abnormality in calcium homeostasis. However, calcitonin may play a more important role in bone accretion in the fetus and growing neonate.

Calcitonin, a polypeptide hormone like PTH, does not cross the placenta.[20] Calcitonin levels in the plasma of the fetus are, however, elevated above normal adult values. This hormonal response to fetal hyper-calcemia enhances bone accretion and formation of the skeleton. Increased levels of calcitonin in the early neonatal period have been postulated as etiologic in the decrease in ionized calcium levels observed during the first days of life.[21] However, a more likely explanation for the pathologic decrease in ionized calcium levels in the neonatal period is end-organ unresponsiveness to parathyroid hormone due to decreased synthesis of calcitriol during the first days of life.[16]

HYPOCALCEMIA AND HYPERCALCEMIA

The three calcium regulatory hormones maintain the ionized calcium level in plasma within a very narrow range. Pathologic levels of ionized calcium in the plasma, both decreased and elevated, result from abnormalities in the regulatory mechanisms.

Hypocalcemia

Hypocalcemia must be defined in relationship to the plasma ionized calcium level, not the total calcium concentration. Low levels of serum total calcium may be due to a reduction in the serum albumin concentration, which decreases the protein-bound calcium levels without affecting the serum ionized calcium level. Thus, in evaluating any patient with suspected hypocalcemia, either the ionized calcium concentration must be determined or total protein and albumin in plasma must be estimated to confirm the suspicion of hypocalcemia based on a decrease in the total calcium level.

Patients suffering from hypocalcemia usually manifest signs of tetany, i.e., hyperexcitability of the central and peripheral nervous systems. Frank seizures usually of a short generalized tonic and clonic nature are also associated with low plasma calcium levels. However, earlier signs frequently occur, such as spontaneous tonic contractions of the muscles of the upper and lower extremities; specifically, a spasm in which the hand is held with the fingers extended and the wrist flexed, called carpopedal spasm. Tonic and clonic contractions of various muscles can be evoked by the examiner — in the hand by decreasing blood flow to the extremity (Trousseau's sign) and in

Table 8–1. Causes of Disorders Characterized by Hypocalcemia

DECREASED PTH SECRETION	INAPPROPRIATE RESPONSE OF TARGET ORGAN TO PTH
Hypoparathyroidism	Vitamin D deficiency
Hypomagnesemia	Abnormalities in vitamin D metabolism
	Pseudohypoparathyroidism
	Miscellaneous

the facial muscles by brisk percussion of muscles in the distribution of the facial nerve (Chvostek's sign). Hypocalcemia may also cause many nonspecific symptoms such as lethargy, bone pain, and a generalized feeling of debilitation. In the neonate, hypocalcemia can cause apnea, poor feeding, and abdominal distention.

Decreased levels of calcium in plasma do not result from a decreased amount of calcium in the body of the patient; rather, hypocalcemia is the result of an inability to mobilize calcium from bone into the extracellular and intravascular compartments. This failure promptly to maintain calcium levels in plasma is a result either of a failure of secretion of adequate amounts of PTH or of inadequate responsiveness of end-organs to PTH despite adequate secretion of the hormone. Disorders characterized by hypocalcemia can be separated into those that are caused by decreased PTH secretion and those that result from inappropriate responsiveness of target organs to adequate levels of PTH (Table 8–1).

Hypercalcemia

Hypercalcemia is more difficult to diagnose than hypocalcemia because of the nonspecific nature of the symptomatology. Symptoms may include bone pain, fatigue, anorexia, nausea, and vomiting, and particularly important are polyuria and polydipsia. Changes in behavior and frank psychiatric disorders may also be a result of hypercalcemia.

Hypercalcemia is due to either increased intestinal absorption of calcium or increased mobilization of calcium from bone with or without increased absorption of calcium from the intestinal tract. Hypercalcemia may occur in such disorders as hypervitaminosis D, sarcoidosis, hyperparathyroidism, phosphate depletion, and hyperthyroidism; disorders involving tumors that secrete parathyroid-like peptides; disorders in which the patient is immobilized; and idiopathic ailments.

In evaluating a patient with hypercalcemia, it is important to take a careful history of drug and vitamin intake. The major factor determining the efficiency of calcium absorption in the gastrointestinal tract is the level of calcitriol in plasma. Even intakes of calcium greatly exceeding normal requirements do not result in excessive absorption of calcium, or absorption at a rate greater than the rate of removal from the extracellular fluid. However, excessive intake of vitamin D overwhelms the feedback system and can result in absorption of calcium from the gastrointestinal tract that exceeds normal needs.

Prolonged hypercalcemia may result not only in the symptoms described, but also in the precipitation of calcium phosphate in the interstitial tissue of the kidney and metastatic calcifications in other soft tissues. The damage to the renal tissue may be insidious in onset and can progress to severe renal insufficiency.

Patients with hypercalcemia associated with sarcoidosis manifest increased calcium absorption from the gastrointestinal tract and an unusual sensitivity to vitamin D.

Hyperparathyroidism due to generalized hyperplasia of the parathyroid gland or to a localized hypersecreting tumor of the gland is the most common cause of hypercalcemia. However, in evaluating serum calcium levels and making the diagnosis of hyperparathyroidism, it is important to note that growth spurts at certain times during infancy, childhood, and adolescence result in plasma levels of calcium in the high normal or just above normal range. Therefore, in making the diagnosis of hyperparathyroidism, serum phosphate levels and urinary excretion levels of calcium, phosphate, and cyclic AMP, as well as serum levels of immunoreactive parathyroid hormone, must be obtained in order to confirm the clinical impression of hyperparathyroidism.

PHOSPHORUS

Phosphorus, atomic number 15, atomic weight 30.97, accounts for 0.12 per cent (by weight) of the earth's crust. There is a single natural isotope, although four artificial ones have been prepared. The chemical valence may be 3 or 5. In the plasma, inorganic phosphorus appears primarily as a mixture of HPO_4^{2-} and $H_2PO_4^-$ in a ratio of about 4:1. Accordingly, in calculations the valence assigned to phosphate in plasma is 1.8. In body processes, both the inorganic form and organic compounds are highly important. Our concern here is primarily with the inorganic form.

Phosphate is important for multiple metabolic processes and growth. Like calcium, the bulk of phosphate in the body is found in the skeleton. However, more than 15 per cent of the phosphate in the adult is found in the extracellular fluid space and intracellularly in tissues other than bone. Because the phosphate in the plasma is almost entirely inorganic, it is readily diffusible throughout the extracellular space. Cells, however, take up phosphate rapidly. The phosphate can be quickly incorporated into nucleotides and subsequently used in the synthesis of nucleic acids, phospholipids, and phosphoproteins, and in various other steps in intermediary metabolism. Major lipid constituents of cellular membranes are phospholipids. Phosphorylated nucleotides such as ATP are the major repositories and sources of chemical energy for intracellular work.

In spite of this obvious importance of inorganic phosphate in cellular activity and growth, the concentration of inorganic phosphate in the serum varies within a broad range, depending upon the age, diet, and rate of growth of the individual. Normal serum phosphorus levels may range from 2.5 to 8 mg/dl, depending upon multiple metabolic and growth factors.[22]

Most diets are high in inorganic phosphate because of the presence of large amounts of phosphate within all kinds of cells, both vegetable and animal. Milk, as the primary diet of the young infant, contains large amounts of phosphorus, which is consistent with the large need for phosphorus for bone accretion. Intestinal transport of phosphate from the lumen to the intravascular space is enhanced by calcitriol. The exact mechanism for this transport of phosphate is unclear. Low phosphate concentration in plasma enhances formation of calcitriol from 25-hydroxyvitamin D by increasing 1-α-hydroxylase activity in the renal tissue. However, calcitriol is much less important in the gastrointestinal absorption of phosphate than in the absorption of calcium. The important control system in the regulation of inorganic phosphate concentrations in extracellular fluid is in the kidney tubule. Because phosphate is readily diffusible, it is readily filtered by the glomerulus. The renal tubule, then, determines the amount of phosphate that is reabsorbed, and ultimately determines the level of inorganic phosphorus in plasma. The tubular capacity to reabsorb phosphate varies with the glomerular filtration rate. A high phosphorus concentration is maintained during rapid periods of growth in early infancy and adolescence.

PTH is the major regulator of tubular reabsorption of phosphorus. By activating adenyl cyclase and increasing cyclic AMP, PTH inhibits reabsorption of phosphorus and increases phosphorus excretion in the urine. This results in a decrease in the serum and extracellular fluid levels of phosphorus. Calcitriol enhances tubular reabsorption of phosphorus through a mechanism independent of the PTH-mediated cyclic AMP.

Extracellular fluid concentration of inorganic phosphorus is affected by bone accretion and dissolution in much the same manner that calcium is. Inorganic phosphorus, however, is also required in all the cells of the body for vital cellular functions, which also affects extracellular concentrations of phosphorus.

Unlike calcium regulation, which is determined by the amount of calcium absorption, phosphorus regulation is determined by the amount of phosphate reabsorbed from the urine after glomerular filtration. Hyperphosphatemia is caused by decreased glomerular filtration of phosphorus, as in chronic renal disease. Hypophosphatemia is most often caused by enhanced urinary excretion of phosphorus through decreased tubular reabsorption of phosphate. A primary defect in phosphate reabsorption occurs in familial hypophosphatemic rickets, Fanconi's syndrome, and other disorders that involve abnormalities in renal tubular function. Hypophosphatemia can also be the result of primary hyperparathyroidism and is a necessary concomitant of that diagnosis. It should be remembered, however, that the range for serum phosphate is quite wide and that a level of phosphate of 3 to 4 mg/dl in a young infant would indicate hypophosphatemia, whereas a level of 2.5 to 3 mg/dl in an older child would indicate hypophosphatemia. Hypophosphatemia can also be caused by decreased absorption of phosphate in the gastrointestinal tract as a result of chelation of phosphate by aluminum or other cations found in antacids.

MAGNESIUM

Magnesium is a divalent metal accounting for 2.1 per cent (by weight) of the earth's crust. The atomic number is 12; the atomic weight is 24.3. There are three natural isotopes. Magnesium is found in small amounts in the body, but it is essential for the activity of numerous enzymes. It is also required for the synthesis of nucleic acids and many proteins. Normal plasma values for magnesium range from 1.6 to 2.2 mEq/l.[23] This range for magnesium concentration in the extracellular fluid is maintained by a balance of absorption of magnesium from the diet on the one hand and renal excretion of magnesium by the tubules on the other, along with the utilization of magnesium within the cells for enzyme activity and for storage in bone.

The exact mechanism of gastrointestinal absorption of magnesium is unknown. Vitamin D metabolites tend to enhance magnesium absorption, but magnesium can be absorbed at a normal rate in vitamin D-deficient animals.[24] Calcium in the lumen of the intestines tends to inhibit magnesium absorption, suggesting that there may be a competitive mechanism for absorption of calcium and magnesium, with calcium being the more dominantly regulated ion. PTH increases the renal tubular reabsorption of magnesium, resulting in increased magnesium levels in the serum. Conversely, states of hypomagnesemia have been associated with decreased secretion of PTH in response to hypocalcemia.

Magnesium is actively taken up by cells, and the body guards the intracellular concentration even at the expense of extracellular fluid levels of magnesium. Magnesium is necessary intracellularly for the structural integrity of ribosomal particles and is further involved in protein synthesis by contributing to the binding of messenger RNA to the ribosome. It is obvious that magnesium is an extremely important intracellular ion, but the exact methods of regulating intracellular magnesium concentra-

tion and providing for adequate availability of extracellular magnesium to support the intracellular space are unknown.

Hypomagnesemia is a rare disorder. Idiopathic hypomagnesemia caused by an absorptive defect specifically for magnesium does occur and can present as hypoparathyroidism with hypocalcemia.[25] Hypomagnesemia also can be seen as a result of hypoparathyroidism and decreased formation of calcitriol and, therefore, of decreased absorption of both calcium and magnesium.[26] Hypomagnesemia also occurs as a consequence of chronic liver disease.[27] In children, hypomagnesemia is most commonly secondary to chronic diarrheal disease and poor absorption in general.

Hypermagnesemia occurs only as a result of exogenous treatment of patients with magnesium. Newborn infants can develop hypermagnesemia as a result of the use of magnesium sulfate in maternal hypertension in labor. Hypermagnesemia is associated with generalized lethargy and can lead to respiratory arrest.

BONE MINERALIZATION

Bone consists of a matrix or lattice structure called osteoid and a mineral component made up of inorganic crystals. On a dry-weight basis the mineral component of bone constitutes approximately 65 to 70 per cent and osteoid makes up the remaining 30 to 35 per cent. Osteoid is made up almost entirely of collagen, with an additional small amount of mucopolysaccharides and other proteins. The unique nature of the collagen molecules, which consists of multiple polypeptide chains coiled in a lattice structure, allows for the orderly deposition of mineral in this matrix.

The mineral content of bone comprises crystals of hydroxyapatite, a series of calcium-phosphate polymers whose molar ratio varies from 1.3 to 2.0. These hydroxyapatite crystals are deposited on and within specific regions of the collagen structure of the matrix.

We will not discuss in any great detail the metabolism of bone matrix. It should be noted, however, that this matrix is dynamic and is continually being synthesized, mineralized, and dissolved. This is necessary for bone remodeling, restructuring, and growth. Collagen is a complex protein consisting to a large extent of proline and glycine. Thus, dissolution of bone and therefore of collagen results in increased levels of hydroxyproline excreted in the urine.

After bone matrix is synthesized, mineralization must occur. Mineralization of osteoid requires adequate extracellular levels of calcium and phosphate. Because the serum and extracellular levels of ionized calcium are maintained within a very narrow range by multiple regulatory mechanisms, the extracellular level of phosphate often determines the adequacy of mineralization. It appears that membrane vesicles — either derived from intracellular organelles already containing aggregates of calcium and phosphate or extruded from the cells and then accumulating calcium and phosphate from the extracellular fluid — act as nuclei for the growth of calcium-phosphate precipitates in the matrix. The cells that provide these vesicles are osteoblasts. Alkaline phosphatase, the enzyme that is found in the osteoblasts, is concentrated in the membrane and found in the matrix vesicles derived from these membranes. Alkaline phosphatase may function in the transport of calcium and phosphate into the vesicles or in the formation of the hydroxyapatite crystals.

The resorption of bone and the dissolution of bone mineral occur at the same time that new osteoid is created and mineralized. The resorption of bone and the dissolution of bone mineral are the functions of the osteoclast, a multinucleated giant cell. Osteoclastic activity results in the production of organic acids and in a decrease in extracellular pH. This decrease in pH on the surface of bone results in the dissolution of bone mineral. Osteoclasts also secrete proteolytic enzymes that can attack the basic collagen lattice structure of the matrix after bone has been demineralized. The process of demineralization, with the resultant increase in extracellular and plasma levels of ionized calcium, is under the control of parathyroid hormone and calcitriol. The remodeling and increased osteoblastic activity that results in bone accretion is under the control of the extracellular fluid levels of calcium and phosphate as well as of the hormone calcitonin. This dynamic process of bone remodeling allows for the growth of the organism and the necessary remodeling of longitudinal bone.

Careful control of mineralization and dissolution in bone is critical in the maintenance of the ionized calcium level in the serum.

Disorders of matrix formation and bone mineralization are not within the scope of this chapter. The reader is referred to a recent text (reference 28) for further information.

REFERENCES

1. Sorell M, Rosen JF: Ionized calcium: serum levels during symptomatic hypocalcemia. J Pediatr 87:67, 1975.
2. Sherwood LM, Rodman JS, Lundberg WB: Evidence for a precursor to circulating parathyroid hormone. Proc Natl Acad Sci USA 67:1631, 1970.
3. Anast CS, Mohs JM, Kaplan SL, Burns TW: Evidence for parathyroid failure in magnesium deficiency. Science 177:606, 1972.
4. Canterbury JM, Levey GJ, Reiss E: Activation of renal cortical adenylate cyclase by circulating immunoreactive parathyroid hormone fragments. J Clin Invest 52:524, 1973.
5. Haussler MR, McCain TA: Basic and clinical concepts related to vitamin D metabolism and action. N Engl J Med 297:974, 1977.
6. Cushard WG, Creditor MA, Canterbury JM, Reiss E: Physiologic hyperparathyroidism in pregnancy. J Clin Endocrinol Metab 34:767, 1972.
7. Pitkin RM: Calcium metabolism in pregnancy. Am J Obstet Gynecol 121:724, 1975.
8. Tsang RC, Chem IW, Friedman MA, Chen I: Neonatal parathyroid function: role of gestational age and postnatal age. J Pediatr 83:728, 1973.
9. Ponchon G, DeLuca HF: The role of the liver in the metabolism of vitamin D. J Clin Invest 48:1273, 1969.
10. Lawson D, Fraser DR, Kodicek E: Identification of 1,25-dihydroxycholecalciferol: A new kidney hormone controlling calcium metabolism. Nature (London) 230:228, 1971.
11. Fraser DR, Kodicek E: Regulation of 25-hydroxycholecalciferol-1-hydroxylase activity in kidney by parathyroid hormone. Nature New Biol 241:163, 1973.
12. Brumbaugh PF, Hughes MR, Haussler MR: Cytoplasmic and nuclear binding components for 1-α-25-dihydroxyvitamin D_3 in chick parathyroid glands. Proc Natl Acad Sci USA 72:4871, 1975.
13. Markowitz M, Rosen JF, Rotkin L, et al: Twenty-four hour mineral homeostasis and sterol levels in 1,25-dihydroxycholecalciferol-treated hyperparathyroid children. In Cohn DV, Talmage RV, Matthews JL (eds): The Endocrinology of Calcium Regulating Hormones. Excerpta Medica, in press.
14. Fleischman AR, Rosen JF, Nathenson G: 25-hydroxyvitamin D, serum levels and oral administration of calciferol in neonates. Arch Int Med 138:869, 1978.

15. Steichen JJ, Tsang RC, Graton TL, et al: Vitamin D homeostasis in the perinatal period 1,25-(OH)$_2$D in maternal cord and neonatal blood. N Engl J Med 302:315, 1980.
16. Fleischman AR, Rosen JR, Cole J, et al: Maternal and fetal serum 1,25-dihydroxyvitamin D levels at term. J Pediatr 97:640, 1980.
17. Chesney R, Rosen JF, Hamstra AJ, et al: Absence of seasonal variation in serum concentration of 1,25-dihydroxyvitamin D despite a rise in 25-hydroxyvitamin D in summer. J Clin Endocrinol Metab, 53:139, 1981.
18. Haymovits A, Rosen JF: Calcitonin: its nature and role in man. Pediatrics 45:133, 1970.
19. Foster GV: Calcitonin. N Engl J Med 279:349, 1968.
20. Garel JM, Michaud G, Sizonenko PC: Inactivation de la calcitonine porcine par différents organes foetaux et maternels du rat. C R Acad Sci (D) (Paris) 270:2469, 1970.
21. Dirksen C, Anast CS: Hypercalcitoninemia and neonatal hypocalcemia. Pediatr Res 11:424, 1977.
22. Meites S (ed): Pediatric Clinical Chemistry. American Association for Clinical Chemistry, Washington DC, 1977.
23. Wacker WEC, Vallee BL: Magnesium metabolism. N Engl J Med 259:431, 1958.
24. George WK, George WD, Haan CL, Fisher RG: Vitamin D and magnesium. Lancet 1:1300, 1962.
25. Wacker WEC, Parisi AF: Magnesium metabolism. N Engl J Med 278:712, 1968.
26. Jones KH, Fourman P: Effects of infusions of magnesium and of calcium in parathyroid insufficiency. Clin Sci 30:138, 1966.
27. Cohen MI, McNamara H, Finberg L: Serum magnesium in children with cirrhosis. J Pediatr 76:453, 1970.
28. Harrison HE, Harrison HC: Disorders of Calcium and Phosphate Metabolism in Childhood and Adolescence. W.B. Saunders, Philadelphia, 1979.

Chapter 9

ORGANIC MOLECULES IN EXTRACELLULAR FLUID: EFFECTS ON PHYSIOLOGY

Although the chemical anatomy of the body fluids, the extracellular fluid (ECF) in particular, concerns water and inorganic mineral matter for the most part, there are some organic substances whose role is frequently important. Among these are the plasma proteins, urea and glucose. Each of these appears in sufficient concentration, is involved in a number of interactions, and shows sufficient variation to affect water and mineral metabolism. Many other compounds affect important biologic processes at much lower levels of concentration. These concerns are beyond the scope of this work, as is discussion of the complex molecular interactions within cells and on cell membranes.

PLASMA PROTEINS

The total concentration of protein in plasma varies in healthy individuals from about 6.0 to 7.5 gm/dl. Four to five grams of this amount are albumin molecules with molecular weights of about 40,000. The remainder of the protein comprises a variety of globulins and fibrinogen with much larger molecular weights. These larger molecules are much fewer in number and, therefore, have little influence on the oncotic, or Starling, forces. The total concentration of the plasma protein, measured in milliosmols, is less than 2 mOsm/kg of plasma water.

The amount of circulating protein is only about half the total extracellular protein. The noncirculating fraction consists of molecules that, despite low permeability, have leaked through capillary walls into the interstitial fluid. At any given moment these molecules are being transported back to the circulation through the lymphatics or are temporarily sequestered in tissue fluids. When radioactive albumin tracers are injected, two "half-life" times are discernible: a rapid one of about 0.6 day, reflecting mixing, and a longer one of 11.2 days, resulting from metabolism.

The plasma protein constitutes most of the solid phase of plasma, roughly 6 to 7 per cent of the volume. Many physiologic and pharmacologic substances complex with or bind to plasma albumin, defining another important biologic role of this protein. Albumin levels are affected by dietary protein intake and thus represent a measure of adequate nutrition. The remaining proteins of plasma are involved in coagulation and immunologic roles; therefore, they are only very indirectly related to body fluid physiology.

The gradient created by 1.5 to 2 mOsm of albumin is sufficient to generate a colloid oncotic pressure of 36 cm of water. At the arterial end of the capillary bed the hydrostatic pressure is 44 cm of water, creating a filtration pressure of about 8 cm. At the venous end of the network the hydrostatic pressure falls to 17 cm; thus, the filtration pressure is here -19 cm, causing water and permeable salts to re-enter the circulation. These numbers are average and illustrative, subject to systemic and local controlling modulators. For example, blood pressure and tissue pressure are important variables.

UREA

Urea is a small molecule with a molecular weight of 60, which represents the principal end-product of protein (nitrogen) metabolism in mammals. Urea is synthesized from amino acids by deamination and then through the urea cycle of enzymatic steps. Normal levels of urea are expressed usually in milligrams per deciliter (mg/dl) of urea nitrogen (BUN for blood urea nitrogen; more properly SUN, since modern measurement is in serum). For infants and children the range is from 8 to 28 mg/dl. To convert to millimoles per liter (mmol/l), the factor is 0.357.

Urea is highly soluble in water, enabling some species of fish to use this substance as an osmoregulator to achieve concentrations of 350 mmol/l (>1000 mg/dl) in body fluids. Urea also moves freely and quickly across all membranes so that under any physiologic conditions urea levels do not redistribute body water. On the other hand, rapid infusion of hypertonic urea solutions will establish an osmolal gradient for a number of hours. In the mammalian kidney, the countercurrent architecture concentrates urea to levels as high as 1000 mmol/l in the inner medulla, thus aiding the reabsorption of water. In disease states, such as sickle cell anemia where the inner medulla is progressively destroyed, urine can no longer be concentrated, urine flow is high, and urea levels in body fluids are low.

GLUCOSE

Glucose, a simple hexose of molecular weight 180, is a critical molecule in biologic systems because of its role in energy metabolism. Normal fasting levels in blood after the neonatal period are 50 to 90 gm/dl (2.75 to 5.0 mmol/l), higher by two- to three-fold postprandially. In considering the role of glucose in body fluid physiology, a few properties are noteworthy. Although highly soluble, glucose does not enter cells rapidly except when insulin is present to facilitate transport. Therefore, in diabetes, marked elevation of glucose causes a shift of water from cells to the ECF in the same manner as sodium chloride. Insulin reverses this process. Either circumstance, hypoinsulinemia or the sudden addition of insulin, may produce a physiologically significant disturbance of water distribution in addition to other effects. The disturbed states are discussed in the chapters on hypernatremia (Chapter 11), the central nervous system (Chapter 23), and diabetes (Chapter 27).

Sugars that cannot be metabolized, such as mannitol, have the same effect as glucose without insulin; that is, they are confined to the ECF. The rapid administration of a large amount (>10 mmol or 1.8 g/kg) in concentrated form (50 per cent glucose or 25 per cent mannitol) produces the same consequences on the central nervous system (CNS) and cells as hypertonic saline in an equivalent osmolal concentration and amount. An experimental state in dogs induces idiogenic osmol production in the brain.[1] Ethyl alcohol in body fluids depresses the freezing point by markedly increasing osmolality even at low levels of intoxication. It does not affect water distribution, however.

In summary, the status of three kinds of physiologic organic molecules — albumin, urea, and glucose — is of concern to clinicians analyzing and managing patients with problems of body fluid balance. Unphysiologic substances used or abused as drugs or toxins may also have to be considered in appropriate circumstances.

REFERENCES

1. Arieff AI, Guisado R, Lazarowitz VC: The pathophysiology of hyperosmolar states. In Andreoli TE, Grantham JJ, Rector FC Jr (eds): Disturbances in Body Fluid Osmolality, pp. 227–250. American Physiological Society. Williams & Wilkins, Baltimore, 1977.

Pathophysiology and Pathology of Fluid Disturbances: Clinical Understanding

Chapter 10

ISOTONIC AND HYPONATREMIC DEHYDRATION

Dehydration comes from fluid loss in excess of fluid intake — a simple truism. Note that the word "fluid" is used here rather than "water," as ordinary English usage would dictate. Physiologists and clinicians have used dehydration to mean a diminution in volume of the extracellular fluid (ECF); thus, both water and sodium salts (principally chloride) are deficient. This type of dehydration is occasionally called isotonic, isonatremic, or "classical" dehydration, giving symmetry in nomenclature to the altered sodium states. When we wish to denote pure water loss, we say hypernatremic dehydration. That condition is of sufficient clinical importance to warrant a separate chapter (11). Here, after a review of physiologic fluids and sites of loss, the pathophysiology of the various compositional types of dehydration will be reviewed and the quantitative relationships discussed.

Losses of fluid may occur in several ways and from several sites. The foremost is the loss of gastrointestinal tract secretions. The fluid content of the alimentary canal results from a mixture of the secretions from the stomach, the pancreas, the bile, and the various intestinal segments, and, of course, from the diet, from which are subtracted the water and solute absorbed along the canal. The approximate composition and daily volume of the important secretions are shown in Figure 10–1. The resemblance to ECF may be appreciated.

Gastric secretion is, of course, very acidic. It will not be further discussed here, nor will the details of salivary, biliary, or pancreatic secretion, since rarely does their composition or volume determine the type of dehydration. All of these, along with the dietary components, are subject to absorption by the intestine. Further discussion of intestinal secretion and absorption, however, is germane to all the diarrheal diseases, which are the principal cause of infantile dehydration.

Intestinal secretion of ions appears to

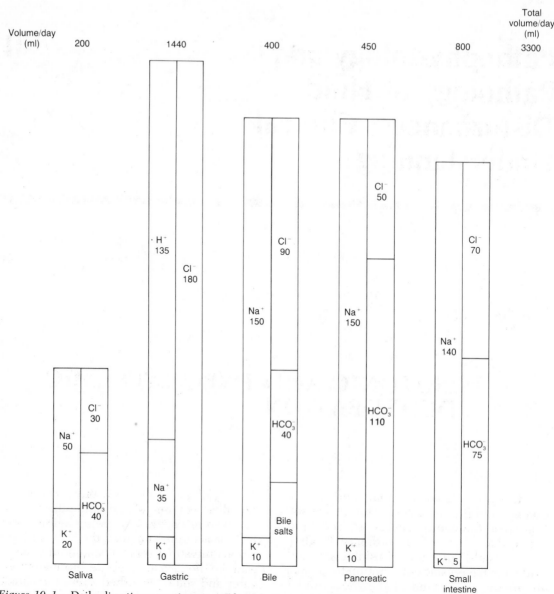

Figure 10–1. Daily digestive secretions in a 7-kg infant: approximate secretory volumes and concentrations of digestive secretions for a 7-kg infant at rest. Both volume and concentration vary; these values are illustrative rather than precise and constant. The values represent a composite from a number of sources; some of the concentration data were derived from adults.

depend upon active electrogenic secretion of chloride ion from serosa to mucosa. The numerous secretagogues that initiate this process are mediated through cyclic AMP, cyclic GMP, or calcium levels that act as intracellular messengers.[1] A number of pathogenic agents also stimulate secretion (see Chapter 20), resulting in high electrolyte losses. High secretory rates (as in cholera) produce the highest sodium and chloride concentrations. Water movement, however, follows osmotic gradients throughout.

Ion absorption from the intestine fol-

lows one of three processes: active sodium transport not coupled to other solute but passively accompanied by chloride; sodium transport coupled to nonelectrolyte solutes such as glucose or amino acids; and sodium absorption coupled to chloride absorption. All these active processes depend upon energy from ATP and upon Na-K-ATPase for hydrolysis. The cotransport of Na^+ and Cl^- is inhibited by elevated cellular levels of cyclic AMP, a factor of importance in the secretory diarrheas.[2] Water, again passively, follows osmotic gradients.

When a secretory process is causing

Table 10–1.   Concentrations of Electrolytes
in Stool Water[3]

ION	RANGE	MEDIAN CONCENTRATION (mEq/l)	MEAN CONCENTRATION (mEq/l)
Na⁺	5.3–150	60.5	65.2
Cl⁻	3.9–129	46.8	50.6
K⁺	11.5–117	41.3	45.0
Na⁺ and K⁺	35 –202	110	110

The concentrations in this table present analyses of stool water obtained on admission from patients presenting with diarrhea and dehydration.[3] Both older studies[4] and more recent ones[5, 6] reveal the same kind of pattern in populations of infants living in various parts of the world.

sodium and chloride loss, losses of water will also be high. In most situations stool losses have less sodium than does ECF, although the range is very large. Table 10–1 shows data on stool electrolyte concentrations from North American infants admitted consecutively to a hospital for diarrhea and dehydration. The most striking feature is the variability. Diet undoubtedly contributes to the finding, but this is not quantifiable from studies done to date. Both older studies[4] and more recent ones[5, 6] have shown similar data.

In general, when an infant has lost high-volume stool for several days while maintaining intake, net salt losses are usually proportionally higher than net water losses. A short illness with early anorexia, on the other hand, most often leads to predominant water loss. Most of the time, in 65 to 70 per cent of infants hospitalized in the United States, water and sodium — thanks to homeostatic compensation — are lost proportionally during enteric disease.

Water and salts may be lost from the gastrointestinal tract through the placement of tubes in the stomach or intestine or from fistulas. The urine may also be the site of abnormal losses in such conditions as diabetes mellitus or diabetes insipidus. These special circumstances will be discussed in the appropriate clinical section.

Whatever the route of loss and whatever the etiology of the disease process producing the loss, dehydration, by definition, results in a loss of body water. This change in volume or deficit is clinically and physiologically the most significant of the changes. Therefore, it is the clinician's first consideration. There may be a change in the relative proportions of the body water compart-

ments as well. This shift of water illustrates the mechanisms of osmolal physiology because of the biologic role of sodium. Henceforth, we shall refer to this type of disturbance as an "osmolal disturbance" — a shorthand way of describing distortions in the body fluid spaces. With more severe degrees of dehydration, changes in hydrogen ion metabolism, cellular ions, and relationships of the ECF to the skeleton will occur. In this chapter and the next, we shall deal only with the disturbances in volume and body fluid compartment distortions (osmolality). In subsequent chapters, the other disturbances will be delineated.

ISOTONIC (ISONATREMIC) DEHYDRATION

As previously mentioned, the word "dehydration" refers primarily to a reduction in ECF (Fig. 10–1). This reduction comes about because physiologic fluids that are lost from the body contain sodium in much the same concentration that ECF does. Moreover, as the pathologic process proceeds, a number of compensating homeostatic mechanisms tend to cause net water and sodium losses to occur in accordance with the proportions of these materials in the extracellular fluid. In recovery, most of the fluid retained goes back to the ECF, as shown in Figure 10–2.

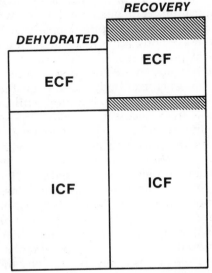

Figure 10–2. Isotonic constriction in enteric disease: distribution of water after hydration (24 hours). The figure traces the water supplied during treatment (together with sodium salts) to its "space" in recovery, indicated by the shaded areas. Note that in isotonic dehydration two thirds of the water goes to the smaller space, the ECF.

Water and sodium salts may be lost from the body to a considerable extent before the loss is detectable by clinical examination. Patients do experience thirst relatively early in a dehydrating process, but this is entirely subjective. The plasma volume as a portion of the ECF is the bodily component of principal vulnerability; thus, the objective signs, when they appear, will relate to circulatory deficiency. The delay in appearance is strong evidence of the effectiveness of the many compensatory mechanisms for sustaining blood pressure and flow even when blood volume is compromised.

It is customary to refer to fluid deficits incurred in acute dehydration as percentages of body mass or weight. Indeed, changes in body weight of more than 1 or 2 per cent within a 24-hour period represent changes in body water, with its small amount of dissolved solute. This makes such a conventional nomenclature justifiable as well as useful. It must be remembered, however, that such changes cannot be added cumulatively over many days, because cell destruction and the tissue loss may then become a sizable portion of the total.

Three clinically significant landmarks may be defined in the course of the pathogenesis of dehydration, corresponding to body weight losses of approximately 5, 10, and 15 per cent. This assumes a patient whose fluids are of approximately average composition. A 5 per cent loss of weight rapidly incurred is approximately a 7 per cent loss of body water in a lean patient. For clinical purposes, all but the most exceptional infant may be considered to have all their mass as lean body mass, even though this is not strictly true. For older children it is sometimes necessary to take adipose tissue into account in making estimates for therapeutic consideration. Obviously, if one knows a patient's weight 24 hours before dehydration begins, it is possible to have a very precise measure of the fluid loss. In practice, this is unlikely, and estimates eventually are made from three levels of circulatory deficiency and other objective manifestations. In the next paragraphs, the three conventional levels of dehydration will be described.

When 5 per cent of the body weight (7 to 8 per cent of body water) has been lost in less than a day, the earliest objective signs of dehydration appear. The first is the presence of a tachycardia. The pulse rate increases 10 to 15 per cent over its usual resting rate. The skin and mucous membranes appear dry and are dry to the touch. The urine becomes concentrated. The infant does not produce tears well while crying. Brachial blood pressure is maintained in the normal range, and if there is no concomitant disturbance from some other aspect of the illness, the patient does not appear seriously impaired. This appearance is deceptive, because from this point on, if the process continues, the infant is particularly vulnerable.

As acute dehydration progresses, circulatory failure will become more clinically manifest. There will be some mottling of the skin of the extremities. The distal portion of the extremities may become cool to the touch, owing to compensatory vasoconstriction. Gradually there will be loss of turgor of the skin, a rather significant sign of circulatory insufficiency. This sign is elicited by pinching a small area of skin between the thumb and forefinger, squeezing the blood from a few centimeters of skin, and then releasing the constriction. In the normal person, the blood flows back into the pinched skin almost immediately, restoring its color. If the blood returns slowly, turgor has been lost. This sign is frequently confused with, but is in fact distinct from, the loss of elasticity of the abdominal skin, which is generally seen only in infants or severely undernourished patients. Loss of turgor may be seen at any age.

The change in the elasticity of the abdominal skin of infants that accompanies dehydration is also a useful sign when the amount of loss approaches 10 per cent of body weight. The sign occurs because the nature of the subcutaneous tissue in infants differs from that in older children; in the dehydrated child, the skin when pinched or folded does not snap back to its normal taut condition but instead stands in folds. As the loss approaches 10 per cent of weight (14 to 15 per cent of body water), the eyeballs appear sunken in the head, and in infants the anterior fontanelle is depressed. Brachial blood pressure is usually still well maintained despite the fact that shock is impending. Oliguria is present, and tears are generally absent. This is perhaps the most common status of dehydrated infants at the moment of admission to the hospital. Homeostasis plus prior efforts (if any) to sustain them clearly have not worked, and this failure has precipitated admission. The patient's vital physiologic functions, while for the most part still intact, are highly vulnerable to disaster.

When the process proceeds beyond this point, all these signs become worse and serious circulatory collapse develops, with loss of blood pressure, damage to renal tubular cells, and potential ischemic damage to all peripheral tissues. This near-moribund state will be present at fluid deficits between 12 and 14 per cent of body weight (21 to 24 per cent of body water). On rare occasions, even more profound deficits have occurred with subsequent survival. The mortality and lasting morbidity are very high for such patients.

From these descriptions, the clinician may make reasonable estimates of the degree of fluid deficit. Since most of this deficit will come from the ECF, it is clear that the sodium concentration of the repair solution should resemble that of extracellular fluid.

HYPONATREMIC (HYPOTONIC) DEHYDRATION

Occasionally, instead of sodium and water being lost in extracellular physiologic proportions, something happens to make these losses disparate. A sodium loss that is proportionally greater generally occurs because, while sodium and water are being lost, water is being replaced by the patient either ingesting salt-free water or having (glucose) water administered by a physician. Under these circumstances, a hyponatremic type of dehydration ensues. Loss of sodium in this fashion causes water to shift to cells, inasmuch as potassium losses usually accumulate more gradually so that an osmotic gradient moves water from ECF to ICF (intracellular fluid). This internal loss of water from the ECF aggravates the circulatory disturbance, so all the manifestations described for isotonic dehydration develop clinically at lesser degrees of deficit. Since the danger to the patients is from the circulatory disturbance, patients with hyponatremic dehydration are in relatively greater jeopardy from any given level of fluid loss. Among hospitalized patients in North America, about 10 per cent of the infants admitted to hospitals for dehydration have the hyponatremic variety of physiologic disturbance. Since sodium is the key to the disturbance, the term "hyponatremic" seems preferable to "hypotonic," although the two terms are used interchangeably.

Another way that hyponatremic states may develop occurs in patients who have tubes draining one of the gastrointestinal fluids. The losses in such drainage will contain sodium as well as water if, when the replacement water is given without sodium, hyponatremia results. This is analogous to the classic experiments of Darrow and Yannet more than 45 years ago.[7]

A larger proportion of patients with diarrheal disease, generally about 25 per cent in North America, will have a hypernatremic dehydration with relative preservation of the ECF. In these patients, as ECF is preserved, circulatory signs are less manifest at any given level of fluid loss. The condition is sufficiently important in pediatrics to warrant an extended discussion, which appears in the next chapter.

REFERENCES

1. Frizzell RA, Heintze K, Stewart CP: Mechanism of intestinal chloride secretion in secretory diarrhea. Field M, Fordtran JS and Schultz SG (eds): Secretory Diarrhea. Williams & Wilkins, Baltimore, 1980.
2. Frizzell R, Field AM, Schultz SG: Sodium-coupled chloride transport by epithelial tissues. Am J Physiol 236:F1, 1979.
3. Finberg L, Cheung CS, Fleischman E: The significance of the concentrations of electrolytes in stool water during infantile diarrhea. Am J Dis Child 100:809, 1960.
4. Holt LE, Courtney AM, Fales HL: The chemical composition of diarrheal as compared with normal stools in infants. Am J Dis Child 9:213, 1915.
5. Sperotto G, Carrazza FR, Marcondes E: Treatment of diarrheal dehydration. Am J Clin Nutr 30:1447, 1977.
6. Nalin DR, Harland E, Ramlal D, et al: Comparison of low and high sodium and potassium content in oral rehydration solutions. J Ped 97:848, 1980.
7. Darrow DC, Yannet H: The changes in the distribution of body water accompanying increase and decrease in extracellular electrolyte. J Clin Invest 14:266, 1935.

Chapter 11

HYPERNATREMIC DEHYDRATION

The role of sodium in life processes is so pervasive that alterations in the concentrations of this ion produce a very wide range of disturbances. Among these, the hypernatremic states have a special place because they were probably not experienced as a disturbance at early levels of evolution. Although many other effects of high sodium levels may eventually be uncovered, the characteristic of sodium that dominates our present understanding is its function as the cation of an electrolyte pair that determines the partitioning of body water in higher animals. This arrangement exists presumably because as very primitive multicellular life forms developed, they took some of the primeval sea as a bathing medium, which was enclosed by an outer integument, so that cell functions would go on in relative tranquility.

Hypernatremic disturbances are not readily corrected by homeostatic systems, since all body secretions have a lower concentration of sodium than does extracellular fluid (ECF). Because virtually every hypernatremic state is also a dehydrated state — special experimental circumstances excepted — hypernatremic *dehydration* is a constant focus. This may occur with a body sodium content that is increased, normal, or decreased. All have been described; decrease is the most common. The following discussion defines the necessary concepts, gives some clinical historical background, touches on etiologic factors, and describes clinical presentations before providing a more detailed examination of pathophysiology and pathology. A discussion of therapeutic approaches is presented in Chapter 19.

INTRODUCTION AND DEFINITIONS

Hypernatremia is a physiologic disturbance arbitrarily defined by a concentration of sodium in serum of 150 mEq/l or greater. This definition is useful to clinicians because this measurement is performed by clinical laboratories. This definition also has been accepted generally by authors, journals, and texts. Certain limitations of the definition for both physiologist and clinician need to be identified, however, for expert evaluation. The first and less important of these is that the measurement of sodium concentrations in serum is not a measure of the chemically and biologically active sodium ion, which is the concentration of sodium in serum water. As discussed in Part I, the non-water portion of serum consists mostly of protein; since protein levels are usually similar, serum concentrations of sodium are comparable to one another even if the numerical values understate the active concentration. The second problem with using an arbitrary serum level stems from the fact that some of the important physiologic changes of hypernatremia result from the imposition of a sudden gradient with the higher concentration on the extracellular (and vascular) fluid side. The rapid adjustment results from the difference in concentrations, not the level. Thus, if a subject has an adaptational sodium concentration of 125 mEq/l and it is changed rapidly to 140 mEq/l, some of the induced disturbances will be the same as if the change had been from 145 to 160 mEq/l.

A change in sodium concentration means, in effect, a change in body fluid

78

osmolality, because the sodium ion, along with a negatively charged ion or ions, is the principal solute of the ECF and because sodium is relatively and actively excluded from most cell water. Thus, sodium salts act as the partitioner of body water between cells and ECF. One central part of the disturbance of hypernatremia is a shrinking of cell water with an expansion of ECF. This may come about because of water loss or sodium gain or both. At steady state the subject may be dehydrated (most commonly), normally hydrated, or (theoretically) overhydrated. Normal hydration or over-hydration is apt to occur only under circumstances of manipulation, such as dialysis or faulty intravenous infusions. The second most important part of the hypernatremic disturbance affects the central nervous system only when the gradient change is rapid (i.e., over hours, not days). The blood vessel changes in the central nervous system (CNS) will not occur if hypernatremia develops slowly. The reasons for this will be discussed later.

HISTORICAL BACKGROUND

When the pioneer chemical anatomist Schmidt[1] described the chemical composition of dehydrated tissue, he recognized two types of dehydration: one, more common, resulting from loss of water and salts, which became the definition of dehydration by physiologists and clinicians, and the other resulting from loss just of water, which has come to be known as hypernatremic dehydration. Between 1915 and 1920, L. H. Weed[2] performed experiments on the effects of hypertonic infusions upon the nervous system, first describing the pressure changes. In the 1940s, Rapoport and Dodd[3] described the "post-acidotic syndrome," an entity resulting in part from generous infusions of sodium bicarbonate. Subsequently, Rapoport[4] described patients with hypernatremia from several causes. Other case reports from neurosurgeons and others also appeared in the 1940s. In the early 1950s, after the widespread use of flame photometry, Finberg and Harrison[5] and Weil and Wallace[6] described large series of infants with hypernatremic dehydration, mostly secondary to enteric (diarrheal) diseases. These papers, first presented at the same meeting (American Pediatric Society, 1954), defined the clinical syndrome in infants and delineated the modern prevalence and importance of the entity. Since that time, additional insights into pathophysiology, pathology, and management have emerged.

IMPORTANCE AND EPIDEMIOLOGY

The importance of hypernatremia in infants emerged from the papers cited in the previous section,[5, 6] which showed an increased mortality of approximately 8 per cent, or fourfold more than that of otherwise similar patients with enteric disease and dehydration but not hypernatremia. An increased morbidity involving the CNS was also appreciated, although follow-up study in the 1960s was carried out in Great Britain, showing residual brain damage in hypernatremic dehydration in excess of other physiologic dehydrating disturbances.[7]

The incidence of hypernatremic dehydration in infants has had to be measured in hospitalized patients as a fraction of all infants hospitalized for dehydration over a given period of time. While not a true incidence, it is a clinically useful index of prevalence and actual incidence. From 1950 to 1980, in the United States the proportion has varied from about 15 to 30 per cent, with most reports between 20 and 25 per cent. Similar data have come from Nigeria,[8] but most workers in the underdeveloped world, where malnutrition is common, report little hypernatremia defined as sodium concentration greater than 150 mEq/l. Most writers do indicate a clear increase in the disturbance in the winter, even in the tropics. This has implications — specific and nonspecific — which are taken up below.

In Great Britain[9] and Spain[10] during the 1960s and early 1970s, there was a sharp increase in the incidence of hypernatremic dehydration in infants. This occurred because in both countries dry milk was made available at low cost. Inappropriate mixing (too much powder for the recommended volume of water) resulted in very high solute intakes and a virtual epidemic of hypernatremia. In Great Britain, the elimination of the dry milk and the introduction of low-solute feedings has been followed by a much lower incidence of hypernatremic dehydration in English infants.[11] A review of the epidemiology of hypernatremic states has recently been published.[12]

ETIOLOGIC FACTORS

The factors that produce a hypernatremic disturbance involve, on the one hand, either failure of intake or abnormal loss of water or, on the other, either excess salt or failure to excrete sodium. These events may occur singly or in any combination. The two simplest events are uncomplicated thirsting and salt poisoning. Thirsting with or without solute intake will in some species (e.g., humans, dogs) produce a hypernatremic state. An extensive literature on shipwreck victims describes the clinical and chemical events in such circumstances.[13] In other species (e.g., rats, mice) cellular breakdown and the release of cell water prevent hypernatremia resulting from simple total thirst. Despite these species differences, death occurs in approximately the same amount of time, suggesting that gradual development of hypernatremia is not the crucial factor in human death from total thirsting. Salt poisoning has occurred in a variety of ways, including suicide in adults and improper mixing of infant formulas usually by accidental substitution of salt for sucrose,[14, 15] and it is the usual method of producing hypernatremic states in experimental animals.

A frequent factor in the production of hypernatremia in certain patients is a diet or fluid intake too high in solutes, exceeding the kidney's capacity to excrete. The human kidney does not defend well against high solute intake; the thirst mechanisms are the primary homeostatic means of defense. It is to be expected, therefore, that the vulnerable individuals are those whose thirst mechanism is either faulty or unable to operate because of a problem of access to water. Small infants,[5] unconscious patients, psychotic patients, and patients with damage to the thirst center[16] all fit this description. Factors that lead to high insensible water loss also increase vulnerability. High environmental temperature, low humidity, high body temperature, small size with a higher ratio of surface area to weight, and hyperventilation[17] are the principal ones encountered. Those conditions that contribute to poor

solute excretion, such as diabetes insipidus (pituitary or renal), renal immaturity (as in small and, especially, prematurely born infants) and renal medullary impairment, also predispose individuals to hypernatremia. Finally, loss of water from the gastrointestinal tract through vomiting and diarrhea usually results in proportionally more water loss (in the physiologic context of the extracellular fluid) than sodium loss. This is not true of the toxigenic diarrheas such as cholera and certain *Escherichia coli* infections, which act on cyclic AMP or cyclic GMP to produce a stool water with high sodium concentration. It is, however, theoretically true of infections, such as that produced by rotavirus, that induce inflammation, malabsorption, and, usually, low-sodium stools. Confirmation that malabsorptive diarrheas predispose to hypernatremia has not been made, probably because of the many variables (most importantly, dietary intake) that affect stool composition. On the other hand, rotaviruses are recovered from patients mostly during winter epidemics when hypernatremia is more prevalent.

In recapitulation, small body size, unconsciousness, irrationality, immaturity, inability to self-regulate water intake, lack of renal water regulation, fast breathing, and sweating all represent patient vulnerabilities. Hot, dry atmosphere, high solute intake, limited water access, and, possibly, enteric infection with organisms causing inflammatory malabsorption constitute the main environmental predisposing events.

CLINICAL SYMPTOMS AND SIGNS

Patients or animals with hypernatremic dehydration have less circulatory disturbance for any given amount of fluid loss than do those with physiologically proportional water and sodium loss, i.e., isonatremic dehydration. The ECF volume, including the plasma volume, is relatively preserved; the cell water volume is relatively reduced. Clinicians accustomed to finding circulatory deficits, therefore, may not appreciate this kind of *inapparent* dehydration. Should the dehydration become very severe — e.g., 12 to 18 per cent of body weight loss in 24 to 36 hours — circulatory signs will appear in addition to those described in the following paragraphs.

Signs indicating nervous system involvement are almost always present in acute hypernatremic states. Disturbance of consciousness is the most constant, thus being an effect as well as a cause. A peculiar state of lethargy or even semi-coma when the patient is not stimulated, coupled with hyperirritability to virtually any stimulus, is the usual clinical state. This picture is perhaps appreciated more readily in infants than in adults or children. Hypertonicity of muscles often occurs, as does hyperreflexia. Nuchal rigidity, as a part of hypertonia, may falsely suggest meningitis, especially in infants. More overt CNS manifestations sometimes occur, including muscle twitchings and either focal or generalized convulsions. Less commonly, hemiparesis or evidence of focal neurologic damage may be seen. Chvostek's sign may occasionally be elicited.

Fever is usual — again a cause and an effect — and in infants, blood-tinged vomitus has often been seen. The skin of infants frequently feels thickened or doughy, although even more frequent is a velvety-soft skin texture.[18] In patients who are given access to water, avid thirst is the rule, unless an underlying illness interferes. In salt poisoning, pulmonary edema may occur early with resultant hyperventilation, which further aggravates the hypernatremia.

In chronic hypernatremic states, including all those in which the phenomenon has occurred gradually, the CNS signs may be absent until the disturbance is extremely severe in terms of sodium concentration or osmolality of plasma (sodium > 175 mEq/l, osmolality > 360 mOsm/kg).[19] At these very high levels, however, CNS symptoms do appear, presumably because of cellular desiccation.

PATHOPHYSIOLOGY

As previously discussed (Chapter 2), the principal role of sodium and chloride in mammalian physiology is to determine the partitioning of body fluid into the cells (as intracellular fluid, or ICF) and outside the cells (as ECF). This role is accomplished because most cells extrude sodium (and an accompanying anion) through a biochemical transport system known as the Na-K-ATPase, or sodium, "pump." Except at great extremes of concentration, this "pump" maintains a low concentration (6 to 8 mEq/l) of sodium in cells. In the muscle cell, the dominant one by mass, chloride is virtually absent in the milliequivalent order of magnitude. There is controversy as to whether the chloride distribution is passive, as in classic theory,[20, 21] or whether other explanations need to be invoked.[22] At present, the preponderance of evidence supports the pump system and a passive role for chloride as the most likely explanation.[23]

The various disturbances of hypernatremia are related to this property of sodium, regardless of the reason for this property. Water moves freely across virtually all the membrane interfaces of the body. Hence, except for some very specialized tissues, osmolality will be the same in all body fluids. When a solute gradient is created, water moves to adjust concentration almost instantly. Specifically, if sodium concentration in the ECF rises, water leaves cells to equilibrate the osmolality. Thus, ECF expands and ICF constricts. This explains why the circulation (plasma volume) is relatively expanded in hypernatremic states. The space disturbance of cellular desiccation can be documented by tracing water during rehydration (Fig. 11–1).

An unexpected phenomenon occurs when mammalian animals are subjected to extreme hypernatremia. Through a variety of experimental approaches,[24-27] it has been demonstrated that osmols are generated within cells, a phenomenon that will reduce the efflux of water. This has been called idiogenic osmol production.[24, 25] A number of theoretic explanations have been offered, most of which may coexist. Water binding by protein (not currently thought likely), osmotic activation of K^+ and Mg^{2+} from binding sites, inorganic PO_4 generation from complex organic phosphates,[28] and a breakdown of both peptides and proteins to amino acids have all been suggested as the source of the idiogenic osmols. At present, the likely source of most of these milliosmols is the breakdown of peptides or protein to release primarily taurine, aspartate, and glutamate, among other amino acids.[29] Figures 11–2, 11–3, and 11–4 illustrate diagrammatically the phenomenon of idiogenic osmol formation. After the addition of NaCl, the system has more osmoles, as amino acids, than the sum of the initial system and the added salt.

Taurine in particular does not diffuse readily from cells, thus increasing the total

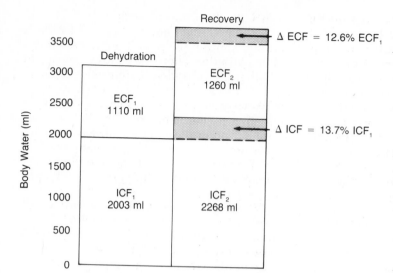

Figure 11–1. Water distribution before and after hydration; recovery weight, 5040 gm. The left side of the diagram shows the calculated compartments of the patient's body water prior to hydration. The right side depicts the assumed total body water and its distribution subsequent to recovery (see text). Areas designated by the symbol Δ indicate the calculated additions to each compartment. ECF = extracellular fluid; ICF = intracellular fluid. (From Finberg L, Harrison HE: Hypernatremia in infants. Pediatrics 16:1, 1955. Copyright © 1955 American Academy of Pediatrics. Used with permission.)

of ICF osmols and preserving cell volume in the presence of an osmotic gradient. There are comparative phylogeny data of considerable interest here. Both in invertebrates[30] and primitive vertebrates,[31] taurine is an osmoregulator for species that inhabit both fresh water and salt water at different times in their life cycle. This ancient life phenomenon of regulation involves mollusks, crabs, fish, and amphibians, and perhaps has been retained by mammals either vestigially or as a useful protective mechanism.[32] Prolactin, a hormone named for a function appearing much later in evolution, seems to be involved in osmoregulation, possibly in taurine metabolism. It should be

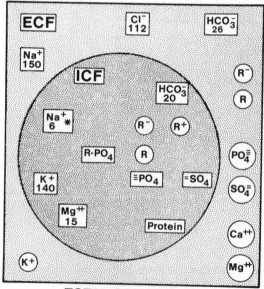

Figure 11–2. Muscle or brain cell in ECF. Initial stage — The diagram shows a cell prior to experiment in a sea of ECF. The concentrations of the principal solutes are indicated in the rectangles, the lower concentrations in circles. The values are given as concentrations in water with a Donnan correction. These values differ slightly from those shown in Figure 3–2 because they come from a particular set of experiments on a group of animals. The total number of osmols in the system is measurable and is indicated by the quantity A.

noted that it takes time to generate "idiogenic" osmols and that, once present, the taurine will remain a cell constituent past the time osmolality has been returned to normal by, for example, an intravenous infusion of water. The brain cells of animals appear to produce more idiogenic (taurine) osmols than do other tissue.[25, 29] Thus, during rapid correction, although all cells may show an increase in volume, the taurine may cause this to be exaggerated for brain cells, resulting in an important increase of brain size.

As previously mentioned, the CNS seems to be a particularly vulnerable tissue for the symptomatic ill effects of hypernatremic states. There are currently three mechanisms known that may account for this. They are, first, hemorrhage and thrombosis; second, idiogenic osmol formation; and, finally, response to a change in calcium concentration in the ECF.

Infants with hypernatremic dehydration following enteritis[33] and salt poisoning[13, 14] have been shown to have hemorrhage and thrombosis in the CNS and not in other tissues (Figs. 11–5 and 11–6). Experimental animals have had similar lesions produced by salt poisoning.[34] Mice, rats, cats, and dogs have all shown the same

phenomenon. When the brains of either the patients[14] or the animals[25, 34] are examined, dilated capillaries and venules are in evidence in addition to hemorrhage and (presumed) secondary thrombosis.

Further experiments[24] have demonstrated that hemorrhage, at least in the animals, was related to cerebrospinal fluid (CSF) pressure changes. When hypertonic (1 M, 20 mOsm/kg) solutions are infused intraperitoneally[25] or intravenously,[35] the CSF pressure falls predictably below atmospheric pressure and stays low for up to 6 hours (Fig. 11–7). If, in the experiments, the pressure is kept above atmospheric pressure by external manipulation of pressure in the monitoring manometer, the hemorrhages do not occur, nor does the capillary dilation.[25, 34]

These last phenomena are explainable by the anatomy and physiology of the blood-

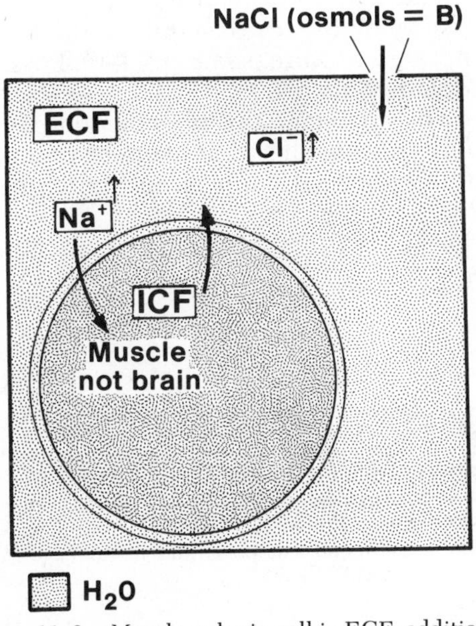

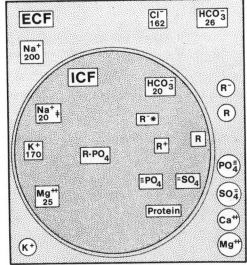

TOTAL OSMOLS = C

‡ **Na⁺ INTRACELLULAR (muscle only)**

*△ **R⁻ = TAURINE ASPARTATE,**
GLUTAMATE = IDIOGENIC OSMOLS

$$A + B < C$$

▨ **H₂O**

Figure 11–4. Muscle or brain cell in ECF: Hypernatremia; idiogenic osmols. Result — Expected increases of sodium and chloride concentrations in ECF (and, in muscle, of sodium concentrations in ICF). Osmols measured are indicated by the quantity C. A + B <C. The system has generated "idiogenic osmols." These appear to be mostly the amino acids taurine, aspartate, and glutamate.[29]

NaCl (osmols = B)

ECF

Cl⁻ ↑

Na⁺ ↑

ICF

Muscle not brain

▨ **H₂O**

Figure 11–3. Muscle or brain cell in ECF: addition of NaCl, 10 mEq/kg. Action — The experiment is conducted by adding a known amount (B) of NaCl osmols to the system. Water leaves the cell and, in muscle (not brain) cell, appreciable sodium enters.

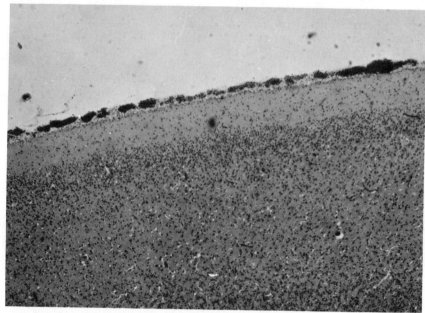

Figure 11–5. A section of brain from an infant dying after hypernatremic dehydration. Hemorrhage is subarachnoid and intracerebral. Note extensive capillary dilatation.

brain and blood-CSF barriers. It is known that both the brain capillary endothelial cells and the cells of the choroid plexuses have tight junctions between them,[36-38] unlike endothelial cells in most tissues. These tight junctions appear to be the basis of the long-known physiologic and pharmacologic phenomena of nondiffusion or slow diffusion from blood to brain or CSF and from brain or CSF to blood. Even the small crystalloid ions, Na^+ and Cl^-, diffuse slowly into and out of the CSF and the brain interstitium; water flows instantly to nullify

any osmolal gradient to a uniform concentration.[25] Thus, when Na^+ concentration in ECF rises rapidly, water leaves the interstitium and the CSF and enters the circulation. This, in turn, drags water from brain cells. The entire brain shrinks away from the cranium, and blood vessels under the pressure of the cardiac pump dilate and sometimes rupture (see Fig. 11–6). Possibly, bridging veins tear.[34, 39]

To understand this phenomenon better, it helps to compare what happens in muscle tissue with what happens in brain when a

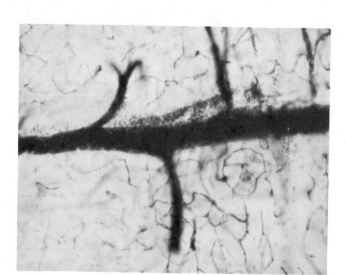

Figure 11–6. A high-powered view of a section from the brain of a patient dying after salt poisoning. The vessel wall is rupturing. (From Finberg L, Kiley J, Luttrell CN: Mass accidental salt poisoning in infancy. JAMA 184:187, 1963.)

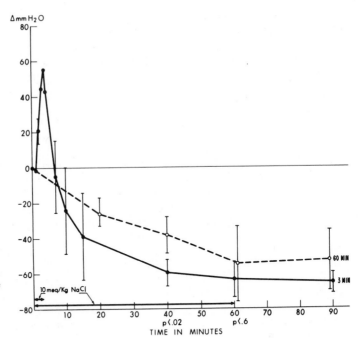

Figure 11–7. Cerebrospinal fluid (CSF) pressure changes versus time after infusion (10 mEq/kg NaCl; 1 mEq/ml). Two experiments are illustrated. In each, 10 mM/kg of NaCl in 1 molar concentration is infused intravenously. In the 3-minute infusion (solid line), the CSF pressure (measured as millimeters of change on the ordinate) shows an upward spike, which corresponds to temporarily increased intracranial blood volume. The pressure then falls below baseline and will remain down for 6 hours.[35] In the second experiment (dotted line), the infusion lasts an hour, and a similar drop in pressure (without prior increase) is noted.

If the infusion were given over a 24-hour period, a straight line from the zero on the ordinate would result. If the same quantity of sodium chloride were given as a $\frac{1}{6}$ molar solution (167 mmol/l), the same straight horizontal line would result.

sudden sodium concentration gradient is created, with plasma greater than ICF. In the muscle the sodium and chloride pass readily through the endothelial "loose" junction to the interstitial fluid. The ions do not, in net, enter muscle cells, which instead lose their water to the interstitium. Thus, cells shrink and interstitial fluid expands; the tissue volume is essentially the same after equilibrium. In the brain the boundary at which water molecules and sodium chloride ions diverge in their diffusion characteristics is the blood vessel wall. Thus, the entire CNS (brain cells, brain interstitial fluid, and CSF) shrinks.

The brain is encased in a rigid skeletal structure, the cranium. The shrinking in volume of the brain creates a lower pressure outside the tissue, including the capillaries, which dilate, sometimes rupture, and sometimes have secondary thrombosis with possible propagation and small or large infarcts.

The evidence for the genesis of idiogenic osmols has already been mentioned. The presence of these particles, perhaps taurine molecules primarily, will, after generation, defend cell volume. More of these particles may be present in brain cells than in muscle cells, as judged from available data.[25] An explanation may be that there is less entry of sodium into brain cells under the pathologic circumstance of hypernatremia. It is known that the muscle cell water concentration of sodium may triple whereas the non-chloride space (not as surely identical to cell water in brain as it is in muscle) of brain may not have any increase in sodium. Alternative explanations are possible from known data, but all require some difference between muscle and brain adaptation.

The experimental animal manifests dramatic CNS symptoms without hemorrhage but only after idiogenic osmols are present. Thus, the change in the colligative nature of the cell material is at least a marker for the electrical disturbances that occur, if indeed it is not the cause. Glutamate and aspartate are known to be involved as neurotransmitters in some circumstances. The role of these molecules in this pathologic state has not yet been explored.

As noted earlier, once taurine is present, it will not be reincorporated into protein quickly, nor will it diffuse well from the cells. Should sufficient (glucose) water be infused, the cells will swell back to a size greater than that prior to the taurine generation. Cerebral swelling is about as risky and certainly just as likely to produce symptoms as cerebral shrinkage. This in turn poses a problem for rapid therapy with dilute solutions.

The final mechanism known to produce CNS symptoms or signs is one involving several metabolic changes. When data from hypernatremic patients are analyzed, it is noted that calcium levels in serum are depressed.[5, 40] Most of the time the change is 1 to 3 mg/dl lower, not enough to cause symptoms even if all the change is in the ionized fraction. Rarely, the level falls to the range of 4 to 5 mg/dl of total calcium, and clinical tetany then occurs. This phenomenon has been reproduced in experimental animals.[41] The mechanism has not yet been very far elucidated. The lowering of calcium does not occur during the experiments on rats loaded with sodium salts if a simultaneous potassium deficiency in the animals is also prevented.[41] These data remain unexplained but have clinical relevance. The evidence indicates that the site of the cause of the disturbance is at the interface of the ECF with the skeleton; neither renal nor intestinal sites of calcium loss need be invoked. In the experimental situation, the lowering is maximal 24 to 48 hours after loading with salt and resolves soon thereafter. Possibly, vitamin D metabolites are involved in regulating the release from bone, but this remains a speculation.

There are two other important metabolic changes in hypernatremic states: changes in glucose homeostasis and in hydrogen ion metabolism. The first recorded data on glucose changes were obtained by Levin and Geller-Bernstein, who found frequent hyperglycemia.[42] Subsequently, a number of authors have confirmed this finding.[43-45] In as many as 25 per cent of infants (data on adults have not been systematically sought, to date), the blood glucose level is greater than 200 mg/dl. In some patients, levels of over 1000 mg/dl have been recorded.[44] In a few studies it has been suggested that insulin levels are well below what would be expected as a normal response to hyperglycemia.[45] Thus, this appears to be a transient diabetic state — transient in that no long-term consequence or later abnormal carbohydrate metabolism has occurred.

The presence of a hyperglycemic and insulinopenic state is of pathophysiologic consequence in worsening brain shrinkage. Physiologic levels of glucose cross the brain vessel endothelium by active transport.[38, 39] One of the functions of insulin is to facilitate glucose transport into cells and possibly into brain. With pathologic high levels of glucose and inadequate insulin, glucose becomes an extracellular obligate osmol in the same way that sodium is, and thus adds its osmolal concentration increment to that of the sodium salts in causing maldistribution of body water.

In severe experimental hypernatremia, cell desiccation causes release of hydrogen with resultant acidemia.[46] In less severe but steady-state circumstances, pH will fall because of an obligatory drop in plasma bicarbonate.[47] In clinical practice, virtually any hydrogen ion disturbance (acidemia to alkalemia) may be seen concomitant with hypernatremia because the number of variables is so great.

In addition to its direct metabolic effects, hypernatremia also modifies renal function. If there is expanded blood volume, osmotic diuresis ensues, so that the $[Na^+]_{urine}/[Na^+]_{plasma}$ ratio falls to unity or even slightly below.[48] If dehydration is present with a low blood volume, oliguria occurs, so that little sodium is excreted. Either way, renal function does not adapt well in order to remove sodium from humans with hypernatremia. In other species, sodium excretion in the urine is vastly more efficient.

Very high sodium concentrations may cause appreciable hemolysis by destroying red cell membranes in shrinking. Coupled with the expanded plasma volume and shrunken red cells, a low hematocrit is common. More recently, rhabdomyolysis has also been demonstrated in patients, with attendant risk for renal injury.[49]

PATHOLOGY

There are three principal sites for gross pathologic change from the physiologic disturbance of hypernatremia. These are the CNS, the kidney, and the skin. Although dehydration is usually also present, the CNS and renal changes can be produced experimentally in animals that are not dehydrated.[48, 50]

In the preceding discussion of pathophysiology in the CNS, hemorrhage and thrombosis are discussed as the source of symptoms. These changes are also the cause of mortality and late morbidity. About one third of patients dying during hypernatremic dehydration following enteritis have extensive hemorrhage or thrombosis. All

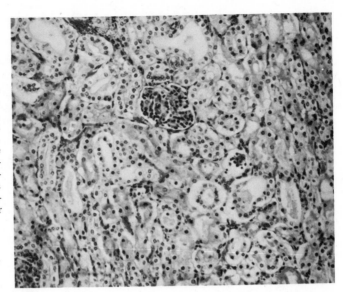

Figure 11–8. Section from autopsy specimen of an infant who died from salt poisoning incurred over three days prior to death, showing extensive sub-basilar vacuolation in renal tubules at all levels of the nephron. Note that the cytoplasm may be lifted off the basement membrane and the lumen obliterated. (Reproduced with permission from Finberg L.: Hypernatremic dehydration. *In* Schulman I, et al (eds): Advances in Pediatrics, Vol 16, p 325. Copyright © 1969 by Year Book Medical Publishers, Inc., Chicago.)

victims of salt poisoning show similar findings.[14] The predilectional sites for hemorrhage are along the sagittal sinus and over the cerebellum. The bleeding may be intracerebral, subarachnoid, subdural, or intradural.[25, 34] In low birth-weight infants subjected to rapidly infused, highly concentrated $NaHCO_3$, intraventricular bleeding may be precipitated.[51,52] Similar (although not intraventricular) changes are seen in adults poisoned[53] or overtreated with hypertonic $NaHCO_3$ during resuscitation. Small hemorrhages are seen following most deaths in hypernatremic states, but these do not cause death. The mechanism for CNS hemorrhage has already been discussed in the section on pathophysiology. Since the brain is very rich in thromboplastic substances, it is not surprising that thrombosis follows hemorrhage.

Renal pathology is primarily in the medulla and involves all the tubular portions of the nephron. The following processes have been commonly seen: vacuolation of the tubular cytoplasm (sometimes the vacuoles coalesce to lift the cell off the basement membrane) with necrosis, eosinophilic debris in tubules (Tamm-Horsfall protein), and medullary necrosis[39] (Fig. 11–8). The lesions can be experimentally produced in dogs without concomitant dehydration.[48] The necrosis appears to be reversible if the animals or patients survive. Renal vein thrombosis has occurred in young infants, hypernatremic secondary to high solute feedings.[10]

Changes in the skin are rare and, when seen, are part of circulatory gangrene of a distal extremity — purpura fulminans. The mechanism is not known, but local endothelial damage in a dehydrated patient seems likely.[54] Hypernatremic rather than isotonic dehydration appears more likely to do this, somewhat surprisingly in view of the relatively expanded blood volume. Perhaps endothelial cell damage together with platelet interaction occurs.

The approach to correction of the pathophysiology described here is given in Chapter 19.

REFERENCES

1. Schmidt C: Charakteristik der epidemischen Cholera gegenüber verwandten Transsudationsanomalieen. G. A. Rehyer, Leipzig, 1850.
2. Weed LH, McKibben PS: Pressure changes in the cerebrospinal fluid following intravenous injection of solutions of various concentrations. Am J Physiol 48:512, 1919.
3. Rapoport S, Dodd K, Clark M, Syllm I: Postacidotic state of infantile diarrhea: symptoms and chemical data. Am J Dis Child 73:391, 1947.
4. Rapoport S: Hyperosmolarity and hyperelectrolytemia in pathologic conditions of childhood. Am J Dis Child 74:682, 1947.
5. Finberg L, Harrison HE: Hypernatremia in infants. Pediatrics 16:1, 1955.
6. Weil WB, Wallace WM: Hypertonic dehydration in infancy. Pediatrics 17:171, 1956.
7. Macaulay D, Watson M: Hypernatremia in infants as a cause of brain damage. Arch Dis Child 42:485, 1967.

8. Ahmed I, Agusto-Odutola TB: Hypernatremia in diarrheal infants in Lagos. Arch Dis Child 45:97, 1970.

9. Taitz LS, Byers HD: High calorie/osmolar feeding and hypertonic dehydration. Arch Dis Child 47:257, 1972.

10. Rodrigo F, Ruza FJ: Deshidratacion hipertonica en la infancia: fisiopatologia y pautas de tratomiento. Rev Esp Pediatr 174:865, 1973.

11. Davies DP, Ansari BM, Mandal BK: The declining incidence of infantile hypernatremic dehydration in Great Britain. Am J Dis Child 133:148, 1979.

12. Wolf AV: Thirst. Charles C Thomas, Springfield IL. 1958, Part I, chap. V and Part II.

13. Paneth N: Hypernatremic dehydration. Am J Dis Child 134:785, 1980.

14. Miller N, Finberg L: Peritoneal dialysis for salt poisoning. New Engl J Med 263:1347, 1960.

15. Finberg L, Kiley J, Luttrell CN: Mass accidental salt poisoning in infancy. A study of a hospital disaster. JAMA 184:187, 1963.

16. Segar WE: Chronic hyperosmolality. Am J Dis Child 112:318, 1966.

17. Rapoport S: The role of overventilation in diseases of infancy. Ann Paediatr 176:137, 1951.

18. Harrison HE, Finberg L: Hypernatremic dehydration. Pediatr Clin North Am 11:955, 1964.

19. Crigler JF, Suh S: Hyperosmolarity in patients following radical treatment of craniopharyngioma. Am J Dis Child 102:469, 1961.

20. Ussing HH, Erlij D, Lassen U: Transport pathways in biologic membranes. Am Rev Physiol 36:17, 1974.

21. Sweadner KJ, Goldin SM: Active transport of sodium and potassium ions. New Engl J Med 14:777, 1980.

22. Ling G, Ochsenfeld MM: Studies on ion accumulation in muscle cells. J Gen Physiol 49:819, 1966.

23. Gulati J, Palmer LG: Potassium accumulation in frog muscle: the association-induction hypothesis versus the membrane theory. Science 198:1281, 1977.

24. McDowell ME, Wolff AV, Steer O: Osmotic volumes of distribution. Am J Physiol 180:545, 1955.

25. Finberg L, Luttrell C, Redd H: Pathogenesis of lesions in the nervous system in hypernatremic states. II. Experimental studies of gross anatomic changes and alterations of chemical composition of the tissues. Pediatrics 23:46, 1959.

26. Arieff AI, Kleeman CR: Studies on mechanisms of cerebral edema in diabetic comas: effects of hyperglycemia and rapid lowering of plasma glucose in normal rabbits. J Clin Invest 52:571, 1973.

27. Holiday MA, Kalayci MN, Harrah J: Factors that limit brain volume changes in response to acute and sustained hyper- and hyponatremia. J Clin Invest 47:1916, 1968.

28. Nitowsky HM, Herz F, Geller S: Induction of alkaline phosphatase in dispersed cell cultures by changes in osmolarity. Biochem Biophys Res Commun 12:293, 1963.

29. Thurston JH, Hauhart RE, Dirges JA: Taurine: a role in osmotic regulation of mammalian brain and possible clinical significance. Life Sci 26:1561, 1980.

30. Bedford JJ, Leader JP: Hyperosmotic readjustment of the crab, *Hemigrapsus edwardsi*. J Comp Physiol 128:147, 1978.

31. Gordon MS: Intracellular osmoregulation in skeletal muscle during salinity adaptation in two species of toads. Biol Bull 128:218, 1965.

32. Jacobsen JG, Smith LH Jr.: Biochemistry and physiology of taurine and taurine derivatives. Physiol Rev 48:424, 1968.

33. Finberg L, Harrison HE: Hypernatremia in infants. An evaluation of the clinical and biochemical findings accompanying this state. Pediatrics 16:1, 1955.

34. Luttrell CN, Finberg L, Drawdy L: Hemorrhagic encephalopathy induced by hypernatremia. II. Experimental observations of hyperosmolarity in cats. AMA Arch Neur Psychiat 1:153, 1959.

35. Kravath RE, Aharon AS, Abal G, Finberg L: Clinically significant physiologic danger from rapidly administered hypertonic solutions: acute osmol poisoning. Pediatrics 46:267, 1970.

36. Reese TS, Karnovsky MJ: Fine structural localization of a blood-brain barrier to exogenous peroxidase. J Cell Biol 34:207, 1967.

37. Spector R: Vitamin homeostasis in the central nervous system. New Engl J Med 296:1393, 1977.

38. Goldstein GW: Pathogenesis of brain edema and hemorrhage: role of the brain capillary. Pediatrics 64:357, 1979.

39. Finberg L: Hypernatremic dehydration. Adv Pediatr 16:325, 1969.

40. Finberg L: Pathogenesis of lesions in the nervous system in hypernatremic states. Pediatrics 23:40, 1959.

41. Finberg L: Experimental studies of the mechanism producing hypocalcemia in hypernatremic states. J Clin Invest 36:434, 1957.

42. Levin S, Geller-Bernstein C: Alimentary hyperglycemia simulating diabetic ketosis. Lancet 2:595, 1964.

43. Stevenson RE, Bowyer FP: Hyperglycemia with hyperosmolal dehydration in nondiabetic infants. J Pediatr 77:818, 1970.

44. Finberg L: Current Concepts: hypernatremic (hypertonic) dehydration in infants. New Engl J Med 289:196, 1973.

45. Mandell F and Fellers FX: Hyperglycemia in hypernatremic dehydration. Clin Pediatr 13:367, 1974.

46. Sotos JF, Dodge PR, Talbot NB: Studies in experimental hypertonicity. II. Hypertonicity of body fluids as a cause of acidosis. Pediatrics 30:180, 1962.

47. Winters RW, et al: The mechanism of acidosis produced by hyperosmotic infusions. J Clin Invest 43:647, 1964.

48. Finberg L, Rush BF, Cheung CS: Experimental observations of the renal excretion of sodium during hypernatremia. Am J Dis Child 107:483, 1964.

49. Opas LM, Adler R, Robinson R, Lieberman E: Rhabdomyolysis with severe hypernatremia. J Pediatr 90:713, 1977.

50. Rush BF, Finberg L, Daviglus GF, Cheung CS: Pathologic lesions in experimental hypernatremia induced by extracorporeal dialysis. Surgery 50:359, 1961.

51. Papile L, Burstein J, Burstein R, et al: Relationship

of intravenous sodium bicarbonate infusions and cerebral intraventricular hemorrhage. J Pediatr 93:834, 1978.

52. Volpe JJ: Intracranial hemorrhage in the newborn: current understanding and dilemmas. Neurology 29:632, 1979.

53. Johnston JG, Robertson WO: Fatal ingestion of table salt by an adult. West J Med 126:141, 1977.

54. Comay SC, Karabus CD: Peripheral gangrene in hypernatremic dehydration of infancy. Arch Dis Child 50:646, 1975.

Chapter 12

PATHOPHYSIOLOGY OF HYDROGEN ION DISTURBANCE

Disorders of H^+ metabolism result from two types of physiologic disturbances: acidosis and alkalosis. Actual changes in blood pH resulting from these disturbances are called acidemia when there is a fall in pH, and alkalemia when there is a rise in pH. When the disturbance is due to a primary change in PCO_2, it is termed respiratory. All other primary changes are called metabolic. Thus, four primary categories of disturbances of acid-base equilibrium are recognized: respiratory acidosis, metabolic acidosis, respiratory alkalosis, and metabolic alkalosis.

RESPIRATORY ACIDOSIS

Respiratory acidosis is a result of pulmonary alveolar hypoventilation so that, by definition, CO_2 production exceeds CO_2 excretion. Carbon dioxide traverses tissue fluids extremely rapidly, so clinically significant accumulation in the body will only occur if CO_2 accumulates in the alveolar air. Severe uncomplicated pure respiratory acidosis occurs relatively uncommonly in childhood, since the anoxia invariably associated with it when a child is breathing room air quickly leads to the production of a superimposed metabolic acidosis. Less severe respiratory acidosis, when chronic, is usually compensated.

Respiratory acidosis occurs in almost all newborn infants during delivery and may become persistent in depressed infants. It is also seen with severe pulmonary diseases such as hyaline membrane disease, pleural effusions, pneumothorax, phrenic palsy, status asthmaticus, cystic fibrosis, and bronchiolitis; and with croup and deformities of the chest wall as well as with sleep apnea, neuromuscular disease, paralysis, sedation, and cardiac arrest. It is particularly dangerous in patients with cerebral edema, since the increased blood volume in the cranium produced by the CO_2-induced vasodilation may increase the intracranial pressure to a great extent and cause brain herniation.

Clinical Manifestations

The manifestations of respiratory acidosis with acidemia depend upon three factors: (1) how long the acidosis has been present and the degree of compensation, (2) the severity of the acidosis, and (3) the state of the patient's central nervous system.

Patients with intact central nervous systems and acute mild to moderately severe acidosis who are not sedated are extremely unhappy about the condition and tend to devote all their faculties to concern about this one aspect of disordered physiology. This should be recognized as an almost pathognomonic sign of respiratory acidosis. These patients will be noted to be making forceful efforts to breathe, although with only limited success, so that use of the accessory muscles of respiration is obvious, as are retractions and bulgings of the chest wall, neck, and trachea. If they are breathing room air, their degree of hypoxia will at least parallel their degree of hypercapnia, and they will show increasing cyanosis as the respiratory acidosis worsens. Giving them oxygen to breathe, while correcting the hypoxia and preventing further development of metabolic acidosis, may also correct the cyanosis, thus obscuring this useful sign of hypoventilation. In a patient with long-standing respiratory acidosis with metabolic compensation, the effect of elevated carbon dioxide as a respiratory stimulant may have been lost, and such a patient may be functioning on hypoxia alone to provide respiratory drive. Giving such a patient oxygen will eliminate the residual respiratory drive due to hypoxia and will precipitate even worse hypoventilation and respiratory acidosis, which may prove lethal. This is not to say that such patients should never be given oxygen, but they require very careful observation, frequent determinations of blood gases and pH, and cautious administration of relatively low concentrations of oxygen.

Carbon dioxide, although usually an excellent respiratory stimulant, is a general central nervous system depressant when present in marked excess. Therefore, a patient who may be trying very hard to breathe at a PCO_2 of 60 mm Hg may look very comfortable at a PCO_2 of 100 mm Hg and may go to sleep and die. Unfortunately, in such a patient there are no reliable signs of impending death except the rising PCO_2 and falling pH, although decreasing breath sounds may be apparent. Vital signs such as pulse, respiratory rate, and blood pressure may show no abnormal trends before dropping to zero.

Therefore, although a *moderate* degree of respiratory acidosis in a patient with otherwise intact physiologic responses is very easy to diagnose, *severe* respiratory acidosis is much harder to diagnose, because those who have it may look comfortably asleep. This is unlike most other diseases and physiologic disturbances, which become easier to diagnose as they become worse.

If compensation for the respiratory acidosis has occurred, if respiratory acidosis is combined with metabolic alkalosis, if the patient is comatose, if neuromuscular disease or sedation are present, or if muscle relaxants have been administered, then diagnosis is also very difficult, since signs will be minimal. Carbon dioxide is an excellent vasodilator and therefore may produce a red flush of the skin. Dilation of blood vessels in the brain may increase intracranial pressure to the point of papilledema. Chronic hypoventilation will also produce an adaptive increase in hemoglobin and hematocrit. It also causes pulmonary hypertension, which may induce right

heart failure and signs of right atrial and ventricular hypertrophy on physical examination, electrocardiogram, and chest x-ray.

The physiologic mechanism is relatively simple. Retention of CO_2 leads to a shift of the carbon dioxide-bicarbonate equilibrium reaction in the direction of bicarbonate and H^+ formation, by the law of mass action. Thus, alveolar hypoventilation leads to the following changes:

$$CO_2 + H_2O \underset{\text{carbonic anhydrase}}{\overset{}{\rightleftharpoons}} H_2CO_3 \rightleftharpoons H^+ + HCO_3^-$$

Hydrogen ion is released with a potentially resulting acidemia, but all but about 0.00016667 per cent of it is buffered by nonbicarbonate buffers. Respiratory acidosis thus produces an immediate small increase in hydrogen ions and bicarbonate.

This rise in bicarbonate is relatively small in magnitude, as can be seen from the Siggaard-Andersen alignment nomogram (Fig. 12–1) by choosing any base excess (BE) at a given hemoglobin value and keeping it fixed as the point of rotation of a straightedge, then rotating the straightedge from a given PCO_2 to any other PCO_2, and reading the effect from the bicarbonate line. For example, if one starts with pH 7.4, PCO_2 40 mm Hg, HCO_3^- 24.5 mEq/l, and base excess 0 mEq/l at hemoglobin 10 g/100 ml (Line 1) and rotates the line around the point at base excess 0/hemoglobin 10 to PCO_2 60 mm Hg (Line 2), it can be seen that the HCO_3^- will rise to 27.5/mEq/l. At PCO_2 80 mm Hg (Line 3), the HCO_3^- is 29.5 mEq/l. If one corrects for the expected fall in base excess of 2 mEq/l for each 20 mm Hg increase in PCO_2, owing to the shift from blood to interstitial fluid of some bicarbonate (see Chapter 6, p. 48) by lowering the base excess/hemoglobin rotation point accordingly (to base excess −2/hemoglobin 10), the HCO_3^- at a PCO_2 of 60 mm Hg becomes 25.5 mEq/l (Line 4). At a PCO_2 of 80 mm Hg (base excess −4/hemoglobin 10), the HCO_3^- becomes 26 mEq/l (Line 5).

This relatively small increase in bicarbonate as the PCO_2 doubles is surprising at first, but it is a consequence of the large amount of bicarbonate already present. Although the amount of bicarbonate generated by the PCO_2 rising abruptly to 80 mm Hg from 40 mm Hg is a small percent-

SIGGAARD-ANDERSEN ALIGNMENT NOMOGRAM

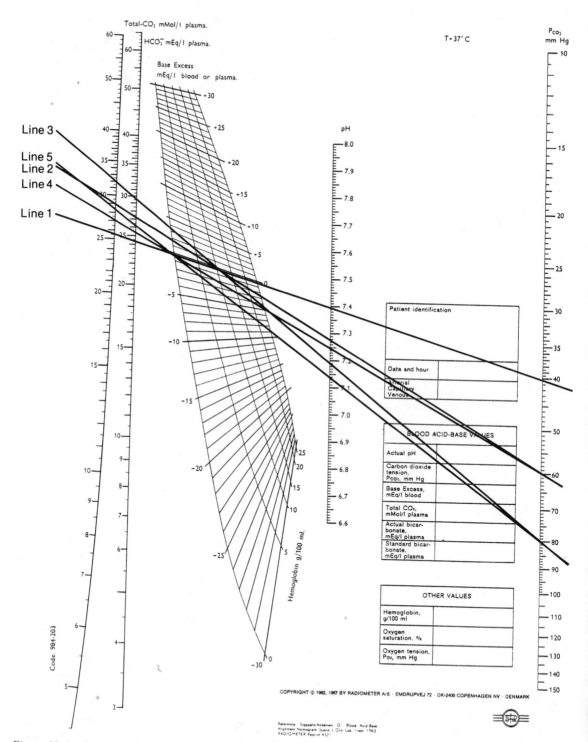

Figure 12–1. Siggaard-Andersen alignment nomogram. (See text.) (From Siggaard-Andersen O: Blood acid-base alignment nomogram. Scand J Clin Lab Invest 15:211, 1963. Radiometer Reprint AS21. Copyright © 1962, 1967 by Radiometer A/S. Used with permission.)

age of the total bicarbonate, it should be noted that for each HCO_3^- ion produced, a H^+ ion is also produced. Although 1.2 mmol/l of HCO_3^- does not seem like much, 1.2 mmol/l is quite a lot of H^+ compared with the normal amount of $10^{-7.4}$ mol/l. Almost all this new H^+ is buffered in the nonbicarbonate buffer system. In fact, as the PCO_2 increases 40 mm Hg and the H_2CO_3 and dissolved CO_2 increase 1.2 mmol/l, the H^+ concentration increases only 0.000042 mmol/l.

The effects of compensatory mechanisms take hours to develop. Urine will be produced with increased titratable acidity, and therefore virtually no bicarbonate, and with increasing levels of ammonium. The reabsorption of the filtered bicarbonate will further increase serum bicarbonate concentration, which will shift the carbonic acid equilibrium reaction to decrease H^+ concentration. The excretion of the H^+ in the urine will lessen the degree of acidosis and also shift the equilibrium in the direction to produce new bicarbonate. The degree of metabolic compensation is indicated by the degree of increase in base excess. This compensation is not generally complete, and therefore a mild acidemia usually persists.

In addition to the buffering of most of the H^+ in the nonbicarbonate blood buffers such as hemoglobin, serum protein, and phosphate, there is also buffering in the form of exchange of H^+ for Na^+, K^+, and Ca^{2+} from cells and bone. Correction of the disturbance takes place with an increase in alveolar ventilation (or conceivably a decrease in CO_2 production).

Therapy

Treatment of respiratory acidosis should be directed at correction of the ventilation problem. The rapid administration of sodium bicarbonate will increase the PCO_2 and may make matters worse, since the newly formed CO_2 will enter cells more rapidly than the bicarbonate, lowering intracellular pH and also imposing sodium, volume, and osmolal loads, but it may be temporarily useful on occasion. Tris(hydroxymethyl)aminomethane (THAM) can also quickly raise the pH, with an advantage over $NaHCO_3$ in that it will lower rather than raise the PCO_2, but has the drawback that its use may be followed by apnea.[2,3] It

has not been found to be of much more use than sodium bicarbonate, since it shares the other hazards of that compound. It may have an occasional role in the treatment of extremely severe, imminently life-threatening respiratory acidosis when rapid CO_2 excretion cannot be otherwise accomplished.

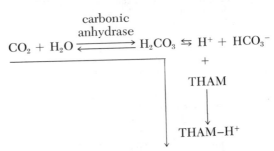

THAM combines with H^+, shifting the equilibrium to the right. It also removes H^+ from the nonbicarbonate buffers. For every molecule of THAM–H^+ produced from CO_2 and H_2O, one molecule of HCO_3^- is produced. Tham–H^+ is excreted in the urine.

Typical arterial blood gases in acute uncomplicated respiratory acidosis are pH 7.15, PCO_2 80 mm Hg, PO_2 40 mm Hg, and base excess −3 mEq/l. With metabolic compensation pH would be 7.35, PCO_2 80 mm Hg, PO_2 40 mm Hg, and BE + 15 mEq/l.

METABOLIC ACIDOSIS

Metabolic acidosis results from one or more of the mechanisms shown in Table 12–1. The degree of metabolic acidosis is indicated by the amount of the fall in base excess. Compensation begins immediately and takes the form of hyperventilation with compensatory respiratory alkalosis, owing to direct stimulation of respiratory chemoreceptors by the increased H^+ concentration.

In experimental animals there is a delay of several hours before maximal respiratory compensation occurs, owing to the lag of pH changes in the cerebrospinal fluid (CSF) behind those induced in the blood by the acidic infusions designed to lower the pH.[4] A similar lag time is noted after alkaline infusions. This is thought to be due to the blood-brain barrier, which delays the passage of H^+ or base into the CSF. This effect of the blood-brain barrier is not seen when changes in CO_2 or in acid or base production occur in the brain itself, since

Table 12–1.   Mechanisms of Metabolic Acidosis

A. Increased production of H^+ by the cells, which occurs as a result of the following mechanisms:
 1. Overall increase in the metabolic rate due to fever, convulsions, respiratory distress, etc.
 2. Interference with normal metabolism resulting in the production of excess quantities of organic acid rather than volatile CO_2, which is easily removed by the lungs. This occurs in the following states:
  a. Severe tissue hypoxia from hypoperfusion, as in diarrheal dehydration with lactic and pyruvic acids released by anaerobic metabolism
  b. Ketosis (due to starvation, ethanol and methanol ingestion, diabetes mellitus, glycogen storage disease, or salicylate and paraldehyde poisoning)
  c. Lactic and pyruvic acidosis from metabolic blocks
  d. Methyl alcohol poisoning (formic acid)
  e. Branched-chain ketonemia
  f. Isovaleric aciduria
  g. Methylmalonic aciduria
  h. Propionic acidemia
  i. Hyperglycinemia
B. Loss of bicarbonate, as in diarrheal stools, ileostomy drainage, ureterosigmoidostomy, ileal bladder, and acetazolamide poisoning.
C. Administration of acids, e.g., HCl, amino acids.
D. Failure of the kidney to excrete a normal acid load. This results from either a fall in glomerular filtration or tubular dysfunction. Renal tubular dysfunction may occur as a primary disease, can follow shock, and is seen in such diseases as Fanconi's syndrome, cystinosis, fructose intolerance, and hypercalcemia. Several factors may play a role, including defective excretion of H^+, a defective carbonic anhydrase mechanism, defective formation of ammonia, and a lowered bicarbonate threshold.
E. Expansion of extracellular fluid and decrease in the concentration of HCO_3^- with maintenance of the previous CO_2 levels, which produces a "dilution acidosis."

the changes in the central nervous system (CNS) would not then lag behind changes in the blood.

Buffering takes place in the bicarbonate and nonbicarbonate systems. Correction takes place by renal H^+ excretion and HCO_3^- retention and by metabolism of organic acids in the tissues. Typical arterial blood gases in metabolic acidosis with respiratory compensation are pH 7.25, PCO_2 20 mm Hg, PO_2 110 mm Hg, and BE −17 mEq/l.

Clinical Manifestations

Air hunger is a prominent finding in metabolic acidosis with acidemia and may be mistaken for respiratory disease. Arterial blood gases easily provide the distinction. Anorexia, nausea, and vomiting may also be manifest. With increasing severity of the acidosis, depression of CNS function occurs, leading to coma and convulsions. Decreased peripheral vascular resistance and decreased cardiac contractility with hypotension, heart failure, and a lowered threshold for ventricular fibrillation may provide a lethal pathway.

The hyperventilation and decreased peripheral resistance are part of the physiologic response to the disturbance and result in increasing transport of oxygen and carbon dioxide. Acidemia also decreases the oxygen affinity of hemoglobin and increases oxygen unloading in the tissues. As a consequence, cyanosis will be more pronounced at any given PO_2.

Endogenous production of metabolic acids in the CNS, as in lactic acidosis from hypoxia, results in a more rapid respiratory response than does exogenous acid administration to the CNS, as in experimental intravenous infusions of acid into animals and in diabetic acidosis in which the keto-acids are produced in the liver. The blood-brain barrier protects the CNS from rapid changes in concentration of metabolic acids in the extracellular fluid.

Some patients with metabolic acidosis have an increased anion gap. The "anion gap" is the difference between the sodium concentration and the sum of the concentrations of Cl^- and HCO_3^-.

$$\text{Anion gap} = [Na^+] - ([HCO_3^-] + [Cl^-])$$

The normal mean gap is 12 mEq/l and when the gap exceeds 16 mEq/l it is considered increased. The normal anion gap consists of substances not usually measured, such as negatively charged protein molecules and a small amount of other organic anions, sulfates, and phosphates. An increased anion gap is usually due to increases in organic acid anions such as lactate and keto-anions. When HCl or H_2CO_3 is added to blood, there will be no increase in anion gap, since Cl^- and HCO_3^- will increase in concentration and be measured. When acids with other anions are added, such as H_2SO_4, to produce acidemia, the concentration of HCO_3^- will be lowered by buffering and the anion (i.e., SO_4^{2-}) although present, will not be measured in the routine clinical laboratory; thus, its concentration will be reflected in the anion gap. In a recent study of adult patients with increased anion gaps, of the 47 who had arterial blood gas and pH analysis only 55 per cent were acidemic, 24 per cent were alkalemic, and 21 per cent had normal pH values.[5] However, a very large anion gap, of over 30 mEq/l, was always associated with organic acidosis. With a smaller anion gap, one cannot assume that an organic metabolic acidosis is present. The discovery of a large anion gap, therefore, should lead to the suspicion of a metabolic acidosis, and analysis of blood gases and pH can clearly define the acid-base disturbance.

Increased H^+ concentration in the extracellular fluid may be followed by intracellular movement of H^+ in exchange for potassium, which moves from the intracellular to the extracellular fluid; thus, acidosis may be associated with elevated serum levels of potassium even though the cells are depleted of potassium. The effect of acidosis on potassium levels may vary with the kind of acid and the way the acidosis was produced.[6] Massive loss of potassium as a consequence of the disease may overwhelm this effect, as in diarrheal dehydration, where K^+ loss in the stool may produce hypokalemia in the presence of a severe acidosis. Treatment and correction of the acidosis will allow potassium to return to the cells and make the potassium deficit more evident.

Therapy

The main course of action should be directed at correcting the underlying problem, whenever possible, by such measures as administering insulin and fluids in diabetes, increasing the plasma volume in dehydration, and giving oxygen for hypoxia. It should not involve misguided attempts at instantaneous pH correction.[7-11] With moderation, the increased H^+ concentration can be ameliorated by the slow administration of dilute base such as sodium lactate or sodium bicarbonate either orally or intravenously and by allowing time for physiologic mechanisms to come into play. Alkali therapy is an additional, usually unnecessary refinement to the basic treatment, i.e., correction of the underlying defect when possible and maintenance of renal function and tissue perfusion by adequate fluid adminis-

tration and other therapeutic measures. The vast majority of patients with acute metabolic acidosis can be well managed without specific attention to the details of its correction as long as circulation, renal function, and pulmonary function are adequate. Indeed, attempts at rapid correction with $NaHCO_3$ may lower intracellular pH even more, since the administered HCO_3^- moves into cells slowly whereas the CO_2 it produces moves very rapidly.

When severe acidosis occurs during cardiac arrest or when cardiac arrest seems imminent, and in other rare instances when rapid pH rise is warranted, it is probably safe to give as much as 3 mEq/kg of 0.9 to 1 molar $NaHCO_3$ solution intravenously one time only over a period of about ten minutes. This can safely be followed by an isotonic solution of sodium bicarbonate ($\sim$ 150 mEq/l) at the intravenous rate calculated to provide the patient's water requirement. Frequently repeated assessments of blood gases and pH permit the $NaHCO_3$ infusion to be stopped as the patient's pH is titrated toward normal. If organic acids are present, an increasingly severe metabolic alkalosis may develop as they are oxidized over the next one or two days.

Repeated rapid infusions of hypertonic sodium bicarbonate have a multiplicity of adverse effects and should be avoided, even though they may, deceptively, make the patient look better for a short period of time. One group of these adverse effects is related to the hyperosmolality of the solution and is similar to hypertonic dehydration.[12] Since the frequently used solutions of $NaHCO_3$ are 0.9 to 1 molar and have about six times the normal osmolality of body fluids, they will shift water by osmosis from cells into the extracellular fluid as the $NaHCO_3$ solution dilutes itself sixfold. Owing to the tight cell junctions of the capillaries of the brain, which act in this respect as cell membranes, $NaHCO_3$ remains within the capillaries rather than leaking out into the interstitial fluid of the brain, as it does in other tissue. The extravascular water of the brain acts, therefore, as if it were all intracellular, and it will move into the vascular compartment by osmosis. Since the brain is enclosed in a rigid skull, this drop in volume will be accompanied by a drop in pressure. At the same time, capillary pressure will be normal or may even be elevated by the increase in blood volume produced as water shifts into the vascular compartment. The capillaries and other intracranial blood vessels therefore become distended and can rupture, owing to the increased pressure gradient across them (see Chapter 11, p. 84).

The rapid blood volume expansion can itself produce adverse circulatory effects. The shifts of water to the plasma will cause a drop in hemoglobin and an even more exaggerated drop in hematocrit, since water leaves the red blood cells as well. Use of isotonic solutions prevents these problems, since such solutions do not cause major shifts in water. However, certain hazards cannot be avoided by avoiding concentrated solutions of sodium bicarbonate, since they are a function of the amount of $NaHCO_3$ given and not the concentration.

Administered HCO_3^- is rapidly converted to CO_2 and H_2O:

$$HCO_3^- + H^+ \leftrightarrows H_2CO_3 \xrightarrow[\text{anhydrase}]{\text{carbonic}} H_2O + CO_2$$

This conversion will directly elevate the PCO_2, particularly if ventilation is inadequate. The PCO_2 may be raised indirectly even further, since the respiratory drive will be decreased as the pH is elevated. The carbon dioxide so produced will diffuse rapidly into cells and also readily cross the blood-brain barrier. On the other hand, the administered HCO_3^- will tend to remain extracellular, since it moves slowly across cell membranes and capillaries with tight junctions into cells and the brain. The CO_2 entering the cells and the brain will combine with H_2O to produce increased amounts of hydrogen ion:

$$CO_2 + H_2O \xrightarrow[\text{anhydrase}]{\text{carbonic}} H_2CO_3 \leftrightarrows H^+ + HCO_3^-$$

This lowering of the pH of cells and the brain may be dangerous. Thus, rapid infusions of even isotonic $NaHCO_3$, while raising the pH of the extracellular fluid, may paradoxically lower intracellular and brain fluid pH.

Another potentially adverse effect of a rapid bicarbonate infusion is mediated through changing the affinity of hemoglobin for oxygen. By the Bohr effect, an increase in pH will increase the affinity of the hemo-

globin for oxygen, which decreases the unloading of oxygen in the tissues, where it is needed. The patient, as a result, may even become less cyanotic because of this effect and also because of the decrease in hemoglobin concentration, even though oxygen delivery to tissues has been impaired and hypoxia worsened.

Similar difficulties are expected in the use of tris(hydroxymethyl)aminomethane (THAM) in attempting rapid pH correction of acidemia, with the additional problems of hypoglycemia and production of apnea.[2, 3] The use of THAM has remained very limited even though it has the major therapeutic advantage of increasing pH while decreasing PCO_2. When given rapidly, THAM can substantially decrease PCO_2 (thence, the apnea) and increase HCO_3^- markedly (thence, a portion of its osmotic effect).

If excessive dosages of $NaHCO_3$ or other base are given, the patient may become alkalotic and edematous. When organic acids have caused the initial acidosis, they may continue to be metabolized after the pH has been brought back to normal with the administered base, and may produce a worsening metabolic alkalosis.

A formula that assumes a bicarbonate space of one third of body weight can be used for the calculation of the dosage of $NaHCO_3$ required to correct a given degree of metabolic acidosis. The "space" was derived empirically from data obtained in achieving short-term (one-hour) corrections of plasma pH.*

$$NaHCO_3 \text{ required (in mEq)} = \text{patient's weight (in kg)} \times -BE \times \frac{1}{3}$$

If the base excess is -21 mEq in a 10-kg patient:

$$NaHCO_3 = 10 \times 21 \times \frac{1}{3}$$
$$= 70 \text{ mEq}$$

As discussed previously, it would obviously be dangerous and inadvisable to give this dosage rapidly intravenously as a concentrated solution, but the formula may be useful as a rough guide to the maximal amount of base that may be needed. Keep in mind that the usual physiologic mechan-

---

*For full correction (over 12 hours) of acidemia, a space approaching total body water is appropriate but confounded in practice by the many adjustments that simultaneously occur.

isms may be operating to correct the acidosis, so that the entire calculated dosage is not usually needed if the underlying disturbance has been corrected, and great precision in calculations that do not include these physiologic variables is, therefore, not possible. If much larger dosages than calculated continue to be necessary, then the underlying pathologic disturbance has not been corrected and will probably prove fatal unless further steps in the treatment of the underlying problem are effected.

RESPIRATORY ALKALOSIS

Respiratory alkalosis is defined by a low PCO_2 in arterial blood and is a consequence of alveolar hyperventilation with carbon dioxide excretion exceeding carbon dioxide production. The lowering PCO_2 leads to a reduction of H_2CO_3 and a shift to the left of the equilibrium reaction, decreasing H^+ concentration.

$$\uparrow CO_2 + H_2O \underset{\longleftarrow}{\overset{\text{removed in alveolar air}}{\rightleftharpoons}} \overset{\text{carbonic anhydrase}}{H_2CO_3} \rightleftharpoons H^+ + HCO_3^-$$

Buffering takes place in the nonbicarbonate buffer system, metabolic compensation by renal retention of H^+ and excretion of bicarbonate, and correction by retention or increased production of carbon dioxide. Typical arterial blood gases are pH 7.58, PCO_2 20 mm Hg, PO_2 110 mm Hg, and base excess -2 mEq/l.

Arterial blood samples from pediatric patients commonly show respiratory alkalosis as a consequence of the respiratory stimulation produced by the anxiety and pain brought on by the blood drawing, but it can also be seen with pulmonary hypertension, pulmonary emboli, atelectasis, mild asthma, inflammatory lung disease, severe liver disease, fever, hypotension, brain injury, sepsis, salicylate poisoning, and hypoxia. In a patient on a respirator it usually indicates that the settings need to be adjusted to decrease alveolar ventilation, although in patients with cerebral edema, a moderate degree of respiratory alkalosis ($PCO_2 \sim 30$ mm Hg) may be used to decrease intracranial blood volume and decrease intracranial pressure. If the PCO_2 is brought too low, excessive vasoconstriction may occur and brain damage may result from the decreased blood flow. Respiratory alkalosis is also commonly seen as compensation for metabolic acidosis. Respiratory alkalosis has been noted to persist even after the metabolic acidosis that originally induced it has resolved. This persistent respiratory alkalosis is probably a reflection of continuing acid stimulation of the central nervous system that is not reflected in the arterial blood.

Clinical Manifestations

When severe, hyperventilation is obvious even to the casual observer. Milder forms are easy to miss. The alkalemia produced by respiratory alkalosis may produce a feeling of lightheadedness or dizziness as well as numbness and paresthesias of the fingers and toes, and when severe it can produce seizures and coma. Underwater swimmers who purposely hyperventilate and produce respiratory alkalosis and alkalemia to prolong underwater times are taking a lethal risk, since they may lose consciousness from hypoxia before feeling the need to surface. Hypoxia is not so strong a respiratory stimulus as is hypercapnia.

Therapy

Specific treatment of respiratory alkalosis is not usually necessary, except as adjustments to decrease the tidal volume or respiratory frequency in those on respirators. For those with hyperventilation syndrome due to anxiety, rebreathing into a paper bag is very effective. Attempts to raise the PCO_2 in patients with the respiratory alkalosis of liver disease have produced clinical deterioration.[13]

METABOLIC ALKALOSIS

Metabolic alkalosis is a clinically significant disturbance[14] and, surprisingly, has been found to be the most common acid-base abnormality seen in a general hospital population, occurring in 51 per cent of those with abnormal acid-base states.[15] It is not so common in children. Metabolic alkalosis is seen in the following circumstances:

1. Removal of H^+, Cl^-, and K^+ from the stomach by vomiting, as in pyloric stenosis, or nasogastric drainage.

2. Loss of potassium in the urine, as by diuretics, or in the gastrointestinal tract.

3. Administration of alkali.

4. Feeding of inadequate amounts of chloride or excess loss of chloride in stool or urine.

5. As compensation for chronic respiratory acidosis.

6. Contraction of extracellular fluid volume.

7. Hyperaldosteronism.

8. Bartter syndrome.

9. Cushing syndrome.

10. Licorice poisoning.

11. Cystic fibrosis.

Clinical Manifestation

Uncomplicated metabolic alkalosis with alkalemia decreases the concentration of ionized calcium, increasing neuromuscular excitability and producing muscle spasm, tetany, and seizures that may be accompanied by apnea. Respiratory compensation for the metabolic alkalosis takes the form of hypoventilation, which, unfortunately, in a patient breathing room air, produces a drop in PO_2 approximately equal to the rise in PCO_2. This decreased respiratory drive predisposes to atelectasis and may even precipitate severe ventilatory failure.[15] Alkalemia increases hemoglobin affinity for oxygen. This will decrease the amount of oxygen delivered to the tissues and at the same time tend deceptively to ameliorate cyanosis while lowering PO_2 by hypoventilation and atelectasis.

With severe metabolic alkalosis and alkalemia, cardiac output falls, peripheral resistance increases, and refractory cardiac arrhythmias may occur, particularly when K^+ or Mg^{2+} is depleted or when the patient is on digitalis.

During pregnancy chronic respiratory alkalosis with PCO_2 around 30 mm Hg is present, probably as a consequence of respiratory stimulation by progesterone. This may represent an adaptive response in allowing the fetus to have a more "physiologic" PCO_2 and pH than if the maternal pH and PCO_2 were "normal."

Mechanisms

The loss of hydrochloric acid, sodium, potassium, and water from the stomach sets off a chain of events that may culminate in hypochloremic metabolic alkalosis with a paradoxic acid urine. Acid formation in the stomach is similar to that in the kidney, involving production of H^+ and HCO_3^- from CO_2 in the presence of carbonic anhydrase in the gastric cells, with secretion of H^+ and Cl^- into the stomach and release of bicarbonate into the bloodstream producing the short-term postprandial alkalosis. This alkalosis is normally short-lived, because the secretin mechanism leads to the formation of copious quantities of a highly alkaline pancreatic juice that neutralizes the gastric contents.

When the gastric contents are removed by vomiting or external drainage, this mechanism cannot come into play. The effect is then physiologically identical to bicarbonate formation in the renal tubule, where H^+ is excreted in the urine instead of being vomited. This mild alkalosis is initially corrected by the excretion of HCO_3^- in the urine along with Na^+, but as hypovolemia progresses, sodium retention is mandated and K^+ is then excreted in its stead. In

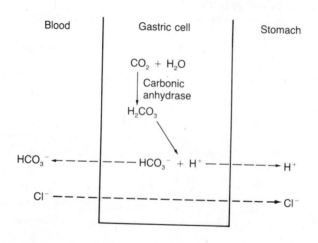

addition, potassium and sodium as well as H$^+$, chloride, and water continue to be lost in the vomitus.

The loss of chloride results in decreased chloride levels in serum and thus in the glomerular filtrate. Chloride accompanied by Na$^+$ is actively absorbed in the loop of Henle. With a deficit of chloride, more Na$^+$ escapes reabsorption at this site and travels down the tubules to the site where reabsorption of Na$^+$ takes place via exchange for potassium. The increased load of Na$^+$ for reabsorption thus increases K$^+$ excretion. Potassium loss may be exacerbated even more by the effect of increased aldosterone secretion produced in response to hypovolemia. In addition to augmenting the excretion of K$^+$, the continuing need for conservation of Na$^+$ as potassium stores drop then augments exchange of Na$^+$ for H$^+$ with loss of H$^+$ in the urine. This paradoxically acid urine then potentiates and perpetuates the metabolic alkalosis.

The process is completed by the development of alveolar hypoventilation as partial respiratory compensation. Respiratory compensation is quite variable and is in part limited by the hypoxia that develops with hypoventilation in room air.

When the deficits of Na$^+$, K$^+$, Cl$^-$, and H$_2$O are corrected, there will be less need for H$^+$ for exchange and renal correction can occur. The degree of metabolic alkalosis is reflected in the increase in base excess. Typical arterial blood gases for metabolic alkalosis with compensation are pH 7.56, PCO$_2$ 58 mm Hg, PO$_2$ 65 mm Hg, and BE +18 mEq/l.

An anion gap is occasionally seen in patients with metabolic alkalosis,[17] which is thought to be due to an increased negative charge on the plasma proteins owing to their decreased association with H$^+$ because of the lower H$^+$ concentration and to increased concentration of protein due to extracellular volume contraction.

Metabolic alkalosis is sometimes produced by the overenthusiastic administration of alkali. This is seen when acidosis is treated with intravenous lactate and bicarbonate, and it may lead to the production of alkalotic tetany.[18] Metabolic alkalosis due to inadequate amounts of chloride in soybean-derived infant feedings has recently been reported[19] and is discussed in Chapter 28.

In a patient with metabolic alkalosis of inapparent cause, chronic hypoventilation occurring during sleep should be considered a possible etiology.[20] Patients who hypoventilate only during sleep may show, while awake, the residual renal compensation for the respiratory acidosis during sleep. This occurs because it takes longer for the kidney to correct the compensatory metabolic alkalosis when it is no longer needed than for the lung to correct the primary respiratory acidosis when the patient wakes and breathes more easily. In patients with undiagnosed metabolic alkalosis, sleep apnea and hypoventilation during sleep should, therefore, be considered.

Therapy

The correct therapy of metabolic alkalosis is to relieve the cause of the original disturbance where possible and to administer sodium and potassium chloride.[21] This will reverse the abnormal renal tubule exchange and permit the formation of an alkaline urine. On rare occasions with severe, life-threatening alkalemia, administration of an acid such as ammonium chloride, lysine hydrochloride, or arginine hydrochloride may be necessary.

Potassium should be administered slowly and preferably orally in sufficiently large doses to replace both extracellular and intracellular losses. A reasonable dosage is 6 mEq/kg/day. The usual maximal safe concentration of potassium in intravenous fluids is 40 mEq/l at a rate of 1 mEq/kg hour.* Too-rapid administration may cause cardiac arrest, particularly if the patient is oliguric. It is important to remember that total body potassium may not be reflected by the serum K$^+$, since alkalosis may cause a shift of potassium into cells and acidosis a shift outward.

MIXED DISTURBANCES

Four possible combinations of these primary disturbances can occur — metabolic acidosis with respiratory acidosis or respiratory alkalosis, and metabolic alkalosis with respiratory acidosis or respiratory al-

---

*Under unusual conditions of severe depletion or continuing heavy K$^+$ losses, higher concentrations and rates may be required, although great caution in administration will be needed, such as close monitoring by ECG.

kalosis — but the most important combination in pediatric patients is mixed respiratory and metabolic acidosis. This occurs as hypoventilation in room air raises the PCO_2 and a base deficit is created by the production of organic acids, such as lactic and pyruvic acids, as a result of anaerobic metabolism owing to hypoxia. An extreme example of this process occurs during cardiac arrest.[22] Arterial blood gases show an elevated PCO_2 and a negative base excess. Typical arterial blood gases are pH 7.0, PCO_2 80 mm Hg, PO_2 40 mm Hg, and base excess -13 mEq/l. Similar findings could occur in a patient with pneumonia and concurrent diabetic acidosis or diarrheal dehydration. This is easy to diagnose, since the metabolic component is reflected in the fall in base excess and the respiratory component in the elevated PCO_2. When both disturbances tend to move the pH in the same direction as in metabolic and respiratory acidosis and in metabolic and respiratory alkalosis, it is obvious that these are not compensatory changes and are, therefore, mixed primary disturbances. Since metabolic alkalosis and respiratory alkalosis both tend to elevate the pH, the fact that they are mixed primary disturbances is apparent as soon as the decreased PCO_2 and the increased base excess are observed. When the changes noted in PCO_2 and base excess have opposite effects on the pH, it is more difficult to determine whether one is compensating for the other or whether they represent mixed primary disturbances. For example, simultaneous respiratory acidosis with a PCO_2 of 60 mm Hg and metabolic alkalosis with a base excess of $+15$ mEq/l could theoretically be either a mixed primary disturbance or a combined primary and compensatory disturbance. Distinction of one from the other will depend upon clinical cues and knowledge of how long it usually takes for compensation to occur. In a previously well patient who just two hours ago developed a pneumothorax and has been treated with a large dose of $NaHCO_3$, a PCO_2 of 55 mm Hg, a base excess of $+15$ mEq/l, and a pH of 7.48 suggest a mixed disturbance, since it is too soon for metabolic compensation for a respiratory acidosis to have occurred and since respiratory compensation for a metabolic alkalosis is not very effective. When respiratory alkalosis is mixed with metabolic acidosis, a similar problem arises, which can be analyzed in a similar manner. Mixed

disturbances of this type, which ameliorate each other, tend to be less of a clinical problem and give the physician time to sit back and think about them.

Another type of complicated disturbance occurs when one cause of metabolic or respiratory disturbance is superimposed on a pre-existing disturbance. This is difficult to diagnose after the fact but is relatively easy to diagnose if blood gases and pH are followed as the changes occur. This is illustrated in the following example; the initial condition and the changes in it are indicated by numbers in parentheses and analyzed in the subsequent paragraphs.

A patient with chronic respiratory acidosis and metabolic compensation (1) suddenly becomes hypoxic and develops more hypercapnia, with metabolic acidosis and worsened respiratory acidosis (2). The patient is treated with $NaHCO_3$ (3) and then placed on a respirator (4).

(1) Initial arterial blood gases show primary respiratory acidosis with partially compensatory metabolic alkalosis and mild acidemia and hypoxia. (pH 7.35, PCO_2 60 mm Hg, PO_2 60 mm Hg, and BE $+5$ mEq/l.)

(2) Worsening hypercapnia with more severe respiratory acidosis now mixed with a metabolic acidosis from hypoxia has been superimposed upon the previous compensatory metabolic alkalosis, reducing the base excess from $+5$ to -5 and producing more severe acidemia. (pH 7.18, PCO_2 90 mm Hg, PO_2 35 mm Hg, and BE -5 mEq/l.)

(3) $NaHCO_3$, 3 mEq/kg of body weight given intravenously, restores the original metabolic alkalosis, makes the respiratory acidosis and hypoxia slightly worse, and relieves the acidemia slightly. The organic acids produced by the hypoxia are still present. (pH 7.18, PCO_2 95 mm Hg, PO_2 30 mm Hg, and BE $+4$ mEq/l.)

(4) The respirator, with 40 per cent oxygen, partially corrects the respiratory acidosis while totally correcting the hypoxia, allowing metabolism of the organic acids, which decreases the H^+ concentration, raising the BE to $+11$ and producing an alkalemia. (pH 7.45, PCO_2 50 mm Hg, PO_2 90 mm Hg, and BE $+11$ mEq/l.)

By following arterial blood gases and pH as the illness progresses, it is easy to see the effects of superimposed disturbances and treatments. After the patient has been on the respirator for several days, if ade-

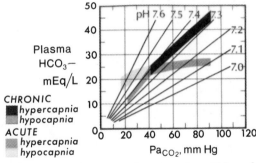

Plasma HCO₃⁻ mEq/L

CHRONIC
■ hypercapnia
hypocapnia
ACUTE
hypercapnia
hypocapnia

The radial lines are isopleths of pH. The shaded bands indicate 95% confidence limits of data obtained from patients with acute and chronic respiratory alkalosis and acidosis.

If measurement of pH, HCO₃⁻ and Pa_{CO_2} (or any two of these) indicate a point lying outside the confidence bands, there is probably either a mixed respiratory and metabolic disorder, or a transition between acute and chronic states.

Figure 12–2. Respiratory alterations in acid-base balance. (Prepared for the American Lung Association by Thomas K. C. King, M.D. Copyright © 1976 American Thoracic Society — Medical Section of the American Lung Association. Used with permission.)

quate water, sodium, potassium, and chloride are given, blood gases and pH may return to normal.

One way to distinguish between compensation and a mixed disturbance is by using equations or nomograms[23, 25] such as that shown in Figure 12–2, to see whether the degree of compensation for the primary disturbance is in the expected range. If it is not, then a mixed disturbance is likely.

A rough guide to the expected degree of compensation for the common disorders for which there is the most reliable and consistent data is shown in Table 12–2. If compensatory changes are greater or less than expected from the table, then either compensation is incomplete or excessive, or a mixed disturbance is present. If the changes are exactly as indicated, it is likely but not certain that a primary disturbance with compensation exists. A mixed disturbance may fall within these limits by chance.

Another clue that a more complicated disturbance exists may be provided by the pH. In a primary disturbance with compensation, the arterial pH should remain on the same side of 7.4 as it would in a primary disturbance without compensation — i.e., compensation should not overcompensate. For example, in a patient with primary respiratory acidosis with compensatory metabolic alkalosis, the pH should remain below 7.4. If it is higher, then a mixed disturbance is likely.

Fortunately for the clinician, it is rarely necessary to make a diagnosis of brain damage, pneumonia, or renal failure solely on the basis of the discovery of a mixed disturbance from analysis of the blood gases and pH. Usually these diagnoses are somewhat obvious, which makes the blood gases and pH easy to interpret even in the most complicated disturbances if one also considers information from the patient's history and physical examination and other laboratory data.

Treatment

The treatment of simple disturbances in acid-base balance is relatively straightforward. If the PCO_2 is 80 mm Hg, the pH 7.2, and the base excess 0 mEq/l in a patient on a respirator, the elevated PCO_2 is corrected by adjusting the ventilator to double alveolar ventilation, bringing the PCO_2 to 40 mm Hg. On the other hand, treatment of a patient with more complicated disturbances seems much more complex. What should be done if this patient also has a severe metabolic acidosis, so that the arterial blood gases are pH 6.95, PCO_2 80 mm Hg, PO_2 30 mm Hg, and base excess − 16 mEq/l

Table 12–2. Expected Changes in Metabolic and Respiratory Acidoses

	For each decrease in BE of 10 mEq/l:	
	pH falls	*PCO₂ falls (mm Hg)*
METABOLIC ACIDOSIS		
without compensation	0.16	0
with compensation	0.10 ± .05	10 ± 3

	For each increase in PCO₂ of 20 mmHg:	
	pH falls	*BE changes (mEq/l)*
RESPIRATORY ACIDOSIS		
without compensation	0.12	− 2
with compensation	0.03	+ 6 ± 3

SIGGAARD-ANDERSEN ALIGNMENT NOMOGRAM

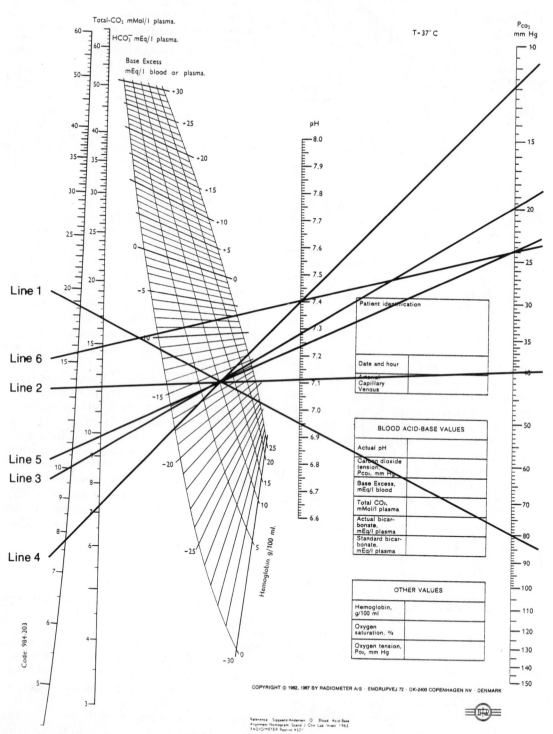

Figure 12–3.   Siggaard-Andersen alignment nomogram. (See text.) (From Siggaard-Andersen O: Blood acid-base alignment nomogram. Scand J Clin Lab Invest 15:211, 1963. Radiometer Reprint AS21. Copyright © 1962, 1967 by Radiometer A/S. Used with permission.)

with a hemoglobin concentration of 10 gm/100 ml? Should the respirator be adjusted to bring the PCO_2 to 40 mm Hg, a normal PCO_2? To estimate the effect of such a maneuver, one can use the Siggaard-Andersen alignment nomogram (Fig. 12–3), keeping in mind that the relationships shown on the nomogram were determined on blood and only approximate those for the body as a whole. A straight-edge should be placed on the points on the nomogram specified for this patient (pH 6.95, PCO_2 80 mm Hg and base excess – 16 mEq/l at hemoglobin 10 gm/100 ml) (Line 1). Since we are referring to respiratory changes, let us assume (acknowledging that the assumption is not totally correct) that the base excess will not change much in the time it takes to readjust the ventilation and change the PCO_2. Therefore, we can use the point where the straight-edge crosses the line through base excess – 16 mEq/l (at hemoglobin 10 gm/100 ml) as the point of rotation, and rotate the straightedge from PCO_2 80 mm Hg to PCO_2 40 mm Hg (Line 2). This new line, going from PCO_2 40 mm Hg to base excess – 16/hemoglobin 10, intersects the pH line at 7.11. This indicates that the patient will still be severely acidemic even at the normal PCO_2. If we continue to rotate the straightedge around the same base excess/hemoglobin point to a PCO_2 of 20 mm Hg (Line 3), we will find a pH-intersect at 7.28, which indicates still significant acidemia. We need to bring the PCO_2 all the way down to 12 mm Hg (Line 4) before the pH will be normal at 7.4. Since the alveolar ventilation and PCO_2 are roughly inversely proportional in the physiologic range, doubling the alveolar ventilation will halve the PCO_2 and halving it will double the PCO_2. To go from a PCO_2 of 80 to 40 mm Hg requires a doubling of alveolar ventilation; from 40 to 20 mm Hg, another doubling; and from 20 to 12 mm Hg, almost another doubling.

Each doubling of alveolar ventilation and halving of PCO_2 produces an increase in pH of almost 0.17. Each time alveolar ventilation is doubled and redoubled, the actual volumes required go up markedly, so that the point of diminishing return is quickly reached; beyond this point the risk of pneumothorax and decreased cardiac output will become a greater problem than the acidemia itself. The physiologic response of a normal human to a metabolic acidosis of

this degree would bring the PCO_2 down to around 24 mm Hg (see Table 12–2). If a PCO_2 of about 24 mm Hg in our problem patient could be achieved without excessively high pressures on the ventilator, then it might be reasonable to adjust the ventilator to give a PCO_2 of 24 mm Hg and a pH of 7.23 (Line 5) and to increase the inspired oxygen concentration. This approximates what the patient's own physiologic responses might produce in the way of an expected degree of compensatory respiratory alkalosis if the patient were able to ventilate adequately on his own.

At the new respirator settings, the improved oxygenation of tissues will halt the production of organic acids and will enable the organic acids already present to be metabolized. These factors, combined with urinary excretion of H^+ and retention of HCO_3^-, will tend to return the pH to normal. Under these circumstances one may choose to allow physiologic correction of the disturbance and not attempt specific correction of the metabolic acidosis by administering base. However, if this patient also has cyanotic congenital heart disease and renal failure, waiting for physiologic responses may not be appropriate and treatment with base may be indicated.

Assuming that the PCO_2 will be brought to 24 mm Hg with the respirator, can we estimate the dosage of $NaHCO_3$ needed to bring the pH to 7.4? A straight-edge placed along the line from PCO_2 24 mm Hg to base excess – 16 mEq/l (at hemoglobin 10 gm/100 ml) intersects pH at 7.23 (Line 5). If we hold PCO_2 constant and rotate the straightedge around this point (PCO_2 24 mm Hg) until it intersects pH at 7.4, we see that the new line intersects the line for base excess (at hemoglobin 10 gm/100 ml) at – 8.5 mEq/l (Line 6). This indicates that if the base excess were raised from – 16 to – 8.5 mEq/l, or 7.5 mEq/l, the pH would become normal at a PCO_2 of 24 mm Hg.

If we rearrange the formula for determining the dosage of $NaHCO_3$ required for acute correction —

Dosage of $NaHCO_3$ (in mEq)

= patient's weight (in kg) $\times$ – BE $\times$ 1/3

— to get

Dosage of $NaHCO_3$ (in mEq/kg) = – BE $\times$ 1/3

and replace $-BE$ with ΔBE, which represents the desired change in base excess, we get

Dosage of $NaHCO_3$ (in mEq/kg) $= \dfrac{\Delta BE}{3}$.

To raise the base excess 7.5 mEq/l, we calculate as follows:

Dosage of $NaHCO_3$ (in mEq/kg) $= \dfrac{7.5}{3}$

$= 2.5$ mEq/kg

This is a relatively small dosage and could probably be given safely even to this patient. One half of the dose could be given over one half-hour period as an isotonic solution (150 mEq/l) of $NaHCO_3$ (~ 8 ml/kg) and then the blood gases repeated to see what should be done next. If the pH is close to 7.3 or higher, the $NaHCO_3$ infusion can be discontinued. If the pH remains low, the infusion may be continued.

This represents what we consider to be a reasonable and safe approach to managing such patients. In contrast, one could theoretically consider treating such a patient with a dosage, calculated to bring the pH to normal, of sodium bicarbonate given rapidly intravenously without correction of the respiratory acidosis. If we start again (Fig. 12–4) with our line in the original position at pH 6.95, PCO_2 80 mm Hg, and base excess -16 mEq/l at hemoglobin 10 gm/100 ml (Line 1), hold the PCO_2 constant (assuming that the respiratory acidosis will not worsen during the infusion), and rotate the line around this point until the line intersects the pH line at 7.4, we find that the new line (Line 2) intersects the base excess line at $+20$ mEq/l (at hemoglobin 10).

If the patient's base excess could be brought to $+20$ mEq/l, the pH would be 7.4 if the PCO_2 remained at 80 mm Hg. This would require an increase in base excess from -16 to $+20$ mEq/l, or 36 mEq/l.

Dosage of $NaHCO_3$ (in mEq/kg) $= \dfrac{\Delta BE}{3}$

$= \dfrac{36}{3} = 12$ mEq/kg

A dosage of 12 mEq/kg given rapidly intravenously as either a hypertonic (12 ml/kg of a 1 molar solution) or isotonic solution (~ 80 ml/kg) would almost certainly be quickly lethal by mechanisms discussed previously. The increase in extracellular fluid volume from either an isotonic or hypertonic infusion would probably be intolerable in itself.

Twelve mEq/kg of a solution containing 150 mEq/l would require 80 ml/kg of solution. A more concentrated solution might seem better, since its volume looks less "impressive" in a syringe, but it will produce almost the same increase in extracellular fluid volume by causing an osmotic shift of water from cells, adding another injury without helping in any known way. A rapid infusion of $NaHCO_3$ will increase PCO_2 and lower intracellular pH and will not be effective in treating acidosis as much as might be expected in any case. This should, therefore, be considered an unreasoned, dangerous, and abhorrent approach to treatment.

Another important example of the use of the Siggaard-Andersen nomogram in the management of a complicated disturbance is with chronic compensated respiratory acidosis with superimposed acute respiratory acidosis. For example, in a patient whose arterial blood has a pH of 7.33, a PCO_2 of 80 mm Hg, a PO_2 of 60 mm Hg, and a base excess of $+12$ mEq/l, at a hemoglobin of 10 gm/100 ml (Line 1, Fig. 12–5), a sudden rise in PCO_2 to 110 mm Hg and a fall in pH to 7.20 with a base excess of $+10$ mEq/l requires the use of a ventilator. What PCO_2 should the ventilator be set to provide? If the PCO_2 is brought to normal (Line 3), the pH would become 7.54, an unphysiologic level of alkalemia, which is undesirable. A PCO_2 of 60 mm Hg (Line 4) would provide a pH of 7.4. This is far easier to achieve with the ventilator and would initially be more physiologic for this patient. Later on, it may be desirable to lower the PCO_2 gradually toward 40 mm Hg.

In this way the Siggaard-Andersen alignment nomogram can be used to analyze the management of complicated disturbances, if it is kept in mind that these are only approximations of reality and that precise application is neither possible nor necessary in most cases, since physiologic treatment with frequent re-evaluations of the arterial blood gases and of the patient's clinical status is far more important. We

SIGGAARD-ANDERSEN ALIGNMENT NOMOGRAM

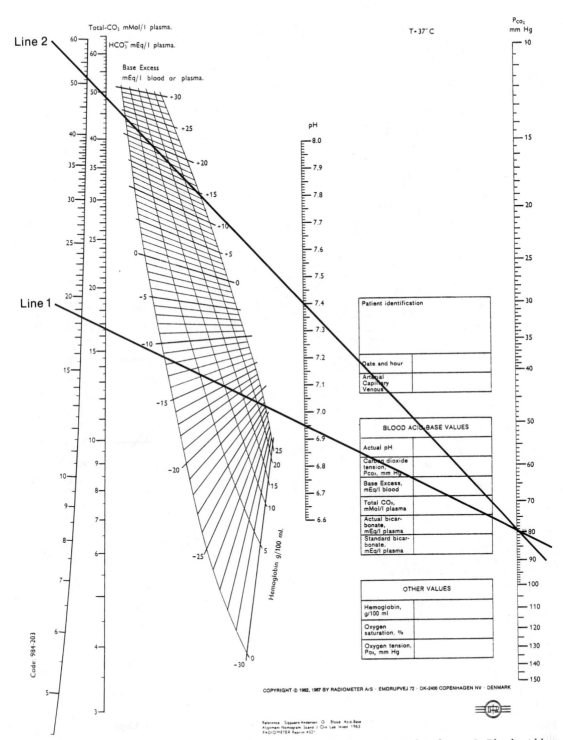

Figure 12–4. Siggaard-Andersen alignment nomogram. (See text.) (From Siggaard-Andersen O: Blood acid-base alignment nomogram. Scand J Clin Lab Invest 15:211, 1963. Radiometer Reprint AS21. Copyright © 1962, 1967 by Radiometer A/S. Used with permission.)

SIGGAARD-ANDERSEN ALIGNMENT NOMOGRAM

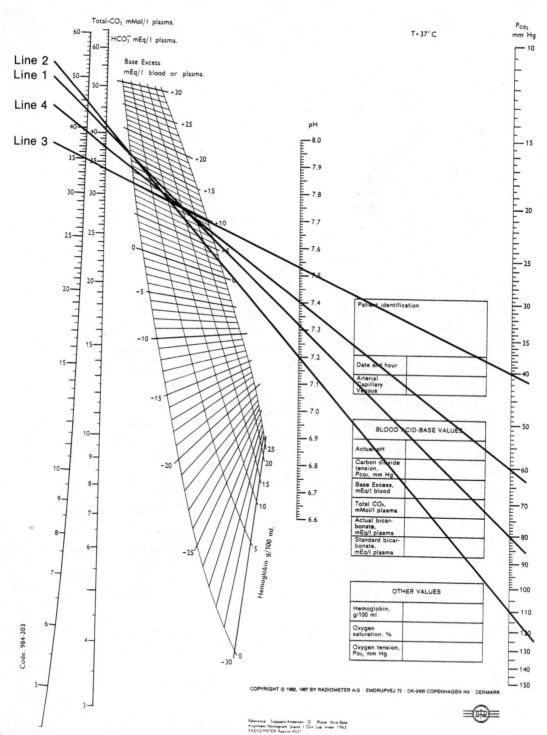

Figure 12–5.   Siggaard-Andersen alignment nomogram. (See text.) (From Siggaard-Andersen O: Blood acid-base alignment nomogram. Scand J Clin Lab Invest 15:211, 1963. Radiometer Reprint AS21. Copyright © 1962, 1967 by Radiometer A/S. Used with permission.)

have not yet reached that degree of refinement that will allow us to treat such patients from an armchair or by computer.

REFERENCES

1. Siggaard-Andersen O.: Blood acid-base alignment nomogram. Scand J Clin Lab Invest 15:211, 1963.
2. Strauss J: Tris(hydroxymethyl)aminomethane (THAM): a pediatric evaluation. Pediatrics 41:667, 1968.
3. Roberton NRC: Apnea after THAM administration in the newborn. Arch Dis Child 45:206, 1970.
4. Bureau MA, Ouellet G, Begin R, et al: Dynamics of the control of ventilation during metabolic acidosis and its correction. Am Rev Respir Dis 119:933, 1979.
5. Gabow PA, Kaehny WD, Fennessey PV, et al: Diagnostic importance of an increased anion gap. N Engl J Med 303:854, 1980.
6. Fulop M: Serum potassium in lactic acidosis and ketoacidosis. N Engl J Med 300:1087, 1979.
7. Finberg L: Dangers to infants caused by changes in osmolal concentration. Pediatrics 40:1031, 1967.
8. Kravath RE, Aharon AS, Abal G, Finberg L: Clinically significant physiologic changes from rapidly administered hypertonic solutions: acute osmol poisoning. Pediatrics 46:267, 1970.
9. Papile L, Burstein J, Burstein R, et al: Relationship of intravenous sodium bicarbonate infusions and cerebral intraventricular hemorrhage. J Pediat 93:834, 1978.
10. Seigel SR, Phelps DL, Leake RD, Oh W: The effects of rapid infusion of hypertonic sodium bicarbonate in infants with respiratory distress. Pediatrics 51:651, 1973.
11. Douglas ME, Downs JB, Mantini EL, Ruiz C: Alteration of oxygen tension and oxyhemoglobin saturation. A hazard of sodium bicarbonate administration. Arch Surg 114:326, 1979.
12. Finberg L: Pathogenesis of lesions in the nervous system in hypernatremic states. I. Clinical observation of infants. Pediatrics 23:40, 1959.
13. Posner JB, Plum F: The toxic effects of carbon dioxide and acetazolamide in hepatic encephalopathy. J Clin Invest 39:1246, 1960.
14. Coe FL: Metabolic alkalosis. JAMA 238:2288, 1977.
15. Hodgkin JE, Soeprono FF, Chan DM: Incidence of metabolic alkalemia in hospitalized patients. Crit Care Med 8:725, 1980.
16. Saunders NA, Carter J, Scamps P, Vandenberg R: Severe hypercapnia associated with metabolic alkalosis due to pyloric stenosis. Aust NZ J Med 4:385, 1974.
17. Madias NE, Ayus JC, Adrogué HJ: Increased anion gap in metabolic alkalosis. N Engl J Med 300:1421, 1979.
18. Feldman W, Stevens DGH, Beaudry PH: Severe metabolic acidemia in infants: clinical and therapeutic aspects. Can Med Assoc J 94:328, 1966.
19. Wolfsdorf JI, Senior B: Failure to thrive and metabolic alkalosis. Adverse effects of a chloride-deficient formula in two infants. JAMA 243:1068, 1980.
20. Kravath RE, Pollak CP, Borowiecki B: Hypoventilation during sleep in children who have lymphoid airway obstruction treated by nasopharyngeal tube and T and A. Pediatrics 59:865, 1977.
21. Schwartz WB, van Ypersele de Strihou C, Kassirer JP: Role of anions in metabolic alkalosis and potassium deficiency. N Engl J Med 279:630, 1968.
22. Fillmore SJ, Shapiro M, Killip T: Serial blood gas studies during cardiopulmonary resuscitation. Ann Intern Med 72:465, 1970.
23. Arbus GS: An in vivo acid-base nomogram for clinical use. Can Med Assoc J 109:291, 1973.
24. Narins RG, Emmett M: Simple and mixed acid-base disorders: a practical approach. Medicine 59:161, 1980.
25. Albert MS, Dell RB, Winters RW: Quantitative displacement of acid-base equilibrium in metabolic acidosis. Ann Intern Med 66:312, 1967.

Chapter 13

PATHOPHYSIOLOGY OF EDEMA, WITH A NOTE ON THE MODE OF ACTION OF DIURETICS

Most of the problems of hydration in pediatrics concern dehydration in its various guises. Overhydration, although less common, is also an important aberration of body water and mineral metabolism. In this chapter, we will describe the pathophysiology of edema, which we will define as an *increase in interstitial fluid volume*. In calculations, overhydration or edema may be looked upon as the algebraic opposite of a deficit.

Edema defined in this way is to be distinguished from the swelling of cells. That process, which also may be important, will be dealt with in subsequent chapters. Interstitial fluid may expand with a concomitant increase in plasma volume or with a reduction in plasma volume. Thus, the two major subcompartments of the extracellular fluid may be disparate in their volume changes in edematous states. Edema may be either generalized or localized to a tissue or anatomic region. The local causes of edema may be secondary to local inflammation or to obstruction of veins or lymphatics that drain a region or an organ. We shall confine the discussion here to generalized, or systemic, edema.

PATHOPHYSIOLOGY OF EDEMA

Edema is caused by a wide variety of disturbances and diseases; in particular, diseases of the heart, kidney, and liver may produce edematous states. In this discussion, we will approach the origin of edema from its pathophysiologic antecedents

under four categories: heart failure, portal obstruction, hypoproteinemic states, and hypervolemic states.

HEART FAILURE

In discussion of cardiac failure, it will be seen that edema formation is both simple and complex. Complexities involve changes in physical forces, hemodynamic changes, neurogenic influences, and humoral effects. Each of these contributes to the final disturbance. The circulation may be looked upon as a closed circle with an efferent arc, or loop, originating from the ventricles and closing via an afferent loop to the atria.

In simplest terms, when the heart muscle is failing as a pump, there is reduced cardiac output. The body senses a change in volume at this efferent end of the circuit. Neither the entire extracellular fluid nor even the entire plasma volume is sensed, but rather a fraction of the plasma volume, which is usually referred to as the *effective (blood) plasma volume*. Ultimately, as the process proceeds, there will be renal retention of sodium and water, although the primary stimulus clearly is the decrease in the arteries of the effective plasma volume.

Leaving the efferent side of the circuit momentarily, consider the afferent loop, where changes in physical forces predominate the pathophysiology and are the first mechanism of edema formation. With cardiac output reduced, the atrium fails to receive venous blood, leading to an increase in venous pressure. With the passage of time, hydrostatic pressure exceeds Starling forces in the involved tissues, with resultant interstitial or pulmonary edema or both.

Three other mechanisms on the efferent side may be described. It is clear that a reduced effective plasma volume reduces renal blood flow. This, in turn, activates secretion of renin and the renin-angiotensin system becomes operative, altering internal renal hemodynamics. Renal vascular resistance rises, thus causing a rise in the filtration fraction. This imbalance leads to sodium and water retention and acts as a rapid system for retaining body fluid under the threat of volume depletion.

Simultaneously, a second rapid system is also initiated by neural stimulus to the kidney from the receptors sensing a volume drop. These receptors initiate a neural increase in symptomatic tone and the release of catecholamines. These, in turn, now through two pathways (neural and renin-angiotensin), lead to the release of aldosterone, the third compensatory mechanism. This somewhat slower humeral mechanism now augments the retention of sodium and water by the kidney. These events produce an increased plasma volume on the venous side, which further enhances the afferent loop process described previously. The net result of these four mechanisms is an accumulation of fluid as a compensatory homeostatic system for increasing a reduced effective plasma volume.

In summary, physical forces, hemodynamic events, neural induction of rapid messenger hormones, and a slower humoral system combine in edema formation of cardiac origin.

PORTAL OBSTRUCTION

When liver disease or disease of the veins of the portal system cause obstruction in that vascular bed, there is an increase in hydrostatic pressure in its distal portions, which results in hydrostatic exudation of a protein-rich fluid. When the production of this fluid exceeds the capacity of the lymphatics to drain the abdomen, ascites results. The associated withdrawal of venous return from the portal system leads to reduced cardiac output, which now sets into motion all the edema-generating processes associated with heart failure. Thus, generalized edema may accompany the regional

problem of ascites. In addition, the loss of protein may lead to the reduction of albumin in plasma and overlap with the third etiologic factor of our classification.

HYPOPROTEINEMIC EDEMA

Hypoproteinemia, specifically hypoalbuminemia, may result from inadequate production of albumin, as in malnutrition, or from excessive losses of albumin in the urine (nephrotic syndrome) or the alimentary tract (protein-losing enteropathy, Menetrier's disease). The loss of albumin results in the reduction of Starling forces, so that hydrostatic pressure increases the interstitial volume up to the point where tissue back-pressure equals the hydrostatic pressure. Inasmuch as tissue is elastic, slow but constant readjustment occurs; as long as the albumin remains low, interstitial fluid volume increases continually until the elasticity is exhausted. This varies from tissue to tissue. In some tissues, of course, the pressure may be very damaging, and skin rupture of the abdomen, scrotum, or vulva may occur before a steady state is reached. The usual critical level of albumin below which this process starts is approximately 2.4 gm/dl. The dynamics of the process sometimes permit this concentration to be maintained at a plateau with no edema or with maximal edema, depending on when the observation is made.

The reduction in plasma volume that characterizes this form of edema even with maximal compensation from tissue pressure results in reduced cardiac output and sets into motion all the mechanisms for promoting the renal retention of salt and water described in the previous sections. In the very rare condition of congenital analbuminemia, the edematous state is mild, so effective are the compensatory forces in patients with this condition. The reasons for this interesting exception are not fully understood.

HYPERVOLEMIC EDEMA

In advanced renal failure or acute renal shutdown either from glomerular inflammation or tubular necrosis, excretion of water through the urine markedly lessens or ceases and any intake exceeding insensible

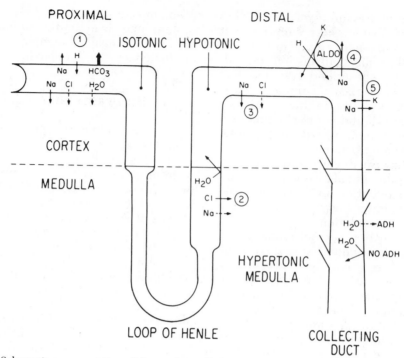

Figure 13–1. Schematic representation of the nephron illustrating the handling of water and electrolytes by the different segments and the major nephron sites of diuretic action. The solid arrows indicate active transport; interrupted arrows, passive transport. (From Kaloyanides GJ. *In* Maxwell MH, and Kleeman CR (eds): Clinical Disorders of Fluid and Electrolyte Metabolism, 3rd ed. McGraw-Hill Book Co., New York, 1980, Chapter 13, p. 669. Used with permission.)

losses of water adds to the body's fluid volume. Plasma volume is thus usually increased in such renal failure. Plasma volume may also be increased when there is an A-V fistula, in hyperthyroid states, and in severe anemias. These states of high-plasma-volume heart failure differ from the low output cardiac failure described above. The main danger to the patient is that the increased pressure in the pulmonary circuit will lead to pulmonary edema, which will interfere with gaseous exchange, leading to severe compromise and possibly death. Clearly, it is important that the clinician recognize and distinguish the high-plasma-volume form of edema and its pathogenesis from the low(or normal)-plasma-volume forms described above.

The foregoing four varieties are the most important types of systemic edema. Some other types, such as the edema of hypothyroidism, are seen only rarely in pediatrics or else they are not germane to the context of this discussion.

MODE OF ACTION OF DIURETICS

In this section, the clinical management of edema will be anticipated somewhat by a review of the mode of action of diuretic drugs at several sites along the nephron. Before going on to discuss drug action, however, it should be pointed out that water functions as a diuretic by increasing plasma volume, that osmotic agents including sodium salts may cause osmotic diuresis, and that antidiuretic hormone inhibition may be involved in any process leading to water excretion.

Diuretic drugs act at one of five sites along the nephron. Figure 13–1 illustrates this clearly. These five sites are the proximal tubule, the ascending loop of Henle, and three regions of cortical distal tubule.

Proximal Tubule (1)*

In this section of the nephron much of

---

*Numbers following headings refer to numbers circled in Figure 13–1.

the active transport is mediated by the enzyme carbonic anhydrase. It is here that 90 per cent of the bicarbonate is normally reabsorbed. Thus, a carbonic anhydrase inhibitor such as acetazolamide will lead to diuresis, with the urine being alkaline from its high bicarbonate content. In actual clinical experience, the effect of acetazolamide is sustained for a matter only of days.

The Ascending Loop of Henle (2)

At this site, where the actively transported substance is chloride ion, molecules that inhibit its reabsorption are extremely effective diuretics. These include mercury compounds, furosemide, and ethacrynic acid. Mercury compounds, described earliest, have sufficiently dangerous side effects that they are now rarely used. Furosemide and ethacrynic acid are both very potent diuretics that not only cause sodium and chloride loss but, because of very high water flow, carry potassium and calcium ions along as well.

Cortical Distal Tubule (3)

At this site, substances that inhibit sodium reabsorption, and thereby chloride as well, induce satisfactory diuresis. This describes the thiazide group of drugs, which act to inhibit sodium transport. High potassium losses occur with these agents, again because of high urine flow.

Terminal Distal Tubule (4)

This is the section of the nephron where aldosterone inhibits sodium-potassium exchange. Thus, anything that inhibits aldosterone will produce increased sodium excretion. Spironolactone is such a substance, although after several days its inhibitory effect wanes.

Terminal Distal Tubule (5)

At this site, certain compounds again inhibit sodium-potassium exchange directly without affecting aldosterone. Triamterene is such a substance, leading to diuresis without the high potassium loss characterized by diuretics acting at the ascending loop of Henle and the cortical distal tubule.

Chapter 14

PATHOPHYSIOLOGY OF HYPONATREMIC STATES

Hyponatremic states appear in a variety of clinical settings and have varying clinical significance. One of the first questions that must be asked is whether the hyponatremia in fact represents the concentration of sodium in plasma water, or whether because of the technique of measurement there is an appearance of a hyponatremic state that in physical-chemical or physiologic terms does not exist. The difficulty arises because clinicians receive measures of the concentration of sodium in serum. Serum has non-aqueous constituents including protein and lipid. Sodium does not distribute in the volume of these organic phases. Thus, if either protein or lipid, particularly lipid, is present in unusual degree, sodium concentration will be reported at low values when, in fact, its physiologic concentration may be entirely normal. Another apparent hyponatremic state occurs when there are high concentrations of glucose, mannitol, or some other osmotically active molecule that is restricted to the extracellular fluid. Glucose in hyperglycemic states, for example, pulls water into the extracellular fluid sufficiently that for each excess 100 mg/dl of glucose in plasma, sodium concentration is reduced 1.6 mEq/l. These last conditions, of course, are associated with an increased osmolality of serum or plasma. These apparent hyponatremias have no physiologic significance, although the condition creating them may.

Hyponatremic states, like hypernatremic states, tend to be symptomatic if they develop rapidly. They may be asymptomatic if the disturbance takes days to develop. Among the symptoms seen in rapidly developing hyponatremias are lethargy, muscle cramps, anorexia, nausea and vomiting, and,

finally, agitation and disorientation. Clinical signs relating largely to the nervous system may accompany these symptoms. These may include changes in sensorium, decreased tendon reflexes, hypothermia, seizures, and coma. The involvement of the nervous system relates in part to special features of the brain described in some detail in Chapter 11 on hypernatremia. The hyponatremic states are, of course, characterized by cell swelling and by a relative dearth of interstitial fluid.

There are a number of ways to classify the hyponatremic states, none of them entirely satisfactory. Quite arbitrarily, we will discuss them under six headings. The first of these represents a dehydrated state. The second, third, and fourth represent states of overhydration or sometimes normal hydration, and the last two are puzzling conditions in which the hydration is generally normal but may vary with circumstance in accordance with the external water and salt balance.

HYPONATREMIC DEHYDRATION

As the name suggests, hyponatremic dehydration involves a reduction in body water volume but a proportionately greater reduction in body sodium content. This usually comes about when the patient has lost both water and salt by a pathologic process and has received partial replacement of water with either insufficient or no salt. Since the body water will shift from extracellular fluid to the cells under these circumstances, circulatory disturbances occur at relatively small degrees of dehydration and may easily become profound.[1]

DILUTIONAL HYPONATREMIA OR SODIUM DEPRIVATION

Dilutional hyponatremia may occur in either of two obvious ways. The patient may drink an excessive amount of water without appropriate salt intake or there may be a normal water intake coupled with salt deprivation. The first of these is more common. When the process goes forth very rapidly, i.e., over a few hours, it is called water intoxication. The condition is characterized by cerebral swelling and convulsions may occur during treatment of dehydration or independently from abnormal water administration. If an adequate history is available, diagnosis is generally not difficult. Salt depletion states are also possible. McCance described the process by deliberately depriving himself and another volunteer of salt for several days.[2] A somewhat similar situation may arise from overuse of diuretics with inappropriate replacement of salt. Potassium losses may, by reducing cellular osmolal concentration, be the genesis of this type of hyponatremia.[3] The urine in patients with such conditions will show very low concentrations of sodium unless a specific renal disease is present.

For reasons not fully understood, low birthweight infants excrete more sodium in the urine than would be predicted from studies on older infants and children. This may lead to a hyponatremic state.[4]

EDEMATOUS STATES

Any of the causes of edema described in the preceding chapter may be complicated by the development of hyponatremia. In essence, the kidney has an absolute or relative ability to excrete a water load under the pathophysiologic disturbance of edema formation. The urine will have a low sodium concentration — for instance, less than 10 mEq/l. The patient will be overhydrated, although the plasma volume may be either increased or decreased depending on the etiology of the edema.

SYNDROME OF INAPPROPRIATE SECRETION OF ANTIDIURETIC HORMONE (SIADH)

This categorization of disorders is somewhat confusing and moderately controversial. The terminology was first advocated by Schwartz, Bennet, Curelop, and Bartter in their description of some hyponatremic patients. They used the word "appropriate" to refer to antidiuretic hormone (ADH) secretion in response to plasma osmolality.[5] Thus, they described circumstances in which, despite the lowered plasma osmolality, ADH is produced in response to another stimulus. Such patients will have a urine osmolality significantly greater than plasma osmolality and generally will have urine sodium concentrations greater than 20 mEq/l.

ADH is released in response to the reduction of effective plasma volume, which may occur in a wide variety of circumstances. ADH is also released in response to the stimuli of pain and anxiety, which, again, affect a wide variety of patients. Finally, a number of drugs stimulate ADH release. All these circumstances usually result in hyponatremia. The multiplicity of responses involving ADH release makes the use of the designation SIADH somewhat confusing, and it has been suggested that the terminology be abandoned for conditions described previously in this text and that we substitute the description of the physiologic disturbance.[6] We concur.

In one situation that might be called a true SIADH, neoplasms of several different varieties have been reported to release a polypeptide that has ADH acitvity. This release occurs independently of all the usual stimuli for ADH release and is truly a syndrome of inappropriate ADH.[7] This phenomenon has also been reported with ADH emanating from lung tissue infected by tubercle bacilli.[8]

INFECTION

Both acute and chronic infections in children have been associated with asymptomatic hyponatremic states. Severe infections causing marked systemic response are more apt to be so associated than are milder ones — bacterial infections more so than viral, but viral infections may also show the same phenomenon.[9] Animal studies have duplicated clinical observation in patients.[10] In addition to hyponatremia, there frequently are reduced concentrations of calcium and phosphorus in serum in the same patients. The mechanism is not well understood, although in some instances, at least, the observed patient will meet the criteria for so-called SIADH. What is certainly clear is that such patients have trouble delivering a water load. It makes them vulnerable to water intoxication if water loads easily tolerated by most patients are given to them rapidly. Bacterial meningitis has been singled out for this effect because cerebral swelling on an inflammatory basis is already present and the vulnerability of water intoxication is thereby enhanced. In fact, this same phenomenon is seen in non-CNS infections as well.

Chronic infection of the meninges with tuberculosis produces a chronic hyponatremic state. This is the basis of the clinical laboratory observation that chloride concentration is low in the spinal fluid of patients with tuberculosis meningitis. This finding actually reflects a low concentration of sodium chloride in the extracellular fluid generally. Patients are adapted to their low body fluid osmolality and have what is sometimes referred to as a lowered "osmostat." When the tissue of such patients has been analyzed, it has been shown that sodium has entered cell water and displaced potassium.[11] Thus, the body content of both sodium and water is normal, but a potassium deficiency is present and a redistribution of sodium has occurred. Whether there is any relation between the acute changes in the infections described previously and this chronic tuberculous state is not known.

MALNUTRITION

Infants in the state of severe malnutrition frequently are hyponatremic, and they function by means of physiologic adaptation to the lowered osmolality. This is almost always true in kwashiorkor and is usually true in marasmic infants, although there are a significant number of exceptions. Whether this dilutional state relates to a reduction in cellular protein as some sort of adaptation or to other factors as yet undiscovered cannot be stated. The hyponatremia is asymptomatic and when corrected does not improve the patient's status; in fact, a relative hypernatremia may develop, with all of the problems associated with hyponatremic states. Thus, the definition of hypernatremia for the malnourished child cannot be the same as the arbitrary definition (Na > 150 mEq/l in serum) of hypernatremia in the adequately nourished.

The management of these various disturbances will be taken up in the clinical sections of this book. The external balance of water and salt may always be manipulated to change the laboratory values!

REFERENCES

1. Darrow DC, Yannet H: The changes in the distribution of body water accompanying increase and decrease in extracellular electrolyte. J Clin Invest 14:266, 1935.
2. McCance RA: Experimental sodium chloride deficiency in man. Proc R Soc Med 119:245, 1936.
3. Fichman MP, Vorherr H, Kleeman CR, Telfer N: Diuretic-induced hyponatremia. Ann Intern Med 75:853, 1971.
4. Roy RN, Chance W, Radde I, et al: Late hyponatremia in very low birthweight infants (< 1.3 kg). Pediatr Res 10:526, 1976.
5. Schwartz WB, Bennett W, Curelop E, Bartter FC: A syndrome of renal sodium loss and hyponatremia probably resulting from inappropriate secretion of antidiuretic hormone. Am J Med 23:529, 1959.
6. Friedman AL, Segar WE: Antidiuretic hormone excess. J Pediatr 94:521, 1979.
7. George JM, Capen OC, Phillips AS: Biosynthesis of vasopressin in vitro and ultra structure of a bronchogenic carcinoma. J Clin Invest 51:141, 1972.
8. Vorherr H, Massry SG, Fallet R, et al: Antidiuretic principle in tuberculous lung tissue of a patient with pulmonary tuberculosis and hyponatremia. Ann Intern Med 72:383, 1970.
9. Gonzalez CF, Finberg L, Bluestein DD: Electrolyte concentration during acute infection. Am J Dis Child 107:476, 1964.
10. Finberg L, Gonzalez C: Experimental studies on the hyponatremia of acute infection. Metabolism 14:693, 1965.
11. Harrison HE, Finberg L, Fleishman E: Disturbances of ionic equilibrium of intracellular and extracellular electrolytes in patients with tuberculous meningitis. J Clin Invest 31:300, 1952.

Clinical Implementation: Diagnosis, Assessment, and Treatment of Dehydration

III

Chapter 15

CLINICAL EVALUATION OF DEHYDRATION

Dehydration, regardless of the etiologic factors that produce it, is a physiologic disturbance of clinical importance. Proper assessment will lead to appropriate therapy when treatment is required. In any clinical evaluation, the tools are the clinical history, the examination of the patient, and a review of laboratory data. Then, a systematic analysis of the problem should lead to a diagnosis of the physiologic disturbance and suggest the nature of therapeutic intervention, if any. Each of these points will be taken up in turn in this chapter.

HISTORY

In obtaining the history from the patient or, more likely in pediatrics, from members of the patient's family, a number of points need special emphasis. Clearly, these points bear upon the intake of fluid and mineral and on unusual losses of these materials. Since most pediatric patients who develop serious dehydration are infants, discussion in this chapter will stress their evaluation. However differences in the evaluation of infants and children will be noted as we go along.

A recent weight of the patient, when it can be obtained from the history, may prove useful as a bench mark. Much attention should be given to obtaining a history of the recent feeding, including and even stressing the intake of liquids. This should include the usual feeding pattern, the specific feeding pattern prior to the onset of illness, and the feeding and liquid (water) intake since the onset of illness. The presence of fever and its type and duration, if possible, are clearly important. A description of the patient's environment in regard to temperature and humidity should be at least approximated. Any evidence of infection, local or systemic, is also of importance because of the influence of infection on catabolism as well as of the implications of infection for physiologic change. A history of drug inges-

115

tion is potentially useful. The most common drug of importance is aspirin or another salicylate. It should be remembered that a number of substances not thought of as medicine may contain salicylate.

Intensive questioning should focus on the site of fluid loss and the type and amount of loss. Since most fluids are lost from the gastrointestinal tract, this is usually the focus, but fluid loss can occur into a tissue or in the urine as well. In fact, even when the fluid is lost from another site, the history of the urine output over the past 24 hours may be illuminating. It is also useful to know, whether the baby is producing tears while crying. If the illness is characterized by diarrhea, it is important to try to characterize that symptom quantitatively, if possible, and qualitatively as well. The type and color of stool, the duration of the abnormal purging, and the presence of blood and mucus are useful pieces of information.

The symptoms of anorexia and vomiting are of special importance in infancy, because a high oral intake of liquid is so immediately essential to life processes, all the more so during a catabolic state. Indeed, the advent of vomiting in an infant with diarrhea is what usually precipitates admission to the hospital, since under most circumstances this symptom ends the ability of the family to manage the baby.

Beyond the historical data bearing upon the disturbance, a skilled physician will also direct questions that may lead to discovery of the etiology of the underlying disease. These matters are not taken up here.

Examination

In examining an infant for dehydration, the most important single determination is the patient's weight. This measurement should always be obtained with great care and precision. Failure to do so jeopardizes the therapeutic plan more than any other error that the clinician can make. Body temperature is another objective measurement that can be made. With these two data in hand, one can proceed to inspection. A look at the facies determines whether the patient is alert or lethargic and, indeed, whether anxiety or even coma has been induced by physiologic disturbance. If the patient is lethargic, it is important to deter-

mine also whether irritability is present either without stimulus or in response to such stimuli as sound, light, and touch. Unusual body movements or convulsive twitchings can be noticed. One can ascertain objectively whether tears are produced.

The skin provides many clues to the state of hydration. This is particularly true in infants up to the age of 1 or 2 years. In older children, examination of the skin is less useful in determining the state of hydration. Two signs that are looked for in particular are changes in elasticity and in turgor. When pinched, the abdominal skin of normal infants will snap back promptly on release. When dehydration has progressed to a serious point, pinched skin will remain standing in folds when elasticity has been lost. This sign may also be seen, however, in patients with serious undernutrition without dehydration. In older children and adults, the nature of the subcutaneous tissue is different and this loss of elasticity will not be elicited when they are dehydrated. The presence of turgor is a sign of circulatory adequacy. One examines for it by pinching the skin and squeezing out the blood from the pinched area, thereby causing a color change. In the normal patient, the color returns almost instantaneously upon release. Slowness in the return of color denotes a loss of turgor. Very slow return in the absence of a local skin problem (or edema) means shock.

In the seriously dehydrated infant the fontanelle, when open, tends to be depressed. In patients of any age, serious dehydration causes the eyeballs to sink in their sockets, although this may not be apparent unless the patient has been seen in his or her normal state. In older children, the eyeballs are often soft in acidemic states. This last sign is not reliable, however. The lips and tongue will be dry and little saliva will be seen when dehydration is serious. Finally, before leaving inspection, one can watch breathing movements of the chest with respect to both rate and depth, and a look at the anus is in order, especially if there has been a history of blood in the stool.

The next steps in the examination are palpation and auscultation. Pulse rate and pressure are most important determinations, since tachycardia is the first manifestation of dehydration. Palpation of the abdomen for masses or tenderness is always important, because the symptoms of diarrhea and vomiting occur in several conditions that are surgical emergencies. The most important of these is intussusception. It should be remembered that diarrhea often antecedes intussusception and rather commonly is present even after the intussusception has occurred.

The examination of the muscle tone, including checking for nuchal rigidity and testing the deep tendon reflexes, is a helpful assessment, as will be discussed below. Auscultation of the heart and lungs gives information on the quality of the heart sounds and confirms the observations with respect to the rate and depth of breathing.

LABORATORY STUDIES

The routine laboratory studies in dehydration should include those generally routine studies of hematocrit and urinalysis. The presence of anemia or polycythemia will be relevant to many of the later decisions. Routine urinalysis is also useful, checking for the presence of glucose or protein and cellular elements. The presence of cellular elements indicates that primary renal disease may be involved. The osmolality of the urine is a particularly sensitive measure of renal function, and the specific gravity determination gives an approximation of osmolality if one bears in mind the possible influence of glucose and protein on this measurement. The presence of ketones in urine and the urine pH are useful to know.

In addition to these routine studies, one should obtain blood from a dehydrated patient and, at the very least, have the serum analyzed for the urea nitrogen level and for the electrolytes sodium, potassium, chloride, and bicarbonate. If a more extensive analysis is desired, the blood gases may be measured, as may calcium, phosphorus, magnesium, glucose, and albumin. Most patients do not require such an extensive workup. For complicated or unusual patients, however, such studies can be quite valuable.

X-ray examinations are not generally required to assess dehydration. If, however, a radiograph of the chest is obtained for some other reason, it should be noted that dehydration does produce a small cardiac shadow and a diminution of vascular markings in the chest.

ASSESSMENT

Having obtained the data base from history, examination, and preliminary laboratory data, the next step is a systematic analysis of certain cardinal clinical points. There are five of these that are definable. Each should be reviewed in assessing the patient's status. In the sickest patients, one may initially have to forgo laboratory information altogether because of the urgency of the problem. The five points we have designated are (1) volume, (2) osmolality, (3) hydrogen ion disturbance, (4) intracellular ion losses, and (5) calcium homeostasis (skeletal ions). Each of these will be discussed in detail. Together, they should enable the analyst to define the degree of dehydration, the distortion of body water distribution, and the metabolic disturbances arising from effects upon hydrogen, potassium, and calcium ions. The first two points of assessment are more important than the last three if the patient has potentially adequate renal and pulmonary function. The homeostatic mechanisms of kidneys and lungs will correct the metabolic disturbances if the volume and space disturbances are quickly and appropriately corrected. Patients with impaired renal or pulmonary function will require careful attention to all five points of assessment.

As we go through these assessments, we will also be determining whether an emergency state exists. We will classify the dehydration by the determinant of water distribution, the sodium concentration, into hypernatremic, isonatremic, or hyponatremic states. Finally, the metabolic disturbances, including those of hydrogen ion, will be taken into account.

Volume

There are three considerations for the therapist with respect to the assessment of volume. The first of these is the degree of deficit. This, of course, is a change in composition and can be expressed as a number of milliliters per kilogram of weight or as a percentage of weight loss. In jargon, it is often designated as, for example, "5 or 10 per cent dehydration," by which is meant 5 or 10 per cent body weight loss. The least objectively detectable deficit is about 50 ml/kg (5 per cent acute weight loss). Elevated pulse rate, diminished pulse pressure, and diminished output of tears and urine may be the only manifestations. When a deficit of about 100 ml/kg exists, a constellation of clinical signs is usually present. These include a depressed fontanelle in infants and sunken eyeballs in patients of any age, loss of elasticity and of turgor of the skin, and other evidences of circulatory deficit, such as coolness and acrocyanosis or mottling of the skin of the extremities, feeble heart tones, and a weak, rapid pulse. The brachial blood pressure is usually maintained. When dehydration has progressed to this point, the patient is in medical shock from the loss of extracellular fluid. Between the above two landmarks — mild (50 ml/kg) and moderately severe (100 ml/kg) dehydration — one can interpolate intermediate degrees of deficit but not with precision. As has been noted in the chapter on pathophysiology, when the deficit over a short period of time approaches 15 per cent of the body weight, blood pressure drops and a moribund state ensues.

In estimating the volume of deficit, we have used the dehydrated weight as our basis rather than calculating the hydrated weight and using it. We compensate for this "error" in the clinical calculations by also ignoring the water of oxidation produced by the patient in each time period, an "error" in the opposite direction. The result in most patients is that these two omissions cancel each other out when the time period of therapy is short, i.e., a day or two. For more precise work, research, or the establishment of long-term regimens for precariously ill patients, the calculations should be refined.

The volume of fluid estimated as the *deficit* should be thought of as deficit primarily from extracellular fluid. Therefore, the deficit is fluid with a sodium concentration of about 150 mEq/l, chloride 115 to 120 mEq/l, and bicarbonate or other base 25 to 30 mEq/l. After considering the next few analysis points, these estimates may be modified.

While assessing the deficit it is also appropriate to consider the fluid volume needed by the patient to replace ongoing obligatory losses. This fluid volume is sometimes referred to as maintenance fluid. One assesses the metabolic state of the patient to estimate these ongoing losses. We have previously indicated that at basal conditions there is an age- or size-dependent caloric expenditure that determines water expenditure. Deviations from the basal state include body temperature changes, ventilation changes, and changes resulting from muscular movement. Included in this last group are shivering, which has an appreciable impact on caloric expenditure, and sweating if present. At average clinical conditions of normal body temperature (37° ± 1° C) with a slight increase in ventilation and with normal movement in bed, the caloric and water expenditure are about one and one half times the basal amount. Although one can, on an experimental basis, define rather precise increments in caloric expenditure for any of the abnormalities described, this is not practical clinically nor does such detailed calculation prove to be even advisable. A margin of safety of ± 10 per cent makes such precision unnecessary. A marked increase in any one of the three important variables — high fever, hyperventilation, or continued convulsive movements — will increase the ongoing obligatory losses to about double the basal expenditure. Should all three be increased, the effect would be to triple the basal expenditure. From these guidelines, reasonable estimates may be readily made by the clinician. The water estimated here is considered free of electrolyte.

A final concern in the assessment of volume relates to continued abnormal losses. In a few diseases, such as Asiatic cholera, these can be estimated from empirical data, but for most etiologies causing diarrheal disease or other problems, the abnormal losses will have to be ascertained by continuing direct observation of the clinician or his assistants. The electrolyte composition of abnormal losses varies with the etiology and the site of loss, as discussed previously.

It is important to point out that the measurement most useful in analysis of volume, that is, the most important of the five elements, is accurate assessment of the patient's weight. Failure to recognize this makes an expensive laboratory of little value.

Osmolality

The term "osmolality" as used here is a one-word, shorthand way of indicating an assessment of a disturbance of the distribution of water among the body spaces. The principal goal at this point in the analysis is to determine whether the patient is hyponatremic, with a relative preponderance of water in the cells at the expense of extracellular fluid; isonatremic, with a proportionate constriction of body fluids; or hypernatremic, with relative cellular dessication, the displaced water being found in the extracellular space.

The patient's history is helpful in making these distinctions. If purging has progressed for a number of days, sodium losses will be high, particularly if no sodium intake has occurred during this period. In fact, if relatively mineral-free water has been offered by any route, a hyponatremic state will result. If, following regular food intake that has been well maintained by the patient, an abrupt cessation of intake with or without vomiting occurs, then water losses will tend to predominate and hypernatremia will result. The presence of any factor that predisposes to insensible water loss — high ambient temperature or low humidity, fever (especially high fever), and hyperventilation — predisposes to hypernatremia.

On examination, deficient circulation indicates loss of extracellular fluid. If the circulation is not severely impaired but signs referable to the nervous system can be identified, particularly the combination of lethargy when the patient is unstimulated and hyperirritability to virtually any stimulus, a hypernatremic state should be suspected. Hypernatremic patients, instead of losing dermal elasticity in the usual fashion, often present with abdominal skin that has a doughy feel. Even more commonly, the skin will have a somewhat velvety feel, which we have found more reliable as an indicator of hypernatremia than the doughy feel. In hypernatremic states, there will be increased muscle tone, often including a very mild nuchal rigidity, which is occasionally mistaken for the nuchal rigidity of meningitis.

The definitive measurement for this assessment is the level of sodium in the serum. This is a better measurement than the osmolality per se, because some substances that affect osmolality, e.g., urea, do not influence body water distribution.

This assessment point permits assignment of a sodium concentration to the *deficit* portion of the repair solution. For patients with isonatremic dehydration, this will be 140 to 160 mEq/l. More sodium should be given if hyponatremia is diagnosed and less if hypernatremia is present. Each of these states is discussed in examples in the succeeding chapters.

Hydrogen Ion Disturbance

The patient's history is helpful in assessing hydrogen ion disturbance. In infancy, unless there has been vomiting with high obstruction, almost all disturbances produce acidosis and then acidemia. As discussed in other chapters, diarrhea is particularly likely to cause this type of disturbance. The degree of acidosis or acidemia is not easily gauged without laboratory data. Hyperpnea is evidence of a compensatory phenomenon and suggests the disturbance. The presence of ketones in the urine is similarly helpful in assessment. It should be remembered, however, that ketonuria does not appear in infants under the age of 5 months as a result of starvation or dehydration or both. Ketonuria in the infant under 5 months of age usually means metabolic disease, such as diabetes or one of the aminoacidopathies.

The symptoms of diarrhea and unobstructed vomiting lead to metabolic acidosis and sometimes acidemia by five mechanisms (see also Table 12–1, p. 94): (1) bicarbonate is lost in excessive stool losses, (2) increased intestinal lumen fermentation may lead to absorption of H^+, (3) inanition leads to gluconeogenesis and lipolysis, producing organic acids, (4) diminished perfusion of muscle tissue initiates lactic acid production, and (5) hypovolemia causes diminished glomerular filtration and oliguria, which decreases acid excretion. The first four mechanisms are readily compensated by increased ventilation, and are corrected by renal excretion of acid until the fifth mechanism supervenes. For the dehydration of enteric disease, then, hypovolemia is the most important factor in the pathogenesis of acidemia. Vomiting from high intestinal obstruction leads to alkalosis and sometimes alkalemia through loss of hydrochloric acid without intestinal bicarbonate. The history of the illness, the physical examination, and inspection of the vomitus for bile facilitate the clinical diagnosis of the qualitative acid-base status.

Measurement of the bicarbonate ion or the complete blood gas battery indicates the quantitative dimensions of hydrogen ion disturbance. Although therapy can and sometimes should take hydrogen ion disturbance into account, adequate attention to volume and correction of the maldistribution of water will usually enable the kidney and lung to do this task quite satisfactorily. During therapy, the cations and anions selected should be slowly corrective or, at least, should not worsen the hydrogen ion disturbance. Remember that the normal pH of plasma and extracellular fluid is alkaline, not neutral; therefore, some base is usually properly included even in "maintenance" solutions.

Intracellular Ion Losses

Although intracellular ion losses include the loss of potassium, magnesium, and phosphate, usually only the potassium is important from a solely clinical point of view. Whenever there are losses of gastrointestinal secretions, significant potassium losses are likely to occur. The extent of these losses is known from empirical data rather than from analyses obtained from clinical laboratories, since there is currently no easy method of either estimating or measuring the losses. When the patient has had longstanding diarrhea or vomiting, the potassium losses will be large. If there has been polyuria, potassium losses will be predictably large as well. Measurement of the potassium level in the serum may be deceptive, because any diminution in the glomerular filtration will cause the potassium level to rise even when the total body potassium is low. A high bicarbonate and a low chloride in serum suggest potassium deficit. This is true in relative as well as absolute terms, so that the experienced clinician is occasionally given a clue by what seems an inappropriate ratio of bicarbonate to chloride. Unfortunately, the electrocardiogram reflects only the extracellular value of potassium and so adds no quantitative information. Phosphate and magnesium levels are discussed in other sections of the book and, as indicated earlier, are only occasionally of clinical importance in states of dehydration.

The clinical principle of importance here is that potassium must be provided to replace tissue losses produced by disease and by the anticipated high urine output during therapy.

Calcium Homeostasis (Skeletal Ions)

Although phosphate and magnesium may be also included among the skeletal ions, it is really the calcium ion that is of importance. Infants in the first week or two of life frequently have impaired calcium homeostasis, so that superimposed dehydration may tip them to hypocalcemia. As discussed elsewhere, hypernatremic states frequently produce mild hypocalcemia; uncommonly, they may produce significant hypocalcemia. Other factors that may do this include high phosphate levels (often because of renal insufficiency) and alkalemia, which is unusual. Relative alkalemia, however, can be produced by treatment of acidemia or acidosis, and rapid hydration may also produce a dilutional state. Either of these may predispose to hypocalcemia, although not commonly. In summary, the neonatal period in general and hypernatremic states in particular are the factors of most importance in calcium disturbances during dehydration.

The preferred measurement is that of ionized calcium, which is the physiologically active modality. This measurement is still not obtainable everywhere, and total calcium levels must often suffice. Interpretation is enhanced if the pH of the serum and the albumin concentration are also known, since both factors affect the level of ionized calcium.

Only in a few situations will calcium salts have to be given during therapy. When this is necessary, however, they must be given by *continuous* intravenous administration, so avid is the skeleton in picking up any bolus that might be administered.

Chapter 16

THERAPY OF DEHYDRATION RESULTING FROM GASTROINTESTINAL FLUID LOSS

IMPLEMENTATION IN ISONATREMIC AND HYPONATREMIC DEHYDRATION

The clinical analyses reviewed in the preceding chapter enable one to know both qualitatively and quantitatively the amount of fluid required for repair and for other needs during the next period of time, which we will arbitrarily place at one day. Before implementation, this information must be translated into a plan for the rate of administration and into a decision whether the components of therapy are to be emphasized equally over the course of the day or whether special emphasis will be given at certain times to a specific element of therapy. This chapter will consider therapy of the first 24 hours in patients with isotonic constriction of body fluids (isonatremia) and in those requiring slight modification because of a hyponatremic state.

PHASES OF THERAPY

It is useful to divide therapy into phases, each with its own time segment within the 24 hours. We have divided the day into three phases, namely, Emergency, Repletion, and Early Recovery. When water is lost from the body through the gastrointestinal tract, the loss ultimately involves all body compartments to some degree. It fol-

lows, then, that water given during treatment must wind up in the various body compartments as well.

The most urgent need of a dehydrated patient is for replacement of the plasma volume when it has been compromised. The blood carries oxygen and nutrients to tissues and removes waste products. Without adequate oxygen and glucose, the tissues will die. Thus, restitution of this subcompartment of extracellular fluid (ECF), when sufficiently depleted, requires urgent attention. The emergency phase, then, has as its emphasis replacement of plasma volume.

Most of the water loss in isonatremic dehydration is from the ECF. Aside from the plasma, the other component of this water is the interstitial fluid, which serves as the transport medium for virtually all substances active in bodily functions. This space needs early repletion (the second phase) so that metabolic processes may proceed normally.

Finally, water and salts from cells (intracellular fluid, or ICF) will need to be replaced to ensure proper cellular function. Each of the three body spaces roughly corresponds, then, to the emphasis of each of three phases of therapy. Each phase is discussed in this chapter in general terms, and then examples of clinical situations are given, illustrating the type of clinical analysis discussed previously and delineating each phase of hydration.

From the clinical assessment scheme described in the previous chapter, the volume of fluid needed to repair the deficit may be estimated with the volume required to recover obligatory ongoing losses. Empirical data have indicated that it is appropriate to give this combined volume of fluid to the usual dehydrated patient within the first 24 hours. We thus have a tentative estimate of volume to use in planning therapy; this volume can be supplemented by that of any continuing abnormal losses. From consideration of the pathogenesis of dehydration, discussed previously, we also know how much sodium should be given during the first day and approximately how much base, potassium, and calcium are needed. It remains, now, to quantitate each element specifically and to apportion the administration of fluids in the several phases.

I. EMERGENCY

An emergency phase is to be implemented only if there is significant circulatory deficit. If this is not present, the emergency phase involves only a more rapid rate of initial infusion during the repletion phase, or it may even be omitted if no circulatory manifestations are detectable. The emphasis during the emergency phase is on restoration of the plasma volume. The simplest way to restore this volume is to infuse a fluid that contains either protein or other substances that will have the same oncotic properties as plasma albumin. Thus, single-donor plasma, or a solution of 5 per cent albumin, or any other analogous fluid is ideal. The volume of water in this infusion will, at least for an appreciable period of time, remain intravascular and accomplish the intended goal. Empirically, we long ago learned that 20 ml/kg of plasma of 5 per cent albumin can be infused in a dehydrated patient without risk of clinical consequence from overexpansion of the plasma volume. This, then, has become one standard way to implement the emergency phase. Subsequently, it was learned that aqueous solutions can also be used for this purpose, thus avoiding the expense and hazards of protein

solutions yet accomplishing the desired goal. In neonates and malnourished infants as well as in hypernatremic patients in shock, the albumin solutions are preferred for the emergency phase.

In other patients, aqueous solutions prove to be equally satisfactory during the emergency phase, but the volume given has to be greater to achieve a similar effect on plasma volume — theoretically, four times greater. Different authorities have recommended somewhat different aqueous solutions. We prefer solutions containing glucose to Ringer's lactate solution, although both have been used successfully. In fact, even when we use an albumin solution, we immediately follow that solution with one of 10 per cent glucose in water, 20 ml/kg, also administered very rapidly. These two infusions can usually be accomplished within an hour, providing a combined volume of 40 ml/kg, which is then subtracted from the proposed total volume for the day to ascertain how much more is needed. If an aqueous solution alone is to be given initially, we recommend a 10 per cent glucose solution to which 75 mEq/l of sodium, 55 mEq/l of chloride, and 20 mEq/l of bicarbonate (or other base) have been added. Forty ml/kg of this solution is administered over approximately the same one-hour interval. Either alternative constitutes the emergency phase.

Those who use Ringer's lactate or 0.9 per cent sodium chloride (so-called normal or physiologic saline) recommend administering 40 to 50 ml/kg again in about an hour. We prefer hypertonic glucose because it not only provides substrate for the nutrition of starving cells but also temporarily pulls additional water to the ECF, even into the vascular fluid, and thus initiates urine formation a bit more rapidly. There has been no detailed comparison of these two approaches, because it is difficult to get comparable patient populations and because it is clear that both approaches have been successful. The earlier presence of urine in the specimen bottle has influenced our choice, as has the relative lack of post-treatment edema in our patients. These observations have led us to prefer this regimen, but the difference in recommendations is not of sufficient importance to warrant quarreling, so long as the therapist understands what he or she is doing.

In assigning the emergency fluid to

either the deficit or the maintenance portion of the allotment, the task is obvious. A simple plasma or albumin solution contains sodium and therefore is assigned to the deficit fraction. Glucose water without sodium belongs to the estimated maintenance portion. A solution containing 75 mEq/l of sodium is half deficit and half maintenance. If Ringer's lactate or 0.9 per cent saline is used, all of it should be assigned to the deficit fraction.

II. Repletion

The duration of the emergency phase, if any, and repletion phase combined should be a third of a day, or eight hours. The emphasis during this phase is on restoration of the interstitial fluid. The volume to be given is such that 50 per cent of the tentatively assigned volume for the day will be administered within eight hours. During this phase, there is no point in using 10 per cent glucose; rather, 5 per cent glucose should be used, which serves well as the stock solution. The sodium content is adjusted according to the estimated sodium need and can range in concentration from 40 to 80 mEq/l. Assuming that urine formation has become clinically visible, it is time to add parenteral potassium. Twenty mEq/l is a safe concentration that will prevent the clinical effects of potassium depletion. Chloride ion and base may be distributed according to the clinical assessment of the hydrogen ion status of the patient.

III. Early recovery

The emphasis during the early recovery phase is on replacement of the intracellular fluid. The rate of infusion should be slowed so that the phase will last for the remaining two thirds of the day, or 16 hours. The fluid composition is similar or identical to that of the preceding phase. Table 16–1 shows the therapeutic scheme for a patient with isotonic dehydration who is presumed to have a deficit of 100 ml/kg (10 per cent of body weight) and who requires an emergency phase.

All examples in this and subsequent chapters are of actual cases. In some, the weight of the patient has been rounded off for quick calculation.

EXAMPLE 1

Infant with Enteritis and Isotonic Dehydration

History. A 3-month-old infant has had loose, watery stools for 3 days, followed by marked anorexia with vomiting four times

Table 16–1. Scheme for First 24 Hours of Rehydration for Isotonic Dehydration of an Infant*

	Phase I	Phase II	Phase III	Total
Phase	Emergency	Repletion	Early recovery	
Duration	½ to 1 hour	6 to 7 hours	16 to 18 hours	24 hours
Emphasis for restoration	Plasma volume	ECF volume	ICF volume	All compartments
Fluid composition	a. Plasma or 5% albumin plus 10% glucose b. 10% glucose with Na$^+$ 75 mEq/l, Cl$^-$ 55 mEq/l, HCO$_3^-$ 20 mEq/l	5% glucose with Na$^+$ 40 mEq/l, K$^+$ 20 mEq/l, Cl$^-$ 40 mEq/l, base$^-$ 20 mEq/l	5% glucose with Na$^+$ 40 mEq/l, K$^+$ 20 mEq/l, Cl$^-$ 40 to 45 mEq/l, base$^-$ 15 to 20 mEq/l	Na$^+$ 9 mEq/kg, K$^+$ 3 mEq/kg, Cl$^-$ 8.5 mEq/kg
Amount in ml/kg of body weight	a. 20 ml/kg of each solution, totaling 40 ml/kg b. 40 ml/kg	60 ml/kg	100 ml/kg, plus any additional abnormal losses	200 ml/kg "plus"

*Estimated deficit: 10 per cent of weight (100 ml/kg)
Estimated ongoing losses: 100 ml/kg

during the last 12 hours. No urine has been seen for 10 hours.

Physical Examination.   Weight 5.0 kg, temperature 37.2° C, pulse 160/min, respiration 60/min, blood pressure 90/58.

Fontanelle and eyes sunken. Extremities are cold and skin over them is mottled. Abdominal skin stands in folds when pinched (loss of elasticity). Color returns to skin poorly after pinching (loss of turgor). No tears. Cry is weak. Reflexes are normal, sensorium is good. Muscle tone is less than normal. Bladder is not palpable. Patient is not observed to void. Few bowel sounds.

Assessment

1. VOLUME

Deficit: On the basis of clinical signs and early shock — 10 per cent of body weight (100 ml/kg), or 500 ml.

Obligatory water losses for 24 hours: Basal expenditure × 1½ = 5.0 × 60 × 1½ = 450 ml. Note that the dehydrated weight has been used, a small "error" offset for clinical purposes by not taking into account the water of metabolic oxidation (12 ml/100 cal), which is a small amount of "error" in the opposite direction.

Abnormal losses: To be observed with the expectation that the fasting state will make them minimal.

Total estimated volume for 24 hours: 500 + 450 = 950 ml.

2. OSMOLALITY.   Illness has been of several days' duration, which suggests loss of electrolyte and water. Physical examination shows circulatory deficit and no CNS signs. Conclusion: Isotonic constriction of body fluids with predominant loss from the ECF.

Question: How much Na^+ should be in the replacement fluid?

Answer: Enough to give a concentration of 150 mEq/l in the deficit fraction of therapy (500 ml), or 75 mEq of sodium.

Question: Why not include electrolyte in the "maintenance" portion of therapy?

Answer: With a large Na^+ deficit being replaced, there is no need to add the very small amount of Na^+ for normal maintenance. The sodium salts scheduled to be given, plus glucose, will protect red cells from hemolysis.

3. HYDROGEN ION.   In enteritis, a mild-to-moderate acidemia may be assumed to be present because of loss of base, acid production secondary to starvation, poor tissue perfusion, and, especially, oliguria. Blood gas determination shows PO_2 90 mm Hg, PCO_2 20 mm Hg, pH 7.28, and CO_2 content (HCO_3^-) 8 mEq/l.

Question: Should IV hypertonic bicarbonate be given stat?

Answer: No! Restoration of volume, especially plasma volume, will enable the kidney and lung to compensate and will correct acidemia of this degree. Give one quarter to one third of anion in therapy as base (HCO_3^-, lactate, or acetate). Patient is sick enough without risking cerebral hemorrhage!

4. ICF ION LOSSES (K^+).   In any enteritis, K^+ losses are of the order of 3 to 10 mEq/kg. Here, the suggestion of hypoactive bowel and poor muscle tone indicates K^+ deficiency.

Plan: Add K^+ as chloride or acetate to IV solution, 3 mEq/kg/day, or 20 mEq/l, as soon as patient voids or has detectable urine in bladder.

5. CALCIUM HOMEOSTASIS.   No special problem is anticipated unless PO_4^- retention proves to be unusual. A high serum urea nitrogen (SUN) may prove to be a marker for this.

Question: What laboratory data should be obtained for additional analysis and confirmation? Weight (mass) has already been measured, as have blood gases.

Answer: Order serum analyses for Na^+, Cl^-, K^+, SUN, and CO_2 content (direct analysis to confirm derived value from blood gas) as a minimum. Save some of the sample for Ca, P, Mg protein, and glucose analyses if additional problems arise. If you automatically receive 18 or more analyses from an autoanalyzer, dividing the sample will not achieve the intended parsimony accomplished by ordering only what is necessary. Someday, health-care economists may insist.

Laboratory results:

Na^+	138	mEq/l
Cl^-	116	mEq/l
HCO_3^-	8	mEq/l
K^+	4.6	mEq/l
SUN	50	mg/dl

Therapeutic Implementation

PHASE I (EMERGENCY).   Duration: 40 min. Two hundred ml (40 ml/kg) to be given. *Step 1* (20 min): Plasma (modified) or 5 per cent albumin — 20 ml/kg, or 100 ml. *Step 2* (20 min): 10 per cent glucose solution — 20 ml/kg, or 100 ml. After Step 2, patient voids 25 ml of urine.

Total volume for Phase I: 40 ml/kg (200 ml) — half for deficit, half for "maintenance" water.

Question: Why Step 2 in Phase I?

Answer: The glucose solution was given to stop ketosis, provide calories, add water to plasma, and provide water for urine formation.

(ALTERNATIVE PHASE I. Ten per cent glucose with Na^+ 80 mEq/l, Cl^- 60 mEq/l, and HCO_3^- 20 mEq/l over 40 min. As before, patient would void 25 ml of urine — easy to specify here in a book, but sometimes missing in real life!)

PHASE II (REPLETION). Duration: 7 hours. IV begun to complete administration of 475 ml (one half of total estimated volume for 24 hours, or 950/2 ml), of which 200 ml has been given. IV solution: 5 per cent glucose with Na^+ 75 to 80 mEq/l, K^+ 20 mEq/l, Cl^- 75 to 80 mEq/l, and acetate 20 mEq/l. If the patient had not produced urine, the potassium acetate would have been temporarily withheld and sodium bicarbonate would have been given, 20 mEq/l, with the Cl^- 55 to 60 mEq/l. Rate of administration: 275 ml in 7 hours = 39 ml/hr = 0.66 ml/min.

PHASE III (EARLY RECOVERY). Duration: 16 hours. Continue administration of Phase II solution at slower rate: 475 ml in 16 hours = 28 ml/hr = 0.5 ml/min. Alternatively, Phase III could be carried out per os, if patient's condition permits or if the IV falls out.

PHASE IV (FULL RECOVERY). See Chapter 20 for details of management. Resumption of oral intake with gradual introduction of infant formula, adding 20 per cent of volume each day with a glucose-electrolyte mixture as the remainder of intake (150 ml/kg/day).

EXAMPLE 2

Hyponatremic Dehydration

History. A 6-week-old infant developed a watery diarrhea (6 to 8 loose stools per day), which has persisted for a week. For the first four days, normal feedings supplemented by plain water were maintained. For the next three days, milk feedings were taken poorly but weak tea and flavored sugar-water were accepted. Since the onset of vomiting 6 hours ago, there has been no fluid or food intake. The last urine that wet the diaper was noted 12 hours ago.

Physical Examination. Weight 4.0 kg, temperature 36.8° C, pulse 180/min, respiration 60/min, blood pressure 80/50.

Fontanelle and eyes sunken. Skin cold and mottled; shows loss of elasticity and turgor. No tears. Cry is weak. Heart tones of poor quality. Infant responds poorly to examiner and to stimuli generally. Tendon reflexes normal. No irritability, although patient is very apathetic.

Assessment

1. VOLUME

Deficit: At least 10 per cent of body weight (100 ml/kg), or 400 ml.

Obligatory water losses for 24 hours: Basal expenditure × 1½ = 4.0 × 60 × 1½ = 360 ml.

Abnormal losses: To be observed.

Total estimated volume for 24 hours: 760 ml.

2. OSMOLALITY. The history suggests loss of water and sodium salts with partial replacement of water only. Circulatory signs marked. The change in sensorium is more likely the result of shock than of hypernatremia. Suspect hyponatremic or isonatremic state with greater than 10 per cent weight loss. Plan to give more sodium than for isonatremic dehydration. Obtain laboratory analyses as quickly as possible.

3. HYDROGEN ION. In a very young patient, anticipate acidosis or acidemia from enteric losses and circulatory deficit. Do not anticipate ketonuria in a patient of this age.

4. ICF ION LOSSES. Long period of stool loss. K^+ deficit will be high. Replace K^+ as soon as possible after urine formation becomes apparent.

5. CALCIUM HOMEOSTASIS. No anticipated problem, but young age of patient makes hypocalcemia a possibility, especially during therapy with base. Watch for high phosphate level in serum despite fasting, if SUN is high.

Laboratory results:

Na^+	128	mEq/l
Cl^-	99	mEq/l
HCO_3^-	12	mEq/l
K^+	3.9	mEq/l
SUN	85	mg/dl

Therapeutic Implementation

PHASE I (EMERGENCY). Duration: 40 to 60 min. *Step 1:* Plasma (modified) or 5 per cent albumin — 20 ml/kg, or 80 ml. *Step 2:* 10 per cent glucose with Na^+ 75 mEq/l, C^- 55 mEq/l, and HCO_3^- 20 mEq/l—20 ml/kg, or 80 ml.

If laboratory data had not been available, the solution in Step 2 might have been given without added sodium salts. No harm would have been likely to occur so long as the next phase compensated.

(ALTERNATIVE PHASE I. Assuming laboratory values were known, 10 per cent glucose with Na^+ 120 mEq/l, Cl^- 110 mEq/l, and HCO_3^- 30 mEq/l — 40 ml/kg, or 160 ml.)

Total volume for Phase I: 160 ml.

PHASE II (REPLETION). Duration: 6 to 7 hours (assumes urine formation during or after Phase I). (If no urine appears withhold potassium and revise maintenance volume to one half of previous allotment.) Five per cent glucose with Na^+ 120 mEq/l, K^+ 20 mEq/l, Cl^- 100 mEq/l, and HCO_3^- lactate, or acetate, singly or combined, 40 mEq/l — 220 ml. The sodium level could range from 100 to 130 mEq/l.

Total volume for Phase II: 220 ml (one half of total estimated volume for 24 hours, or 760/2, minus volume already administered in Phase I).

PHASE III (EARLY RECOVERY). Duration: 16 hours. Same solution as in Phase II — 380 ml — but administered at a slower rate.

PHASE IV (FULL RECOVERY). See Chapter 20.

EXAMPLE 3

Mild Isonatremic Dehydration

History. A 6-month-old infant has had loose stools (4 to 6 per day) for 48 hours. He took liquids fairly well until 4 hours ago, when intake ceased and he vomited twice. Last urine was 4 hours ago.

Physical Examination. Weight 8.0 kg, temperature 37.5° C, pulse 125/min, respiration 45/min, blood pressure 95/60.

No depression of fontanelle or eyeballs. Skin warm and dry; good elasticity and turgor. Tongue and lips dry. Slight tearing noted. Patient alert, although not cheerful. Tendon reflexes normal.

Assessment

1. VOLUME

Deficit: Tachycardia only objective sign of dehydration. Assume loss of 5 per cent of body weight (50 ml/kg), or 400 ml.

Obligatory water losses for 24 hours: Basal expenditure × 1½ = 8.0 × 60 × 1½ = 720 ml.

Abnormal losses: To be observed.

Total estimated volume for 24 hours: 1120 ml.

2. OSMOLALITY. No disturbance anticipated (isonatremic constriction).

3. HYDROGEN ION. Mild acidosis expected.

4. ICF ION LOSSES. Mild K^+ losses expected.

5. CALCIUM HOMEOSTASIS. No anticipated problem.

Therapeutic Implementation

PHASE I (EMERGENCY). No circulatory emergency exists. Omit this phase.

PHASE II (REPLETION). Duration: 6 hours (time period shortened because emergency phase omitted). Five per cent glucose with Na^+ 75 mEq/l, Cl^- 55 mEq/l, HCO_3^- (or lactate) 20 mEq/l. Add potassium acetate, 20 mEq/l, as soon as urine is detected in bladder, bag, or diaper.

Total volume for Phase II: 560 ml.

Comments: (1) The first hour should run more rapidly to ensure urine formation. Failure to do this may result in poor outcome if the diarrhea worsens during the patient's early hours under observation. (2) Phase II can be handled with oral fluids if the patient takes them well.

PHASE III (EARLY RECOVERY). Duration: 18 hours. Same solution as in Phase II, administered at slower rate by vein or by mouth.

Total volume for Phase III: 560 ml.

Comments. This milder degree of dehydration should be taken seriously, especially when vomiting has occurred. The initial rapid administration is important. Failure to observe this point is a common cause of future (next day!) difficulty.

EXAMPLE 4

Severe Hyponatremic Dehydration

History. A small 15-month-old infant receiving pancreatin therapy and antibiotics for confirmed cystic fibrosis developed a febrile illness during a hot week in July. She continued to drink clear liquids and to void urine until about 4 hours prior to admission. She then vomited once and became lethargic, then unresponsive and limp. A few loose stools were passed during the 10 hours before admission. A week previously, while in good condition, the patient weighed 8.3 kg.

Physical Examination. Weight 8.0 kg, temperature 38.5° C, pulse 176/min, respiration 60/min, blood pressure 60/35.

Color pale, Patient rouses to stimuli but is otherwise motionless. Heart sounds have a "tic-tac" quality. Skin turgor poor; elasticity fair. Aside from patient having little adipose tissue, no other findings.

Assessment

1. VOLUME

Deficit: Shock present; ECF losses equal to about 10 per cent of body weight, or 800 ml.

Obligatory water losses for 24 hours: $8.0 \times 50 \times 1\frac{1}{2} = 600$ ml.

Abnormal losses: To be observed.

2. OSMOLALITY. From the prior diagnosis and the environmental circumstances, profuse salt and water loss from sweating seems probable. Patient's intake and weight loss suggest that water was at least partially replaced ($8.3 - 8.0 = 0.3$ kg, or about 4 per cent of weight). Thus, loss of ECF is proportionately much greater than total water loss.

Recalculation of volume requirements for 24 hours: Analysis suggests severe salt loss and hyponatremic dehydration, with a volume requirement for 24 hours of about $600 + 300 = 900$ ml. (The patient's hydrated weight a week ago was 8300 gm compared with the present weight of 8000 gm; the approximate deficit is 300 gm, or 300 ml. The patient's ongoing needs, 600 ml, are unchanged.) Add about 100 ml for anticipated abnormal sweat losses (the hospital air conditioner has broken down).

3. HYDROGEN ION. Not predictable from history as we have it.

4. ICF ION LOSSES. Probably some K+ deficit because of chronic illness. May or may not be severe.

5. CALCIUM HOMEOSTASIS. No anticipated problem.

Summary of clinical analysis: Shock secondary to marked salt depletion with mild water loss — hyponatremic dehydration with marked loss of ECF and with increased relative ICF volume. Clinical emergency present. Obtain blood for analyses and begin emergency phase at once.

Therapeutic Implementation

PHASE I (EMERGENCY). Duration: One hour. *Step 1:* Single-donor plasma, whole blood, or 5 per cent albumin—20 ml/kg in 20 min.

Laboratory results:

Na+	110	mEq/l
Cl−	70	mEq/l
K+	3.9	mEq/l
HCO$_3^-$	22	mEq/l
SUN	95	mg/dl

Re-analysis: Hyponatremic dehydration confirmed and severe.

Na+ deficit calculation:

Total body water (TBW) = $0.7 \times$ weight =
$$0.7 \times 8 \text{ kg} = 5.61$$
$$140 - 110 = 30 \text{ mEq of deficit per liter}$$
$$30 \times 5.6 = 168 \text{ mEq}$$

Question: Why multiply by 0.7 instead of by 0.25, the volume of ECF that contains the sodium?

Answer: For calculation of sodium needs, the proper distribution space is the total body water (the osmotic distribution). Since the sodium remains largely extracellular, water leaves cells, equalizing osmolal concentrations in all body spaces. Therefore, 70 per cent of the lean body mass is the proper distribution space. This thin patient may be considered "lean."

PHASE I (CONTINUED). *Step 2:* Replace half of the deficit with an IV infusion of hypertonic NaCl solution. If the solution is 1 molar (5.8 per cent saline), then administer 84 ml over 30 min. If the solution is $\frac{1}{2}$ molar (3 per cent saline), then administer 168 ml over 45 min.

PHASE II (REPLETION). Continue administration of solution, now of $\frac{1}{6}$ molar (150 mEq/l) balanced sodium salts in 5 per cent glucose at the rate of 60 ml/hr.

Recheck serum analyses in 2 hours. Patient's circulation is now much improved.

Laboratory results:

Na^+	124 mEq/l
Cl^-	85 mEq/l
HCO_3^-	20 mEq/l
SUN	80 mg/dl

Now give the other half of the ½ or 1 molar solution over the next 2 hours. Patient is now very much improved. Continue 5 per cent glucose with Na^+ 75 to 100 mEq/l, Cl^- 75 to 100 mEq/l, K^+ 20 mEq/l, and acetate 20 mEq/l until total volume given equals about 500 ml.

PHASE III (EARLY RECOVERY). Over the next 16 to 18 hours, give another 500 ml of the same solution infusing at the end of the previous (repletion) phase.

Patient should now appear well recovered from dehydration.

Question: Was plasma (albumin) step necessary?

Answer: No. However, one could not quantitate the NaCl deficit without laboratory analyses. The plasma administration bought time without risk and with quick improvement for the patient.

Comments: The repair of the hyponatremia by the administration of hypertonic salt solution was pursued here because the degree of hyponatremia was severe, laboratory results confirmed serious circulatory impairment, and diagnosis of the underlying condition made further sodium losses likely.

Chapter 17

THERAPEUTIC MANAGEMENT OF HYPERNATREMIC DEHYDRATION

The pathophysiology of hypernatremia has distinct features, which differentiate it from the more common forms of dehydration and which the principles of therapy must accommodate. Restoration of hydration follows a different path when moderate hypernatremia is present. The objective of treatment is to replace fluid volume, to restore water distribution, and to correct the complicating disturbances. At first glance, therapy seems to be the simple replacement of water. In fact, careful attention to the content of the solution and the rate of administration used reveals that important special measures must be taken. Two other circumstances also require comment. The presence of oliguria influences decision-making, and salt poisoning should be considered as a separate entity.

Most patients with hypernatremic dehydration are not severely oliguric, owing to a relatively expanded plasma volume. If plain 5 per cent glucose water were to be infused into these patients, the risk would be cerebral swelling — actually, water intoxication. This results from the presence of tight junctions of endothelial cells in the CNS. Just as rapid infusion of hypertonic salt results in brain shrinkage, so does rapid infusion of isotonic glucose water cause brain swelling. Glucose rapidly crosses the blood-CNS barrier by active transport, so that, unlike the red cell, the brain does not recognize glucose as an osmol, at least at physiologic levels of glucose, but it does react to sodium and chloride ions as relatively nondiffusible because of the tight junctions.

When 5 per cent glucose water is infused rapidly intravenously, the cerebrospinal fluid (CSF) pressure rises (Fig. 17–1).

The rise in millimeters of water is the same for a given infused volume and rate regardless of the initial pressure. The increase in pressure results from swelling of the brain cells, not from an increase in interstitial fluid (i.e., edema). Brain swelling affects a number of nervous system functions, frequently resulting in convulsions. For some years after hypernatremic dehydration was described and recognized clinically, convulsions commonly occurred during therapy when rapid water replacement was attempted. This circumstance led many clinicians to suggest adding 75 mEq/l or more of sodium salts to the initial solution. This reduces the risk of convulsions but adds to the sodium burden, frequently while excessive insensible water losses are occurring, and thus aggravates hypernatremia. Such therapy also frequently produces visible edema, prolonging the recovery period. An alternative to increasing the concentration is to slow the rate of infusion, which will also prevent convulsions but at risk of repairing dehydration too slowly, with suboptimal outcome.

We have found a compromise resolution to these problems by considering, in part, that a high potassium intake offsets cerebral swelling and that some potassium enters depleted cells (mostly muscle cells), carrying water into them. At the same time, water is delivered to the patient at a slow, even rate. This regimen is appropriate provided the patient has no initial serious circulatory deficiency. The repair solution is prepared with consideration of the volume to be administered over 48 hours as well as the glucose content, sodium content, potassium content, anion distribution, calcium additive, and rate of administration. The

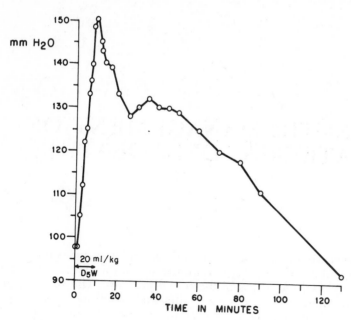

Figure 17–1. Cerebrospinal fluid (CSF) pressure versus time. The effect on CSF pressure of a rapid intravenous infusion of 5 per cent glucose in water (20 ml/kg). The same increase in pressure will occur at any baseline CSF pressure. This phenomenon, when symptomatic, is called water intoxication.

Table 17–1. Regimen for Therapy of Hypernatremic Dehydration

CONSIDERATIONS (in Order)	ACTION
1. *Volume*	a. Estimate the patient's deficit by clinical means, first in milliliters per kilogram, and then multiply by kilograms of weight for total sum. b. Estimate 48 hours' worth of maintenance water following usual clinical rules. c. Add volumes determined in steps a and b for tentative volume of solution for 2 days.
2. *Glucose content*	Use 2½ (2 to 3%) to prevent possible problems with hyperglycemia from arising later.
3. *Sodium content*	Allow 80 to 100 mEq/l for *deficit* fraction of fluid and none for the *maintenance* portion. The resultant concentration is usually 20 to 35 mEq/l. Use this concentration of sodium or simply estimate it at 25 mEq/l.
4. *Potassium content*	Generally, the maximal safe amount for an IV infusion, or about 40 mEq/l.
5. *Anion content*	Advised amount of sodium plus potassium equals 60 to 75 mEq/l of cation. Distribute the anions between chloride and base in accordance with clinical judgment. If desired, start with more base and change to more chloride after 6 to 12 hours. Do not use HCO_3^- as base, since calcium is to be added. Use acetate or lactate along with chloride.
6. *Calcium content*	One ampule of 10 per cent calcium gluconate for every 500 ml of infusate.
7. *Rate of administration*	Administer ¹/₄₈ of volume per hour for 48 hours. In an infant the usual volume will be 275 to 350 ml/kg/48 hours, or about 6 to 7 ml/kg/hour.

regimen shown in Table 17–1 illustrates one method of determining the volume and the amounts of solution appropriate for use in a patient with hypernatremic dehydration who is not in shock and who produces visible urine. The effects of shock, oliguria, and salt poisoning will be considered separately.

Shock

If the patient has circulatory impairment (shock), first infuse 20 ml/kg of 5 per cent albumin solution. (Single donor plasma, plasma without immunoglobulin, and whole blood are all satisfactory.) The sodium content of these fluids up to 140 mEq/l is not important, since nearly the whole volume will remain intravascular. If the patient is producing urine, proceed according to the regimen shown in Table 17–1:

Anuria

If the patient, even though not in hypotensive shock, has no apparent urine, try a rapid infusion of albumin as described under Shock. If urine then enters the bladder, proceed according to the basic regimen. If no urine enters the bladder, give furosemide, 1 mg/kg. If urine flow then occurs, proceed according to the regimen; if not, manage the condition without potassium in the infusion. Increase the sodium concentration to 50 mEq/l and slow the rate by reducing the volume to be administered, subtracting one half of the maintenance allowance from the 48-hour total.

Salt Poisoning

In the event of massive salt poisoning (plasma concentration of sodium greater than 200 mEq/l), use peritoneal dialysis to remove excess sodium chloride. For the dialyzing solution, use 8 per cent glucose with no electrolyte, 100 ml/kg, administering it two or three times approximately one hour apart. Simultaneously, be sure to establish an intravenous solution to deliver a volume of repair and maintenance solution as noted in Table 17–1. The hyperglycemia induced by this method offsets the removal of sodium, preventing water intoxication. As the glucose is metabolized, water slowly enters the cells.

Insulin is not advisable for any hyper-natremic patients with hyperglycemia, because rapid removal of glucose by metabolism is the physiologic equivalent of rapid water infusion.

In summary, treatment seems best handled with a *slow* infusion relatively low in both glucose and sodium and high in potassium with added calcium. For the past 12 years, this regimen has been highly successful and has not produced complicating convulsions.

EXAMPLE 1

Hypernatremic Dehydration of Moderate Severity

History. A 2-month-old infant has had a high fever for 4 days. She took milk formula feedings until 6 hours ago, when she vomited, and she has vomited twice since then, although she seems thirsty. Loose stools began 8 hours ago. The milk feedings were of whole cow's milk.

Physical Examination. Weight 4 kg, temperature 39.5° C, pulse 150/min, respiration 70/min, blood pressure 100/65.

The infant is markedly lethargic, but when stimulated she is overresponsive and very irritable. Her skin is warm and feels velvety smooth but thickened (doughy). Turgor and elasticity are good. Muscle tone is increased; reflexes are very brisk. Neck is slightly resistant to flexion. Fontanelle normal. Patient voids 30 ml of urine during the examination.

Clinical Analysis. A high-solute diet, a prolonged high-grade fever, and the abrupt cessation of intake without much stool loss, plus classical examination findings, suggest hypernatremic dehydration as the probable physiologic disturbance.

Question: What should be done in the emergency phase (Phase I)?

Answer: Skip Phase I! Circulation is good, no physiologic emergency exists, and urine formation has been observed. If patient is not so obliging, start administration of IV solution (described later) without K+ and at an increased rate for 20 to 30 min. That will usually do it. If not, continue to hold the K+ and call a consultant (unless you are one).

Proceed with assessment after drawing

blood for laboratory analyses. Calculate fluid requirements in the usual way.

Assessment

1. VOLUME

Deficit: 100 ml/kg (10%) of body weight, or 400 ml.

Ongoing losses: 4 × 65 × 1½ × 2(days) = 780 ml.

Total estimated volume for 48 hours: Round off 1180 to 1200 ml, which is to be given over 48 hours.

2. OSMOLALITY. Cellular dehydration. Sodium chloride needs are probably small — 2 to 4 mEq/kg, or 8 to 16 mEq total. Use as low a concentration of NaCl as is consistent with avoidance of water intoxication. Patient may be hyperglycemic.

3. HYDROGEN ION. Hypernatremic patients are often acidemic at this age. Blood gases in this patient are found now to be as follows: PO_2 95 mm Hg, PCO_2 30 mm Hg, pH 7.32, and CO_2 content (HCO_3^-) 12 mEq/l. Give half of anion as base.

4. ICF ION LOSSES (K^+). Administration of K^+ salts enables water to be given with low Na^+ concentration and yet avoids water intoxication.

5. CALCIUM HOMEOSTASIS. Young hypernatremic patients frequently have low calcium levels. Plan to add calcium gluconate to the IV solution. This interdicts the use of bicarbonate as an anion because of possible concretions in the tubing. Use lactate or acetate as base.

Summary and Plan. IV solution: 1200 ml of water (2 to 3 per cent glucose) to which has been added, for example, Na^+ 30 mEq/l (20 to 40 mEq/l),* Cl^- 30 mEq/l (20 to 40 mEq/l), K^+ 40 mEq/l (30 to 40 mEq/l), and acetate 40 mEq/l (30 to 40 mEq/l), with calcium gluconate, 20 ml of 10 per cent solution (180 mg of calcium). Rate of administration: 1200 ml in 48 hours, or 25 ml/hr.

Laboratory confirmation: The analyses show

Na^+	160	mEq/l
Cl^-	130	mEq/l
HCO_3^-	12	mEq/l
K^+	4.1	mEq/l
SUN	15	mg/dl
Glucose	250	mg/dl
Calcium	8.0	mg/dl
$[Ca^{++}]$	3.9	mg/dl

*Ranges are given in parentheses.

Question: Why not give simply 2½ per cent glucose, 50 ml/kg, over 6 hours, since water is what the patient really needs?

Answer: Do this only if you are prepared for a lawsuit. A convulsion will probably occur because of brain swelling (water intoxication). We have avoided this complication for 12 years, after years of almost weekly occurrence, by the technique described earlier.

Question: Why not achieve expansion with isotonic or ½ isotonic sodium salt solution (75 to 150 mEq/l)? This will not cause the hypernatremia to worsen or the brain to swell.

Answer: True, but the patient will probably become edematous and, if high insensible water losses continue, her hypernatremia may worsen and hemorrhage may occur! The early observation of this special difficulty in such patients led to systematic studies of hypernatremic dehydration in the early 1950s. Frequently, one may give such therapy without apparent damage, but it involves a small risk of mortality and risk of the morbidity of CNS damage a few years later, which are best avoided.

Question: If the patient had a more extreme hyperglycemia, should she have been given insulin?

Answer: No. Rapid reduction of ECF glucose to physiologic levels is tantamount to rapid water infusion, which causes brain swelling and convulsions. The "diabetic" state is transient and will disappear over a 36-hour period.

EXAMPLE 2

Mild Hypernatremic Dehydration

History. A 7-month-old infant developed explosive diarrhea (which occurred four times) and began to vomit, refusing all feedings, 10 hours before being seen. The patient has had a high fever since that time and also has symptoms of an upper respiratory infection. Urine was noted 1 hour ago.

Physical Examination. Weight 7.2 kg, temperature 39.2° C, pulse 110/min, respiration 50/min, blood pressure 95/60.

An irritable warm infant who prefers to sleep when unstimulated. Cries with tears. Pulse is full. Heart tones strong. Skin warm, dry, and velvety smooth. Deep tendon reflexes are brisk.

Clinical Analysis. Abrupt cessation of intake and impressive history of fluid loss are associated with no clinical evidence of dehydration except for irritability and velvety skin. Condition is probably mild hypernatremic dehydration.

Laboratory analyses (not available at onset of therapy):

Na^+	155 mEq/l
K^+	3.9 mEq/l
Cl^-	120 mEq/l
HCO_3^-	14 mEq/l
SUN	22 mg/dl
Glucose	500 mg/dl

Assessment

1. VOLUME

Deficit: Less than 100 ml/kg; perhaps 50 ml/kg, or 360 ml.

Ongoing losses: Basal expenditure × 1½ for either 24 or 48 hours. (A) For 24 hours: $7.2 \times 60 \times 1\frac{1}{2} = 650$ ml. (B) For 48 hours: 1300 ml.

Abnormal losses: To be observed.

Total estimated volume: (A) For 24-hour regimen: 1000 ml. (B) For 48-hour regimen: 1650 ml.

2. OSMOLALITY. Hypernatremia possible, especially if history is accurate. Condition might also be mild isonatremic dehydration. Plan to manage as hypernatremia, since that is the more dangerous condition.

3. HYDROGEN ION. Give one quarter to one half of anion as base.

4. ICF ION LOSSES. Give K^+ liberally if hypernatremia regimen is followed, and at least 3 mEq/kg if not.

5. CALCIUM HOMEOSTASIS. No problem is likely. If hypernatremia regimen is followed, add 10 ml of calcium gluconate for each 500 ml of fluid administered.

Question: Could patient's condition be managed successfully as a mild isonatremic dehydration (50 mg/kg deficit)?

Answer: Yes. With the regimen recommended by us, he will probably fare well, although he will be a little dry after 24 hours. No great harm is likely in this type of patient when clinical signs are not so clear-cut.

Therapeutic Implementation

EMERGENCY PHASE. None.

REPLETION PHASE. Either give 48-hour volume gradually (this is preferred) or give 24-hour volume as a more rapid infusion over 6 hours.

EARLY RECOVERY PHASE. Follows from above.

EXAMPLE 3

Hypernatremic Dehydration Plus Shock

History. A 3-month-old infant fed whole cow's milk became ill with high fever during the winter. After one day of fever, profuse watery diarrhea began (2 to 3 stools per hour) along with vomiting; the last time he vomited "coffee ground" material. The patient was hospitalized after 16 hours of these symptoms. Urine was last observed 6 hours prior to admission.

Physical Examination. Weight 5.3 kg, temperature 39.1° C, pulse 160/min, respiration 55/min, blood pressure 60/30.

Very sick infant, unaware of surroundings but with increased muscle tone including nuchal resistance to flexion and very brisk deep tendon reflexes. Facies is anxious — staring and unresponsive. Skin shows some loss of elasticity, feels thick or doughy; turgor is fair to poor. Acrocyanosis is present. Pulse rapid, moderate in strength. Heart tones good.

Clinical Analysis. History and findings suggestive of both hypernatremia and shock. Both are probably present. Give immediate emergency infusion of albumin solution, 20 ml/kg, after drawing blood for analyses.

Laboratory analyses:

Na^+	168	mEq/l
Cl^-	139	mEq/l
K^+	5.6	mEq/l
HCO_3^-	8.0	mEq/l
SUN	75	mg/dl
Glucose	420	mg/dl
Ca	7.8	mg/dl

Assessment

1. VOLUME

Deficit: More than 10 per cent of body weight. Tentatively assume 12 per cent — 12 ml/kg × 5.3 kg = 640 ml.

Ongoing losses: $5.3 \times 65 \times 1\frac{1}{2} \times$ 2(days) = 1040 ml.

Abnormal losses: To be observed.

Total volume for 48 hours: 640 + 1040 = 1680 ml.

2. OSMOLALITY. Hypernatremic state.

3. HYDROGEN ION. Acidemia likely.

4. ICF ION LOSSES. Liberal K^+ administration needed.

5. CALCIUM HOMEOSTASIS. Mild hypocalcemia probable. With laboratory data in hand, hyperglycemia also found to be present.

Therapeutic Implementation

EMERGENCY PHASE. Five per cent albumin (20 ml/kg) — 110 ml in 20 min. Patient improved: acrocyanosis gone, turgor good. Urine produced.

REPLETION PHASE. Start hypernatremic regimen with 1570 ml over 48 hours. Solution: 2.5 per cent glucose with Na^+ 25 mEq/l, K^+ 40 mEq/l, Cl^- 25 mEq/l, and acetate 40 mEq/l, to which has been added calcium gluconate, 30 ml of 10 per cent solution. Rate of administration: 33 ml/hour.

Comment: This is a desperately ill infant who would not survive if mishandled and who might easily have CNS complications unless managed very carefully.

EXAMPLE 4

Salt Poisoning[*]

History. A 4-month-old infant had mild diarrhea for a day. The family physician prescribed a homemade salt and sugar mixture for her to take. The mother confused the directions and substituted salt for sugar. A tablespoonful of salt (425 to 510 mmol) was consumed over a 24-hour period ending 12 hours before admission. The patient had been thirsty, drinking avidly during that time. She then became irritable and vomited. The mother noted "stiffenings" of the infant's body. The patient had continued to void urine.

---

[*]This patient was previously reported (Miller and Finberg, 1960; reference 1). The dialysis carried out in 1960 used 5 per cent glucose. From that experience we learned to use 8 per cent glucose to facilitate the recovery of dialysis fluid.

Physical Examination. Weight 7.16 kg, temperature 39.6° C, pulse 152/min, respiration 80/min, blood pressure 85/50.

The patient was comatose and her muscle tone hypertonic. There were brief extensor spasms. DTRs hyperactive with sustained clonus. Skin and oral membranes dry and warm. Turgor excellent. Eyes and fontanelles not sunken.

Laboratory analyses:

Na^+	200+	mEq/l
Cl^-	177	mEq/l
K^+	3.6	mEq/l
HCO_3^-	12	mEq/l
SUN	38	mg/dl

Clinical Analysis. The history indicates salt poisoning; the examination indicates severe hypernatremia; the laboratory results confirm. Here the problem is to remove excess salt without either worsening the cell desiccation or precipitating brain swelling. High fever, hyperventilation, and muscle movements indicate high insensible losses.

Assessment

1. VOLUME

Deficit: Small, perhaps negligible.

Ongoing losses: For first 24 hours: Basal expenditure × 2 = 60 × 7.16 × 2 = 860 ml. For second 24 hours (lower temperature and respiration rate expected): Basal expenditure × 1.5 = 60 × 7.16 × 1.5 = 645 ml. For entire 48 hours: 860 + 645 ≈ 1500 ml.

Abnormal losses: Need to keep balance sheet on dialysis.

2. OSMOLALITY. Severe cellular dehydration with expanded ECF. Dialysis will induce hyperglycemia while reducing NaCl concentration.

3. HYDROGEN ION. Acidemia likely.

4. ICF ION LOSSES. Potassium losses in urine heavy. Be cautious in replacing K^+, because of possible renal damage.

5. CALCIUM HOMEOSTASIS. Probable reduction in ionized calcium.

Therapeutic Implementation

Start IV infusion with 25 mEq of Na^+, 40 mEq of K^+ (as long as urine is present), 25 mEq of Cl^-, and 40 mEq of acetate or lactate. No glucose needed here, but 2 per cent solution would be acceptable.

While IV is being started, prepare to

perform two or three peritoneal dialyses one hour apart, with 100 ml/kg of 8 per cent glucose to be infused and withdrawn.

Question: Will not the rapid removal of sodium chloride cause a shift of water into the brain?

Answer: It would, but the marked hyperglycemia will prevent this.

Question: If the glucose maintains the space disturbance, how is the patient to improve?

Answer: Slow metabolism of the glucose will rehydrate cells slowly, including those in the brain. The potassium provided in the infusion should help.

In actual clinical trials (as well as with laboratory animals) this procedure has worked well.

REFERENCE

1. Miller NL and Finberg L: Peritoneal dialysis for salt poisoning. N Engl J Med 263:1347, 1960.

Chapter 18

INTERPRETATIONS OF
LABORATORY ANALYSES

This material is presented to assist clinicians in interpreting chemical data from the clinical laboratory. It is possible to obtain much useful clinical information from the numbers churned out by the clinical laboratory. In fact, in these days of autoanalyzers with an astonishing number of channels, it is quite possible to get more information than is good to have, sometimes. In most techniques set up to be run in an autoanalyzer, an error of ± 5 per cent is fairly common. This is a bit more than is acceptable in a well-run laboratory that uses manual techniques for electrolytes, but for any individual determination, such an error might be acceptable in clinical work.

One untoward result of the use of autoanalyzers, however, is that 20 determinations are obtained when only four or five were really indicated, and the odds are that one of them will be abnormal because of technical error. It is very difficult, if not impossible, to leave an abnormal laboratory result unchallenged. After the second blood sample is drawn and analyzed, however, if the previously abnormal value is now normal, one still has the problem of knowing which result is correct. That means a third determination must be made. By this time, a few more abnormal results and possibly an indication of iron deficiency may have appeared. The only satisfactory thing to do is to tell the autoanalyzer, in effect, to shut up.

Even before autoanalyzers were widely used, some physicians were induced to make clinical decisions from the laboratory sheet without seeing the patient. This practice must be condemned strongly, because only when laboratory data are coupled with an examination of the patient's status and recent history can one make an interpretation that is maximally free from error.

Almost all determinations useful in the management of water and mineral balance are made on serum. In vivo, of course, the various inorganic molecules are contained in the plasma water. The difference between serum and plasma measurement is of no clinical importance. In previous times some determinations, such as urea and glucose, were made on whole blood. This practice has now largely ceased, and serum is the fluid used. Blood urea nitrogen, abbreviated BUN, is not often determined any more. What is determined is serum urea nitrogen (SUN), although it is a rare laboratory that acknowledges this.

When blood is drawn in order to obtain analyses for electrolytes, it is important that great care be used to prevent mechanical hemolysis. As will be discussed in succeeding paragraphs, hemolysis interferes with the obtaining of accurate information on some of the substances in which we are interested. In general, after admission data have been obtained, it is also desirable to draw blood for chemical analyses only during a fasting state (for infants, 4 hours will usually have to suffice). The postprandial period does present a change in the concentrations of a few important substances.

If immediate analysis is not possible after blood has been drawn, the serum should be separated from the cells by centrifuging the sample and decanting the serum into a clean tube. The tube should then be stoppered with a tight seal and refrigerated (not frozen) until the analyses can be performed. For several days, at least, satisfactory results can be obtained this way, although obviously their interpretation will have to be retrospective.

An accurate laboratory is an enormous aid to a clinician. It should be emphasized, however, that for most problems, a careful history and examination will give sufficient information to carry out initial therapy with considerable success. Only rarely will this not be so. Moreover, total therapy utilizing systematic, physiologically based treatment will be successful in two thirds of infants with dehydration secondary to acute illness, even when no laboratory is available. Obviously, the remaining third of these patients are important also; their particular problems provide intellectual challenge as well as pave the way for new discoveries and insights. One of the joys of treating problems of disturbances of water and electrolytes is that there is a much greater potential for precision in this than in most clinical fields. The laboratory is essential for precision. Just as a good laboratory facilitates and affords precision, however, a bad one is such a catastrophe that the absence of any laboratory is to be preferred.

In the following paragraphs we shall discuss some specific laboratory analyses and stress potential pitfalls in their interpretation.

SODIUM AND CHLORIDE

Sodium and chloride may be discussed together even though the techniques for their analysis are vastly different. Sodium is usually analyzed by flame photometry and chloride most often by an electrochemical technique dependent on a precipitation reaction. Both determinations are extremely accurate and one can expect tolerances of less than 1 per cent.

Normal values for these ions remain fairly constant throughout life.* There are a few situations in which the concentration of these ions may *appear* to be abnormal when there is no actual physiologic problem. The most important of these occurs when there is an unusually high lipid level in the serum. A very high protein concentration can produce the same effect, although this is much less common. Sodium and chloride, of

course, are found in the aqueous phase. Clinical laboratory methods are designed to measure concentrations of ions in a measured volume of serum. Since in the overwhelming majority of instances the non-aqueous portion of serum is a constant proportion, we are accustomed to using concentrations that are, in fact, lower than the true concentration of the ions in serum water, where they dwell and are active. Thus, when there is an abnormally high concentration of lipid, more volume in the serum is taken up by liquid without electrolyte. Concentrations of sodium and chloride will appear low even though in the aqueous phase they are not.

When a substance having the same kind of osmotic effect that sodium and chloride have is also present in a serum in an unusual amount, sodium and chloride concentrations are lowered without any physiologic significance. The only natural substance that is apt to do this is glucose, usually during an insulinopenic state. If the glucose level is very high, sodium and chloride concentrations can be expected to be lowered. Mathematically, for every extra 100 mg/dl of glucose, sodium and chloride concentrations are reduced by 1.6 mEq/l. When the glucose is removed, water will be removed with it, and sodium and chloride concentrations will be restored to their physiologic level.

When serum is not separated from red cells and the blood is allowed to stand, a chloride shift will occur from the change of oxyhemoglobin to its reduced form. The chloride concentration of serum will be reduced. On the other hand, a small amount of hemolysis contaminating serum has no significant effect on sodium and chloride concentrations, nor does the postprandial state influence the concentrations of these ions appreciably.

CO₂ CONTENT, OR BICARBONATE ION

The total content of carbon dioxide is measured (by pressure) after all bicarbonate has been chemically converted to carbon dioxide. Thus, both bicarbonate ion (HCO_3^-) and carbonic acid (H_2CO_3) are included in the (CO_2) analysis. If one knows the pH or the PCO_2, the precise proportion

---

*Na^+, 136–145 mEq/l; Cl^-, 98–106 mEq/l.

of each component may be calculated. If the pH is near normal, the ratio between bicarbonate and carbonic acid is, of course, approximately 20 to 1. Infants, particularly newborn infants, have a lower normal level of bicarbonate than do older children and adults. The normal range for infants is 21 to 24 mEq/l rather than the 24 to 28 mEq/l for adults. Infants, owing to their rapid metabolism, may display very rapid changes in acid-base status, so that levels of bicarbonate as low as 4 to 6 mEq/l may be seen after a short illness without the patient being moribund. Such a rapidly developing acidemia in an adult would be life-threatening because the insult would have to be a more severe one.

The three ions — sodium, chloride, and bicarbonate — may be considered as a group in making useful assessments of both the patient and the laboratory. Prior to the advent of readily accessible blood gas measurements, such assessment was crucial, at least to the laboratory aspect of clinical analyses. It continues to remain useful, in that one can look at the so-called anion gap. The sum of the concentrations of chloride and bicarbonate ions in the normal individual is about 16 to 18 mEq less than the concentration of the sodium ion. An increase in this difference, or gap, indicates either the presence of another anion or a laboratory error. The anions that might cause such an increase in various disease states include ketoacids and lactate ions. When there is clinical reason for one or both of these to be present, the increased gap gives a quantitative estimate of the unanalyzed anions. Diabetic ketoacidosis and acute salicylate poisoning are examples of disorders in which one might expect to see an increased anion gap. The several varieties of lacticacidosis cause a similar gap. When the gap is decreased below credibility (e.g., is less than 10 mEq/l), then laboratory error is surely the basis of the problem. The error, of course, can be in any one of the three ions, in two, or in all three. Common sense plus a little inquiry will usually reveal the source of the difficulty. Repeated errors of this sort should cause one to lose confidence in a laboratory. A sad and repeated experience of many of us is that a bad laboratory leads to worse therapeutic action than does no laboratory.

POTASSIUM

Potassium is determined by flame photometry, and the expected error is less than 1 per cent. The normal potassium level[*] is fairly constant throughout life but can be made to appear artifactitiously high. The most common reason for high potassium as an artifact is hemolysis, since the potassium content of red cells is much higher than that of serum. A meal rich in meat, fruit, and vegetables will cause a postprandial rise in potassium. Patients with high hematocrits, such as newborn infants, also frequently show high potassium concentrations on an artifactitious basis, probably because, in addition to hemolysis, an increased potassium release from the abundant red cells occurs when the blood cools after having been drawn. The potassium level in vivo is dependent in part upon the rate of excretion by the kidney. Even in the face of marked body depletion of potassium, the serum level of this ion may be normal or even abnormally high if there is severe renal impairment. On the other hand, even with very poor renal function, if urine formation proceeds at a normal or increased rate, there will be sufficient potassium excretion so that the serum level will not rise on this account.

BLOOD GASES

The determination of PCO_2 and pH has been discussed in the chapters on hydrogen ion. The technique for rapid determination involves, in fact, the determination by several pHs by a glass electrode at different CO_2 tensions. This enables one to calculate or derive by a nomogram of the Henderson-Hasselbalch equation the three important variables: pH, PCO_2, and bicarbonate. Since PCO_2 and bicarbonate values are derived values, they are a little less precise than electrolyte values. Very slight carelessness in the handling of specimens may lead to rather large errors. The "CO_2 electrode" in current usage works on the same principles; the "calculation" occurs during calibration of the electrode. A value for pH, of course, is a logarithm and as such should not be subjected to ordinary

_____
[*]K^+, 3.5–4.9 mEq/l.

arithmetic computation without prior conversion to the antilog.

SUN AND CREATININE

As previously indicated, what is frequently referred to as BUN is really serum urea nitrogen, or SUN. There are a number of analytic methods for SUN that are quite accurate, with a tolerance of ± 3 per cent. The normal value for newborn infants is 8 to 28 mg/dl (2.9 to 10 mmol/1). For children, the range is 5 to 15 mg/dl (1.8 to 5.4 mmol/l).

There are a few conditions in which the urea nitrogen level may be expected to be low. These include starvation and sickle cell anemia. The first is caused by a low body-intake of protein; the second is caused by a high turnover of urea secondary to a high excretory rate.

The level of urea rises quickly when there is circulatory deficiency, or so-called prerenal azotemia. Urea levels also rise, of course, when there is renal insufficiency.

Another useful indicator of nitrogenous substances in serum is creatinine. The analytic technique for creatinine is less precise than for electrolytes. The creatinine level in each age is proportional to the body muscle mass. Thus, values for infants are lower than those for older children and adults. For infants and children up to 5 years of age, 0.3 to 0.5 mg/dl is normal. For older children, 0.1 mg/dl may be added for each year of life to the age of 10 years or so, when the muscle mass is sufficiently large to give the adult normal level of about 1.0 mg/dl. The level of creatinine will not rise nearly so rapidly as the level of urea nitrogen from prerenal causes—a disparity between urea nitrogen and creatinine that may be useful in clinical analysis. One must be careful to keep in mind, however, that creatinine levels do rise, although more slowly, and that both nitrogenous substances show increased levels during renal insufficiency, of course.

CALCIUM

Calcium is most accurately determined by atomic absorption, but it may also be determined by chemical titrations. Normal levels of total calcium are slightly higher in infants and children than in adults. The physiologically active calcium is found exclusively in the ionized fraction, which in normal serum is about half the total. Determination of ionized calcium can be made directly by several electrodes now available. If these are not available, a McLean-Hastings nomogram can be used to estimate the ionized calcium if the total serum albumin concentration and the pH are known. Even this method is slightly oversimplified, since citrate chelates calcium, which accounts for some of the nonionized fraction, and phosphate and sulfate ions reduce the amount of ionized calcium in fluids by forming ion pairs.

PHOSPHORUS

Phosphorus is measured by chemical titration. The accuracy in most clinical laboratories is ± 5 per cent. Inorganic phosphorus exists in the serum as a mixture of $H_2PO_4^-$, HPO_4^{2-}, and PO_4^{3-}. Within the pH range of serum, most phosphorus is in the form of HPO_4^{2-}, with an average valence of 1.8. The normal levels of this mineral are the most demonstrably age-dependent of those discussed here, as shown in Table 18–1. The phosphate content of the diet also influences the serum concentration.

MAGNESIUM

The measurement of this divalent cation is only occasionally valuable in clinical situations. The normal range is from 1.5 to 2.3 mEq/l.

Table 18–1. Normal Serum Phosphorus Levels at Various Ages

AGE	CONCENTRATION (mg/dl)	(mmol/l)
Newborn	5.6–9.5	1.6–3.0
1 month	5.0–9.5	1.6–3.0
1 year	4.0–6.8	1.3–2.2
2–16 years	4.0–5.7	1.3–1.8
Adult	2.6–5.2	0.8–1.7

TOTAL SERUM PROTEIN: ALBUMIN/GLOBULIN

Albumin and globulin are organic constituents of serum, not electrolytes. The error of the total serum protein measurement is at least ± 5 per cent. It is important that serum protein or albumin be measured, because of the influence of albumin on the plasma volume. As noted previously, albumin also binds calcium, affecting the partitioning of calcium into ionized and nonionized forms.

GLUCOSE

This hexose is worth analyzing in many clinical electrolyte problems because of the interrelationships between carbohydrate metabolism and altered electrolyte states.

Chapter 19

SOLUTIONS AND TECHNIQUES

The drawing of blood specimens, the insertion of arterial and venous lines and their management, and the preparation and administration of solutions are skills. As such, learning them must be accomplished by doing them; reading about them can be only minimally useful. In addition, local styles and customs are quite variable and there are many commercially available brands of supplies and equipment that can be used. It usually is better, therefore, to learn the local customs and to practice them, instead of working up from the theoretic concepts for each technique. The usual way of mastering those skills is to "see one, do one, teach one"; this approach should be tempered with thoughtful skepticism and a mental check against theory.

Arterial blood samples are almost always preferable to venous samples when blood gases and pH are to be analyzed, unless one is interested in local effects such as those of arteriovenous fistulas. Arterial blood samples should be analyzed quickly or kept on ice. Excess heparin dilution should be avoided. Arterial blood samples and venous samples to be analyzed for PO_2, PCO_2, pH, total CO_2, or ionized calcium should not be injected into vacuum tubes, since the gases will tend to be extracted from the specimen and alter these measurements.

Although arterial sampling was initially approached with trepidation, with proper technique it has proved quite safe. By means of small needles, arterial punctures can be made repeatedly on peripheral arteries with exceedingly rare complications. The same cannot be said for indwelling arterial catheters, which have a surprisingly high complication rate and should not be used casually. Arterial lines, when indi-cated, should only be placed in arteries with good supplementary collateral circulation and should be removed if signs of ischemia develop. These indwelling lines can be very useful when multiple samples are required, if it is necessary not to disturb the patient when drawing blood, or when direct blood pressure measurements are also necessary. The smaller, transcutaneous cathe-terization devices now available make it technically possible to insert these lines in small peripheral vessels in small infants without surgical cut-downs.[1, 2]

Our favorite site for arterial puncture is the radial artery. It is easy to find, is not crossed by veins, usually has good collateral circulation that can be checked easily, and is easy to compress both manually and with a pressure dressing to stop bleeding. Other arteries such as the brachial, dorsalis pedis, temporal, and femoral may also be used for puncture, but with caution. Femoral punc-tures, particularly in small infants, may lead to arteriovenous fistulas, damage to the fem-oral head, and septic arthritis. The femoral and brachial arteries have poor collateral circulation, so thrombosis must be avoided. They should never be used with indwelling lines, except in the most unusual circum-stances when one may justify the risk of losing an extremity. The temporal artery is a particularly poor choice for indwelling ar-terial lines, since on flushing the line the infusion solution may flow backward, carry-ing clots into the cerebral circulation and causing brain damage.[3, 4] This will almost certainly be true for any other artery in the head as well, and can even occur with excessively vigorous flushing from the radi-al artery.[5]

Gravity drips are not useful for main-taining flow through arterial lines, since

141

most IV poles and hospital ceilings are not high enough to allow for generation of enough water pressure to counter the arterial blood pressure (100 mm Hg = 1360 mm, or 53.5 inches, of H_2O; 200 mm Hg = 2720 mm, 107 inches, or 8 feet 11 inches, of H_2O). Therefore, pumps, pressure generating devices, or occluding devices with a flushing system are necessary. Great care to avoid injection of air and clots is necessary, since the systemic circulation is not as good at handling emboli as the intact pulmonary circulation is. Heparin to a concentration of 1 to 2 units per milliliter is frequently added to the infusion solutions used to maintain these lines to prevent clotting, but care should be taken to avoid infusing enough heparin to act as a systemic anticoagulant. This can be more of a problem with very small infants or with patients who may otherwise be predisposed to bleeding problems because of liver or hematologic disease or because of concurrent administration of anticoagulants. It is possible, with meticulous care in avoiding clot formation, to infuse through arterial lines solutions that do not contain heparin; this is done using the umbilical artery in neonatal patients.

Infusion pumps are also useful in intravenous infusions to avoid the variable flow rates associated with gravity drips. Changes in the position of the extremity of the patient or in the position of the patient, small clots, crying, and changes in the severity of respiratory distress can influence the rate of flow of gravity drips. This can be very important if high concentrations of glucose are being infused or if intravenous medications such as dopamine are being given with which a constant flow rate is important. Rapid fluctuations in the rate of glucose administration can produce hyperglycemia and hypoglycemia. Pumps are also useful if small volumes of fluid are being administered.

The danger of thrombosis with venous catheterization is less than with arterial lines, owing to the excellent venous collateral circulation and to the rarity of embolic phenomena from superficial phlebitis. There is a significant danger, however, of bacterial and fungal sepsis from both arterial and intravenous lines, particularly catheters,[6, 7] that have been left in place for more than 48 hours; they require antiseptic local care, careful observation with withdrawal at signs of inflammation, and rotation of sites when feasible.[8, 9]

Transcutaneous catheterization of central veins such as the internal jugular and the subclavian has become standard procedure in adults and older children, and the techniques are gradually being extended to younger children and infants. The learning of these skills, as stated earlier, must be by doing and by practicing.

The course taken by long intravenous lines after insertion should be checked, as necessary, by x-ray to determine that the tip of the catheter is actually in a central vein and not in a peripheral one.[10, 11] Otherwise, infusions of hypertonic, hypotonic, or toxic substances undiluted by mixing with the blood may be made directly into an organ, with resulting tissue damage. Care should also be taken to avoid extravasation of these substances into the tissues at the injection site.

Venous samples for electrolytes, calcium, and especially phosphorus should preferably be obtained during the fasting state, since eating and drinking may have a transient effect on their levels. Specimens should not be obtained from the same extremity in which an intravenous infusion is running, since it is possible to contaminate the specimen of blood with the IV fluid, producing very confusing results that are likely to lead to an erroneous diagnosis of diabetes mellitus. If the specimen cannot be sent immediately to the lab, the blood should be spun in a centrifuge, the serum separated, and the test tube sealed and saved. If the sample is to be kept for just a few days, refrigeration is adequate; if longer, the sample should be frozen.

The same devices that permit transcutaneous arterial cannulation even in small infants also permit venous cannulation of tiny veins that previous generations of pediatricians would not have considered feasible for insertion of even the smallest scalp-vein needle.[12] The use of a spring-activated device with disposable needles allows virtually painless sampling of capillary blood. This can be arterialized for approximation of arterial blood by first warming the body part in water at a temperature of 40°C for 5 min. These seemingly minor improvements have made the starting of intravenous and arterial lines and blood sampling so much easier than they used to be that current house-staff members may have little experience with cut-downs or femoral and internal jugular punctures.

When fluids are administered through intravenous or intra-arterial lines, consideration should be given not only to the individual components, such as electrolytes and carbohydrates, but also to the overall osmolality of the solution. Distilled water given intravenously will cause osmotic hemolysis of red blood cells. This can be avoided by administering solutions with at least one-half the osmolality of the blood, which can be accomplished by giving fluids containing appropriate concentrations of glucose, amino acids, or electrolytes, or a combination of these. A common solution for intravenous use contains 5 gm of glucose per 100 ml of fluid, which is also known as D5W, 5 per cent D in W (for 5 per cent dextrose in water) and 5 per cent glucose in water. This solution obviously contains 50 gm of glucose per liter. Since the molecular weight of glucose is 180, this solution has 50/180, or 0.278, of a mole of glucose per liter. Thus, D5W contains 0.278 mole, or 278 mmol, of glucose per liter.

Since a molecule of glucose in solution does not dissociate like NaCl into two particles, for each millimole in solution there is one milliosmole, giving 278 mOsm (without correction for the osmotic coefficient). Since normal serum osmolality is about 280 mOsm/kg H_2O, D5W has almost the same osmolality as plasma and red blood cells and, therefore, should not cause hypotonic hemolysis when infused. However, the red blood cell membrane is permeable to glucose, and glucose should not, therefore, be effective osmotically; thus, red blood cells placed in a solution of 5 per cent glucose in water will hemolyze. This paradox can be resolved by recalling that it takes a number of minutes for the glucose to permeate the red blood cell membrane. As long as the glucose concentration remains substantially higher on the outside of the red blood cell than on the inside, hemolysis will not occur. When the red blood cell is placed into the solution of glucose in water, there is time for permeation of the membrane and equalization of glucose concentration to occur, but when the glucose solution is infused intravenously, it mixes rapidly with the blood and hemolysis does not occur. However, when giving blood to a patient, one should use isotonic (0.9 per cent, 154 mEq/l) NaCl, not glucose solutions without electrolyte, as a flushing solution, since the glucose solution in prolonged contact with blood in the infusion tubing or in a syringe will cause hemolysis.

Aside from not causing hemolysis, solutions with an osmolality close to 280 mOsm/kg H_2O are the most physiologic, since they cause less shifting of water into or from body fluid compartments when administered. Fluids with low concentrations of salts, below 280 mOsm/kg H_2O, cause water to shift intracellularly, and solutions with higher concentrations of electrolyte produce shifts of water from cells, similar to the changes produced by hypotonic and hypertonic dehydration. If the amounts given are small and the patients are otherwise well, no adverse effects will occur. On the other hand, with sick patients or large administered volumes or both, problems often develop. For example, a patient with meningitis and mild brain swelling can develop massive cerebral edema and brain death when given a rapid intravenous push of a solution low in electrolytes (see Fig. 17–1, page 130). A similar course of events can develop with inappropriate treatment of hypertonic dehydration. In addition, the opposite effect can occur. For example, the rapid intravenous infusion of a solution with high osmolality in a newborn infant with minor intracranial hemorrhage can cause a shift of water from the brain into the blood, producing an increase in the pressure gradient across the cerebral blood vessels, and an increase in bleeding by mechanisms outlined in detail in the chapter on hypernatremia.[13] These physiologic changes, as produced in a cat by the rapid infusion of a hypertonic solution, can be seen in Figure 19–1.

Prepared solutions containing concentrations of glucose and electrolyte that approximate those usually needed for maintenance, deficit, and abnormal losses are commercially available under a number of brand names. Alternatively, solutions can be specifically tailored to individual requirements by starting with 5 or 10 per cent glucose in water and adding concentrated solutions of electrolytes ·such as NaCl, $NaHCO_3$, sodium lactate, KCl, and potassium acetate as required by prescription. Ions such as lactate and acetate as salts of sodium

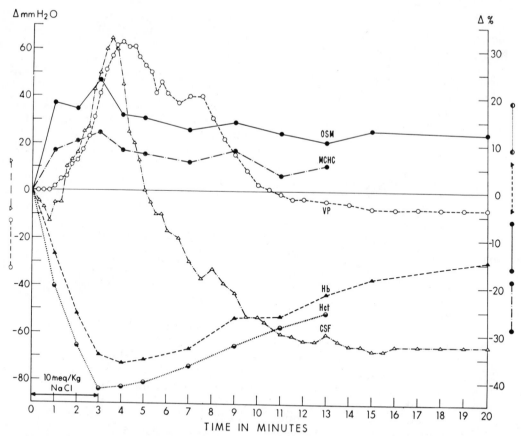

Figure 19–1. Changes in osmolality, mean corpuscular hemoglobin concentration (MCHC), venous pressure, hemoglobin, hematocrit, and cerebrospinal fluid pressure produced in a cat by the rapid intravenous infusion of hypertonic (1 molar) saline solution. Pressure changes should be read on the Δ mm H₂O scale and changes in concentration on the Δ % scale. (From Kravath RE, Aharon AS, Abal G, Finberg L: Clinically significant physiologic changes from rapidly administered hypertonic solutions: acute osmol poisoning. Pediatrics 46:267, 1970.)

or potassium are bases (see Chapter 6, page 41). Even when there is an accumulation of lactic acid from hypoperfusion or another problem, adding lactate will not worsen the acidemia. These anions are not, however, so good as bicarbonate as body fluid buffers (see Chapter 5). Therefore, the immediate effect of administered lactate on pH is less than that of bicarbonate. If there is a significant metabolic block, conversion to the more effective bicarbonate will be delayed.

The adding of concentrated electrolytes to glucose may be safely done as long as sterile technique is used and no major errors in calculations are made. It should be kept in mind that NaHCO₃ should not be mixed with calcium salts lest precipitation of CaCO₃ occur. Except under unusual circumstances the potassium concentration should not exceed 40 mEq/l lest cardiac effects occur.

Gastric feeding tubes and nasoduodenal, nasojejunal, and gastrostomy tubes are occasionally useful for administering fluids. An excellent route for administering water, salt, calories, and other nutrients is by mouth, and this route should not be overlooked by even those most technically proficient.

REFERENCES

1. Barr PA, Sumners J, Wirtschafter D, et al: Percutaneous peripheral arterial cannulation in the neonate. Pediatrics 59:1058, 1977.
2. Johnstone RE, Greenhow DE: Catheterization of the dorsalis pedis artery. Anesthesiology 39:654, 1973.
3. Prian GW, Wright GB, Rumack CM, O'Meara OP: Apparent cerebral embolization after temporal artery catheterization. J Pediatr 93:115, 1978.
4. Simmons MA, Levine RL, Lubchenco LO, Guggenheim MA: Warning: Serious sequelae of

temporal artery catheterization. J Pediatr 92:284, 1978.

5. Lowenstein E, Little JW, Lo HH: Prevention of cerebral embolization from flushing radial artery cannulas. New Engl J Med 285:1414, 1971.

6. Band JD, Maki DG: Infections caused by arterial catheters used for hemodynamic monitoring. Am J Med 67:735, 1979.

7. Maki DG, Goldman DA, Rhame FS: Infection control in intravenous therapy. Ann Intern Med 79:867, 1973.

8. Lowenbraun S, Young V, Kenton D, Serpick AA: Infection from intravenous "scalp-vein" needles in a susceptible population. JAMA 212:451, 1970.

9. Crossley K, Matsen JM: The scalp-vein needle: a prospective study of complications. JAMA 220:985.

10. Rosen MS, Reich SB: Umbilical venous catheterization in the newborn: identification of correct positioning. Radiology 95:335, 1970.

11. Baker DH, Berdon WE, James LS: Proper localization of umbilical arterial and venous catheters by lateral roentgenograms. Pediatrics 43:34, 1969.

12. Tanswell AK: Long-term peripheral intravenous access in the neonate. J Pediatr 94:480, 1979.

13. Kravath RE, Aharon AS, Abal G, Finberg L: Clinically significant physiologic changes from rapidly administered hypertonic solutions: acute osmol poisoning. Pediatrics 46:267, 1970.

Specific Disorders of Water and Mineral Metabolism — Recognition, Prevention, and Management

IV

Chapter 20

DIARRHEAL DISEASE OF INFANCY

The diarrheal diseases of infancy continue to pose a major health problem. For our purposes these diseases of varied etiology are defined by a common symptom, diarrhea. Diarrhea, in turn, is defined simply as liquid stool production. The clinical problem in infancy arises from losses of water and salts in the stool in excess of their intake. Worldwide, over 500 million episodes of diarrhea occur each year in children under 5 years of age, with an associated 6 million deaths, 2.7 million of which are among children under 1 year of age.[1, 2] The association of serious enteritis with poor nutrition and poverty means that the overwhelming majority of deaths occur in malnourished infants. The developing countries account for 99.6 per cent of all deaths from diarrhea.[2] In fact, this combination of malnutrition and diarrheal disease remains the leading cause of infant death in the developing world. In the United States and other "developed" countries, the problem has largely disappeared, although it was similarly severe as recently as 60 years ago in the United States and was present in a number of regions of this country 20 years ago. Even now, in urban North America the inner city population has sufficient incidence of serious diarrhea to have accounted for 2 per cent of admissions (and 5 per cent of hospital days) on a pediatric service (mixed private and public) from 1970 to 1979. The mortality was close to zero and the long-term morbidity slight. For the United States as a whole, however, the diarrheal syndrome continues to be among the first 10 leading causes of death in infants.[2] In this chapter our concern is with acute illness and its continuing subacute sequelae. Chronic inflammatory bowel disease, cystic fibrosis of the pancreas, and other bowel diseases are not discussed here.

ETIOLOGY, EPIDEMIOLOGY, AND PATHOGENESIS

There are a variety of infectious and noninfectious causes of diarrhea. Each cause brings about disease either by inter-

147

fering with digestion and absorption, by stimulating intestinal secretion, or by some combination of these. The most important known etiologies may be divided into viral infections, invasive bacterial infections, bacterial toxin infections, parasitic infections and infestations, and both primary and secondary noninfectious causes. For each major etiologic factor of each type, a description of the agent, the pathology, the immunology, the pathogenetic mechanism, the clinical course, and the implications for therapy are presented in the following discussions.

Etiologic concerns about diarrheal diseases derive significance from three important matters — prevention, pathogenesis, and specific therapy. Some mention will be made of each of these for each known agent. It should be remembered, however, that the successful outcome for the clinical management of dehydrated patients will depend more upon the skill with which the physiologic disturbances are corrected than upon the removal or neutralization of the etiologic agent. Most causes of diarrheal disease are self-limiting infections; the causative agent does not, therefore, persist, even in the absence of specific therapy, although the devastation to the patient may be severe.

VIRAL INFECTIONS

Viruses have been suspected as causes of diarrhea almost since they were first described as "filterable agents" and long before their structure was understood. Only recently have some viruses been firmly established as etiologic for enteritis. Nonetheless, they are listed first here because it now appears that human rotaviruses are the leading cause of infantile diarrhea. The human rotavirus is 70 nm in diameter, is spherical, and has a distinctive double capsid structure. Through the electron microscope it appears something like the thin rim of a wheel with a wide hub and short spokes; hence its name. The genome is a double strand of RNA in 11 segments, and it contains an RNA polymerase. The virus is resistant to heat up to 56°C and to a pH of 3 as well as to most detergents and solvents. Members of the family of Reoviridae, the rotoviruses are a distinct genus. Antigens of the outer capsid appear specific for each

host species. There are at present at least two, and possibly four, antigenically distinct human rotaviruses.[3] The agents have worldwide prevalence.[4] Seasonal incidence shows predominance in winter months in temperate zones and in the dry seasons in tropical areas. By age 2, as many as 90 per cent of infants from various regions show antibodies to the rotavirus. The infection is easily acquired by primary contact from hand to skin to mouth. Outbreaks have occurred in neonates, and nosocomial infection occurs readily, although it is probably preventable by meticulous hand washing.

The virus invades the entire small intestine, probably reaches Peyer's patches through microfold, or "M," cells,[5] and damages the brush border, reducing intestinal enzyme concentrations. It is thought that the mature enterocytes, but not the crypt enterocytes, are infected and destroyed. This pathology will result in malabsorption, which in turn will cause food particles and unbound digestive secretory juices to move downstream, where they will attract water by osmosis and act as irritants to lower intestinal and colonic epithelium. The sodium concentration in the stool water is relatively low, although actual levels will vary considerably because of the contribution of the diet.[6] The stool water in malabsorptive diarrhea usually has an acid pH, unlike the secretory diarrheas described later. This simple test has obvious clinical usefulness.

A specific serum IgM antibody is produced in response to infection, followed by IgG antibody. These antibodies can also be found in human colostrum and milk in sufficient quantities to neutralize the virus in vitro. Thus, breast feeding probably offers protection against rotavirus.[3] Etiologic diagnosis is made by electron microscopic examination of stool or by enzyme-linked immunosorbent assay (ELISA) of stool. These methods are rapid and, in good hands, highly accurate for the presence of the agent. Ascribing causation requires clinical judgment, because the symptom of diarrhea has many causes and most rotavirus infections are either asymptomatic or very mild.

The clinical course of rotavirus illness begins, after about 48 to 72 hours of incubation, with abrupt onset of vomiting and diarrhea. Respiratory symptoms have been noted in 20 to 75 per cent of patients.[7, 8] Fever is a prominent symptom. Note that these are clinical features that favor water loss more than salt loss. To date, however, the etiologic linkage of rotavirus to hypernatremic disturbance has not been made, although seasonal association of the two in North America is certainly present. Characteristically, the illness lasts from two to five days, with viral excretion usually diminished or gone by the eighth day. No specific therapy or preventive measure (other than breast-feeding) is yet known.

Other viruses have been associated with infant diarrheal disease, including parvoviruses,[9] Norwalk virus,[9] adenoviruses,[8] particularly type 38, and possibly coxsackie- and echoviruses.[10] The parvoviruses and Norwalk virus produce disease similar to that produced by rotaviruses. About the others, there are fewer data and less certainty concerning cause and pathogenesis.

INVASIVE BACTERIAL INFECTIONS

Historically, enteric fevers (*Salmonella*) and bacillary dysentery (*Shigella*) are the earliest known identified causal agents of enteritis. Together they account for somewhere between 1 and 10 per cent of cases of diarrhea in infants under 2 years old, depending on the region and perhaps on the vigor and care with which attempts are made to culture fecal specimens.

There are more than 800 species (serotypes) of *Salmonella*. Twenty-three different ones were isolated from 93 patients in a representative report.[11] *S. typhimurium* is the most common isolate in American cities.[10, 11] As the name suggests, mice act as a large reservoir of this species. Pet turtles and products from domestic fowl and contaminated food are important vectors of other salmonellae as well.[12]

The infection rate is highest in warm weather. Salmonellae invade the distal small intestine and the colon, causing diarrhea primarily by malabsorption (osmotic) and increased motility. Toxins may play some role in salmonella infections, but invasiveness appears more important.[13] A number of species of *Salmonella* may penetrate the mucosa, enter the bloodstream, and cause systemic disease. Diagnosis is made by culture of the organism from the stool or, in systemic disease, from the blood and urine. Specific antimicrobial therapy for enteric infections has been disappointing. It is thought to be contraindicated in the ab-

sence of systemic invasion, since such therapy seems to prolong the carrier state, interfering in some way with local immunity.

Shigella organisms from oral-fecal contact invade the small intestine first, perhaps stimulating secretion, but after one or two days all the detectable bacteria have invaded the colon. Although the invasion is superficial, there is intense inflammation and hemorrhage leading to mucoid, bloody stools. There are several toxins, one or more of which may cause the early secretory phase. The exotoxin may also be absorbed from the gut, causing systemic symptoms, but bloodstream invasion by this organism, unlike the salmonella, is rare. After the first day, in some patients the pathogenesis of the diarrhea is malabsorptive (osmotic). Diagnosis is by culture of the organism in the stool. There are several pathogenic species: In the United States, *S. flexneri* and *S. sonnei* are the most prevalent.

The clinical course includes fever, disturbance of consciousness, and explosive bloody, liquid stools. About 10 to 15 per cent of patients have a convulsion, probably from a shigella toxin. The duration of illness is usually a few days, followed by spontaneous resolution, although occasionally the illness lasts up to two weeks. Antimicrobials are effective in eradicating the organism, but they only occasionally shorten the course of illness.

Escherichia coli bacteria have many strains, nonpathogenic and pathogenic. In the next section toxigenic strains will be discussed; in this section we point out that some types of *E. coli* may be invasive and cause malabsorptive diarrhea. These organisms may be identified by serotyping, although some doubt has been cast on the specificity of particular serotypes for invasiveness. One strain of *E. coli* has been shown to adhere tightly to the small bowel mucosa and thus produce diarrhea.[13] The course of illness for the whole group is similar to the mild shigella or salmonella infections.

Several other species of bacteria produce diarrhea in infants by invasiveness; these include *Yersinia enterocolitica* and *Campylobacter fetus*. Both of these organisms are invasive and tend to cause mild diarrhea during an illness characterized by abdominal pain. The seasonal predilection for these as for all other invasive bacteria is summer (or warm weather generally), perhaps because transmission and growth are enhanced then. Examination of the stool for white blood cells, blood, and mucus helps in diagnosing the group of enteritides described in this section.

BACTERIAL TOXIN INFECTIONS

There are two genera of organisms known to produce an enterotoxin that causes diarrhea in infants — *Vibrio cholerae* and enterotoxogenic strains of *E. coli*. Although cholera is rarely seen in North America, it is a disease of primary importance in Asia. Moreover, the discovery of the mechanism of action of cholera toxin foreshadowed our knowledge of toxigenic *E. coli*; the pathogenesis has proved to be similar.

Vibrio cholerae infection requires either the ingestion of enormous numbers of organisms or an achlorhydric state because an acid solution kills the organisms. This illustrates the role of the "gastric acid barrier" as a host defense against enteric infection. If the organisms reach the small intestine, they grow well in its alkaline medium. They then produce a toxin, a protein with a molecular weight of 84,000 with a well defined subunit structure. All cholera organisms produce the same toxin, a chromosomally mediated trait.[15, 16] The toxin rapidly and irreversibly binds to GM_1 monosialogangliosides in the gut cell wall, causing a sustained stimulation of cellular adenylate cyclase production. This in turn increases levels of cellular cyclic adenosine $3',5'$-monophosphate (cAMP), which then causes active secretion of chloride with passive accompaniment of sodium and potassium into the lumen.[15] There is no inflammation, no morphologic change evident by microscopy, and no invasion by the organism. The vibrios may be seen by microscopy in stool specimens and may be cultured on laboratory media.

The onset of the clinical disease is violent, with the passage of stool water equal to about 10 per cent of body weight in the first 12 hours. The chemical composition of the stool resembles interstitial fluid or an ultrafiltrate of plasma.[6, 15] After the first 12 hours, the purging slows but continues for 4 to 5 days and then spontaneously stops in surviving patients. Without antimicrobial therapy the organism disappears from the

intestine in 5 to 7 days. Tetracycline therapy kills the vibrios and shortens the course of illness. The important treatment of the illness, once started, is the management of the physiologic disturbances induced by fluid loss. Therapy may be by parenteral or oral replacement. Vomiting is not a usual symptom in cholera.

Enterotoxigenic *E. coli* is second only to rotavirus as a cause of diarrhea in infants and is probably the leading cause in older individuals. At least two different toxins are produced by different strains of *E. coli* — one that is heat labile and one that is heat stabile.[17] The capacity to produce toxins is mediated by plasmids coded for either or both of the toxins. Thus, the two toxins may be produced in varying proportions by different microorganisms. Some of the toxin-producing strains may also be invasive.[18] It is no wonder, then, that the clinical picture of *E. coli* disease may vary tremendously from the quite mild case to one of cholera-like proportions.

The labile toxin acts similarly to the cholera toxin: it binds to GM_1 gangliosides in the mucosal cell wall and stimulates adenylate cyclase production with the same consequences. The binding, however, is less avid, so the ensuing response is often 10- or 100-fold less severe than that from equimolar doses of cholera toxin. There is also an antigenic cross-linkage to cholera toxin. Stabile toxin does not bind to gangliosides and has a much lower molecular weight (6000).[17] It apparently acts by stimulation of guanylate cyclase, causing accumulation of cyclic guanosine $3',5'$-monophosphate (cGMP) in cells.[19] Most disease-causing strains that have been isolated produce both toxins.[17] Duration of the disease is very short, making antimicrobial therapy of little value, although antimicrobial drugs make excellent preventive agents.

The clinical disease has wide variability, as might be expected. Success in therapy is almost wholly dependent on management of the physiologic disturbances.

Staphylococcus aureus also produces a toxin, usually associated with episodes of food poisoning or postantibiotic enterocolitis. Less is known about the molecular mechanism of action, and this agent is relatively less important for infants. An alga has also been identified as producing a toxin causing diarrhea.[20]

Parasitic Diseases

Giardia lamblia and *Entamoeba histolytica* infections cause a small proportion of diarrhea in infants. The mechanism of virulence for these agents is currently not well understood. Specific treatment is probably of value in eliminating the parasite. Worm infestations may produce diarrhea, but diarrhea is rarely a dominating symptom in such illness.

Noninfectious Primary Irritants

The list of noninfectious primary irritants is virtually endless. It includes anything an infant might ingest, including unwise therapeutic concoctions, poisons, and overgenerous portions of irritant foods. Laxatives, hydrocarbons, drugs, some metals, and soaps are some possibilities. The mechanism of action will vary from osmotic (e.g., $MgSO_4$), to inflammatory and secretory. Removal of the toxin limits the duration. Repair of the physiologic disturbance, once again, is the most important part of therapy in most instances.

Noninfectious Secretory Diarrhea

In this category of illness are included congenital chloride diarrhea, diarrheal diseases secondary to hormone secretion by tumors, and probably the diarrhea that accompanies immunodeficiency diseases. All these disorders may be said to produce diarrhea that is truly intractable, at least until the underlying cause has been removed or countered.

Congenital chloride diarrhea was first described in two separate case reports by the leading electrolyte experts of their time, Gamble and Darrow.[21, 22] In subsequent years the disorder has been found in relatively high frequency in Finland. It demonstrates an autosomal recessive pattern of inheritance. Although early mortality is high, some patients survive with a lifelong disease characterized by watery stools with a chloride concentration around 150 mEq/l. The defect is impaired chloride absorption, probably due to a defect in the chloride-bicarbonate exchange mechanism.[23]

A number of tumors have been described that secrete a substance which in turn stimulates gastrointestinal secretions, the volume of which exceeds the capacity of the ileum and colon to reabsorb the ions and water. Of this group, the tumors most likely to occur in infancy are those arising from the neural crest, e.g., ganglioneuromas. The secretagogue for these tumors is called vasoactive intestinal peptide (VIP). VIP is also produced by non-β islet-cell pancreatic tumors, usually in later life. Pheochromocytoma and bronchogenic carcinoma have also been documented to produce VIP.[24] Tumors that stimulate gastrin or histamine secretion, such as the Zollinger-Ellison lesion, basophilic leukemia, and systemic mastocytosis, also cause more secretion, here from the stomach, than can be absorbed.[25] These rarely are seen in infants. All these lesions plus at least two immunodeficiency states — DiGeorge syndrome and Swiss type agammaglobulinemia — give rise to a perpetual state of watery diarrhea until the underlying problem is resolved.

Noninfectious Secondary Diarrheas

In this category are a variety of intestinal lesions that occur after an enteritis has damaged the gut, removing or diminishing digestive and absorptive enzymes. These include lactase and other disaccharide deficiencies,[26, 27] monosaccharide malabsorption,[28] toddler diarrhea,[29] and the diarrhea promoting effects of unbound bile acids and fatty acids.[30, 31] All these secondary disorders have maldigestive, osmotic, and secretory components from a vicious circle of malabsorption–osmotic load–cell damage, etc. The secretory mechanism is thought to arise from prostaglandin stimulation of adenyl or guanyl cyclase.

Avery defined an entity he called intractable diarrhea of infancy,[32] and recently there has been a report of structural changes in patients with this disorder.[33] In our hands this type of patient, unlike those with tumors or immunodeficiency states, becomes tractable within 10 days or so (no matter how long the previous illness) on a combination of parenteral and oral therapy. The parenteral intake, through peripheral veins, may have to include nutrients, and the oral intake preferably should contain elemental foodstuffs with as low an osmolality as possible.[34, 35] Details of the approach are described in the following section.

THERAPY

The cornerstone of therapy is the correction of the physiologic disturbances of dehydration and its accompanying metabolic derangements. In Chapters 15, 16, and 17 the methods of evaluation and treatment for the first 24 hours or so of therapy have been reviewed, with emphasis on parenteral fluid therapy. It should be pointed out again that oral hydration is equally successful when it is feasible. Contraindications to oral hydration include circulatory failure (shock), unconsciousness, and vomiting severe enough to preclude oral intake. Relative indications include the availability of family members to feed the infant. What is the least expensive, easiest, and preferred method in primitive surroundings, that is, oral rehydration, may be a more expensive method if trained personnel are needed to feed in more institutionally complex situations.

Whichever method is used initially, parenteral or oral, there quickly comes a time for oral intake. Usually this is possible 24 or 36 hours after admission to the hospital, even after the severest shock state. Frequently, the oral phase may begin after 6 hours, even following circulatory failure. Such oral therapy should consist of a glucose-electrolyte solution.

We have seen in previous chapters that parenteral therapy was instituted in 1831 but did not achieve acceptance until about 1910. Oral therapy has much more ancient roots, although not in the quantitative or scientific sense. Breast milk, with its mixture of calories, electrolytes, and antibodies, is acceptable, even optimal, during infantile diarrhea. Folk remedies of cereal waters (rice, barley, gur, etc.) are forerunners of modern oral carbohydrate-electrolyte solutions.[36] During the cholera outbreaks in London in the 1830s, where O'Shaugnessy and Latta (see Chapter 1) foreshadowed modern parenteral therapy, some publications also appeared on the use of oral fluid remedies from this period, but they too were forgotten.[37, 38] Surprisingly, no one developed (or at least published papers on) oral preparations based on the twentieth century advances in electrolyte physiology and clinical care until 1946. At that time, just after Darrow had demonstrated the usefulness of potassium in the therapy of diarrheal dehydration, he and Harold E. Harrison discussed utilizing an oral glucose-electrolyte mixture for two purposes — first, to maintain patients' water and electrolyte needs after parenteral rehydration and, second, to prevent dehydration during the early stages of an enteritis. The initial rationale for the glucose content was to combat ketosis by providing few carbohydrate calories. Harrison's original solution has been modified several times for both practical reasons (its nondeliquescent properties) and theoretical reasons. Table 20–1 illustrates a "descendent" of the original solution, which has been in continual use (with minor changes) for 35 years.

In the 1960s an additional important rationale for the use of glucose was discovered by R.A. Phillips and coworkers.[39, 40] They found that glucose (and other small organic molecules such as amino acids) serves as a carrier molecule, in a 1:1 molecular ratio, and enhances sodium absorption from the small intestine over a range of dilute concentrations. Two per cent glucose (111 mmol/l) proved optimal. Because they were working with cholera patients, mostly adults, they developed oral solutions with high sodium contents (120 mEq/l). They used these solutions for *rehydration*, replacing large deficits of sodium, chloride, and water. For cholera patients and adults,

Table 20–1. Ion Mixture 49–20*

COMPOSITION FOR DILUTION IN 1 LITER		CONCENTRATION AFTER DILUTION	
Sodium chloride	0.61 gm	Na⁺	49 mEq/l
Sodium biphosphate	1.42 gm	K⁺	20 mEq/l
Sodium citrate	2.49 gm	Cl⁻	30 mEq/l
Potassium chloride	1.54 gm	Citrate³⁻	29 mEq/l
Glucose	30.0 gm	H₂PO₄⁻	10 mEq/l
		Glucose	167 mmol/l (3%)

*The glucose-electrolyte solution (modified) in use for 30 years for maintenance and preventive purposes. Powder amounts are shown on left; concentration of solution after dilution to 1 liter is shown on right.

Table 20–2. Oral Rehydration Solution (ORS)*

COMPOSITION FOR DILUTION IN 1 LITER		CONCENTRATION AFTER DILUTION	
Sodium chloride	3.5 gm	Na^+	90 mEq/l
Sodium bicarbonate	2.5 gm	K^+	15 mEq/l
Potassium chloride	1.5 gm	Cl^-	75 mEq/l
Glucose	20.0 gm	HCO_3^-	30 mEq/l
		Glucose	111 mmol/l (2%)

*The left side shows the composition of the powder recommended by the World Health Organization for dilution in 1 liter of clean water, providing the concentration shown on the right.

this was optimal. They later realized that for infants, more water (lower sodium concentration) was desirable because of the high insensible water losses among these young patients.

On the basis of this experience, the solution now recommended by the World Health Organization (WHO), known as the Oral Rehydration Solution (ORS), was developed (Table 20–2). Still later, public health workers utilizing ORS in the field recognized the distinction between rehydration and maintenance and began to recommend supplementation of ORS with plain water or breast milk in a ratio of approximately 2:1, so that hypernatremia would be minimized.[41, 42] The purpose of this approach is to retain the simplicity of a single oral electrolyte-glucose mixture (ORS) because of major problems associated with distributing more than one type of packet of powder worldwide into impoverished areas. We have preferred, in more affluent and better staffed surroundings, to use several different "ion mixtures" for selective purposes. Table 20–1 shows the solution for prevention and maintenance used both for inpatients and outpatients. Tables 20–3 and 20–4 show solutions for rehydration (Table 20–3, deficit repair) and for treatment of hypernatremic patients (Table 20–4), which are recommended *for hospital use* only.

The commercial world has also provided oral electrolyte glucose mixtures. The sodium concentration of these usually is currently 30 mEq/l. This low level probably represents a reaction to earlier difficulties with a solution that had high carbohydrate (8 per cent) and that was prepared to be measured by parents at home, often into various sizes of containers, making final concentrations uncertain. We do not recommend these preparations for very sick infants, although they are adequate for minor illnesses. Whatever the regimen selected, oral electrolyte-glucose solutions or ion mixtures have an important place in the armamentarium.

Currently, controversies rage over sodium content, as indicated earlier, what carbohydrate should be used, and whether homemade salt-sugar mixtures should be used. On the issue of sodium concentration, we have already indicated a preference for the use of several different solutions, each for its selected purpose. This is easily accomplished in a hospital setting but is difficult at home or in primitive surroundings. For home use in the United States, we recommend only the maintenance or preventive ion mixture with about 50 mEq/l of sodium. For situations where large populations of sick infants must be cared for by families or family health workers, the ORS or a similar solution for rehydration fol-

Table 20–3. Ion Mixture 75–15 (Rehydration)

COMPOSITION FOR DILUTION IN 1 LITER		CONCENTRATION AFTER DILUTION	
Sodium chloride	2.63 gm	Na^+	75 mEq/l
Potassium chloride	1.12 gm	K^+	15 mEq/l
Sodium citrate	2.58 gm	Cl^-	60 mEq/l
Glucose	20.0 gm	$Citrate^{3-}$	30 mEq/l
		Glucose	111 mmol/l (2%)

*Oral electrolyte-glucose solution for replacement of deficit in infants. Use is same as that of ORS. Recommended usage in United States: hospital only.

Table 20–4.   Ion Mixture 25–25*

COMPOSITION FOR DILUTION IN 1 LITER		CONCENTRATION AFTER DILUTION	
Sodium chloride	0.58 gm	Na$^+$	25 mEq/l
Potassium chloride	1.86 gm	K$^+$	25 mEq/l
Sodium citrate	1.47 gm	Cl$^-$	35 mEq/l
Glucose	30.0 gm	Citrate^{3-}	15 mEq/l
		Glucose	167 mmol/l (3%)

*An ion mixture for use in infants with hypernatremic dehydration. Hospital use only is recommended.

lowed by the 2:1 alternatives (breast milk or plain boiled water) seems sensible, and it has worked.[42, 43]

Whether the carbohydrate should be glucose, sucrose, a local carbohydrate sweetener, or a glucose polymer is the second problem. The choice should be made on the basis of local availability and economic considerations. All have been successful; if there are no barriers to choice, glucose or glucose polymer (starch) is to be preferred.

Finally, on the issue of homemade mixtures, with which the clear hazard comes from faulty preparation, we think the answer is apparent. In the industrial world, where current mortality from diarrheal disease is negligible and morbidity is low, the use of home preparations is unthinkable. One error in a hundred or even one in a thousand, causing a fatality or brain damage, is a catastrophe. In rural villages where the facts of life are that disease is endemic, costs of prepared powder are too high, distribution facilities are poor, and mortality is high, certainly a homemade mixture will be better than no glucose-electrolyte solution. Moreover, with training, family health workers can keep the rate of error very low.[43] Under these circumstances, one error in a thousand can be tolerated, because of the great saving of life by the program.

Pharmacotherapy

There are two types of drugs that have been used for infant diarrhea. The first type is specific antimicrobials. The usage of these drugs in infant diarrhea evolves from decade to decade and sometimes from year to year. In the sections on bacterial diseases in this chapter, current usage is indicated. The second type of drug includes agents that either afford symptomatic relief or, theoretically, reduce purging. A brief discussion follows. Even the best of these agents have little place in the management of infants with acute dehydration. Some may be useful in subacute or lingering illness.

Agents such as opium and its derivatives (e.g., paregoric), which slow peristalsis, have no place at all in these diseases. Fluid becomes sequestered in the dilated bowel, physiologically outside the body, offering no help and taking away the value of regular weighings. Some of these agents (e.g., Lomotil) may be quite toxic, interfering with respiration. Kaolin or pectin preparations have some aesthetic value in making gels of stool water and may in older children reduce anal irritation, but these too have no place in the management of infants.

Cholestyramine, by binding bile acids, reduces the irritating effect of these molecules and may occasionally be helpful in the subacute phase when there is reason to believe bile acids are present in increased amounts. The drug may also bind toxic molecules, although evidence for this is lacking. Binding of bile acids may also be the mode of action of bismuth salts, although this too is uncertain. Bismuth has been recommended for adults with mild enterotoxigenic E. coli diarrhea, but not for those with serious illness or for infants.

Since prostaglandins stimulate adenyl cyclase systems, inhibitors have been used. In chronic states such drugs, including aspirin, have sometimes been successful, but, once more, they have no place in the treatment of serious levels of acute enteric fluid loss. Other inhibitors of intestinal secretion, including nicotinic acid, propranolol, and phenothiazines, have no place in current therapy, although they provide interesting experimental models in animals.

GENERAL PRINCIPLES OF THERAPY

Before going on to examples of treatment approaches, some general principles of therapy may be offered.

1. Dehydration, if present, should be corrected quickly — circulatory deficits within 1 hour, ECF deficits within 4 to 6 hours or less. When an ECF deficit exists, the initial rate of fluid administration should be rapid even if the deficit is small (see Part III for details).

2. Oral glucose-electrolyte solutions (ion mixtures) may be used at any point at which they will be tolerated, but not for significant circulatory failure and not for preterm infants.

3. If an infant is being breast-fed, try to continue breast-feeding if it is at all possible. Only uncommonly does a breast-fed infant have to be hospitalized.

4. Giving food during periods of malabsorption (e.g., in rotavirus, shigella, salmonella, or invasive *E. coli* infections) will cause osmotic diarrhea. "Resting the gut" is probably of little importance, but diminishing stool volume for a day or two is useful and simplifies therapy. Most infants dehydrated from rotavirus illness will stop defecating when milk intake is curtailed for a few hours. Appropriate glucose-electrolyte solutions do not cause osmotic diarrhea.

5. In oral feeding, amino acids are better tolerated than are whole proteins, which may irritate. Medium-chain triglycerides are better absorbed than are long-chain fats. Starch has fewer osmols than sugar. This makes preparations with the preferred ingredients particularly useful in the recovery phase of very sick or moderately ill infants. Unmodified skim milk has no place in the feeding of these infants. It provides a very high solute load per calorie, thus jeopardizing water balance and predisposing the infant to hypernatremia. (See Table 25–2 on page 190 for comparison of renal solute in various infant feedings.)

Resumption of regular foodstuffs for infants recovering from diarrhea should be very gradual. Food in general and cow's milk in particular markedly increase stool volume. Restoring a few calories is not worth the risk of renewing dehydration or the nuisance of giving parenteral fluids and oral food at the same time. Malnourished infants (see Chapter 21) may need some parenteral nutrients besides glucose; well-nourished ones rarely do. The full caloric load may be resumed over 3 to 5 days — the younger and sicker the patients, the slower this resumption.

6. A brief fast (24 to 36 hours from food, not ion mixtures) is all right, but prolonged or repeated fasting should not be employed. If it is necessary to prevent serious purging, use parenteral nutrition.

7. Almost all infectious and postinfectious diarrheal disease will respond in a few days or, at most, two weeks to the simple measures (not, e.g., total parenteral nutrition) described earlier. Most of what is called intractable is not. When "intractability" is apparent, look for a serious underlying cause such as a tumor or immunodeficiency.

EXAMPLE 1

Enteritis with Vomiting and Moderately Severe Isotonic Dehydration (deficit 100 ml/kg)

(The first day of care for this patient is described in Chapter 16, Example 1, p. 123.)

A 3-month-old infant with a 3-day history of diarrhea weighs 5 kg on admission. After 24 hours of parenteral therapy the patient weighs 5.5 kg and appears hungry.

DAY 2. Discontinue parenteral fluid just after offering the first bottle of "ion mixture 49–20" (Table 20–1) or a similar preparation. Offer at the rate of 150 ml/kg/day.

At the end of 12 hours, substitute 20 per cent of the volume as a balanced milk-type feeding. We have found a casein hydrolysate with starch, glucose, and medium-chain triglycerides (Pregestimil, 0.67 cal/ml) highly satisfactory. This feeding (and similar ones) removes lactose and whole protein molecules from the feed. For most patients this refinement is unnecessary. For a patient in a very expensive hospital bed, however, this regimen will avoid more relapses and cut down on total hospital days at a very slight increase in feeding cost. Note the very slow initial rate of administration. This will keep a few patients in the hospital longer than will a more rapid resumption of calories, but it will reduce the total number of hospital days.

DAY 3. If all goes well (meaning no weight loss and no marked increase in stool losses), increase the feeding fraction of the intake to 40 per cent of volume; the other 60 per cent is the ion mixture.

DAY 4. Again, if all is going well, increase the feeding fraction to 75 per cent of the total volume.

DAY 5. Increase Pregestimil (or equivalent) to 100 per cent of intake (still 150 ml/kg/day). After 12 hours, shift to regular infant formula feeding.

DAY 6. Discharge even if defecation is slightly increased.

Question: Couldn't feedings have been at full caloric intake by Day 3?

Answer: For some infants, yes — but you cannot predict the 30 to 40 per cent who will suffer renewed severe fluid losses. This is how needless "intractable diarrhea" is spawned. This error in management is the most common one seen in modern pediatric services.

Question: Should some babies be kept on a lactose-free feeding?

Answer: Yes, three types of infants should be: (1) those with significant malnutrition or another high-risk problem; (2) very small infants or those with protracted disease prior to admission; and (3) those coming from a population known to have a high prevalence of lactase deficiency.

Question: What about lactose-free soybean feedings instead of animal protein hydrolysate?

Answer: These are probably satisfactory — that is, they work — provided they do not become the sole feeding of the infant for more than a few weeks.

EXAMPLE 2

Mild Diarrhea in a Breast-fed Infant

A 6-week-old infant weighing 3.8 kg who is breast-fed presents in the outpatient department after 12 hours of loose stools. She is not vomiting. Examination reveals slight tachycardia and dry skin and mouth but no circulatory deficit.

This is the ideal time for oral rehydration. Offer 40 to 50 ml of ORS (Table 20–2) "ion mixture 75–15" (Table 20–3) or a similar deficit replacement type of glucose-electrolyte mixture over 60 to 90 min. If the patient takes the fluid, return her to the breast and supply the mother with a maintenance type of ion mixture for supplemental water. Have the patient return in 12 to 24 hours for reweighing and examination. Most of the time, breast-fed infants recover while at the breast.

REFERENCES

1. Rhode JE, Northrup RS: Taking science where diarrhea is. *In* Ciba Foundation (ed): Acute Diarrhea in Childhood. Ciba Foundation Symposium No. 42. Elsevier North-Holland (Excerpta Medica), New York, 1976.
2. Nichols BL, Soriano HA: A critique of oral therapy of dehydration due to diarrheal syndromes. Am J Clin Nutr 30:1457, 1977.
3. Steinhoff MC: Rotavirus: the first five years. J Pediatr 96:611, 1980.
4. Yolken RH, Wyatt RG, Zissis G, et al: Epidemiology of human rotavirus types 1 and 2 as studied by enzyme-linked immunosorbent assay. N Engl J Med 299:1156, 1978.
5. Wolf JL, Rubin DH, Finberg R, et al: Intestinal M cells: a pathway for entry of reovirus into the host. Science 212:471, 1981.
6. Molla AM, Rahman M, Sarker SA, et al: Stool electrolyte content and purging rates in diarrhea caused by rotavirus, enterotoxigenic *E. coli* and *V. cholerae* in children. J. Pediatr. 98:853, 1981.
7. Rodriguez WJ, Kim HW, Arrobio JO, et al: Clinical features of acute gastroenteritis associated with human reovirus-like agent in infants and young children. J Pediatr 91:188, 1977.
8. Hieber JP, Shelton S, Nelson JD, et al: Comparison of human rotavirus disease in tropical and temperate settings. Am J Dis Child 132:853, 1978.
9. Blacklow NR, Cukor G: Viral gastroenteritis. N Engl J Med 304:397, 1981.
10. Moffet HL, Shulenberger HK, Burkholder ER: Epidemiology and etiology of severe infantile diarrhea. J Pediatr 72:1, 1968.
11. Rosenstein BJ: Shigella and salmonella enteritis in infants and children. Bull Johns Hopkins Hospital 115:407, 1964.
12. Fuerst HT: The epidemiology of salmonella infections in the City of New York. Bull NY Acad Med 40:948, 1964.
13. Gianella RA, Gots RE, Charney AN, et al: Pathogenesis of salmonella-mediated intestinal fluid secretion. Gastroenterology 69:1238, 1975.
14. Ulshen MH, Rollo JL: Pathogenesis of *Escherichia coli* gastroenteritis in man — another mechanism. N Engl J Med 302:99, 1980.
15. Carpenter CCJ: Clinical and pathophysiologic features of diarrhea caused by *V. cholera* and *E. coli. In* Field M, Fordtran JS, Schultz SG (eds): Secretory Diarrhea. Williams & Wilkins, Baltimore, 1980.
16. Finkelstein RA: Cholera. CRC Crit Rev Microbiol 2:553, 1973.
17. Sack RB: Human diarrheal disease caused by enterotoxigenic *E. coli.* Annu Rev Microbiol 29:333, 1975.
18. Formal SB, Hornich RB: Invasive *E. coli.* J Infect Dis 137:641, 1978.
19. Hughes JM, Murad F, Chang B, Guerrant RL: Role

of cyclic GMP in the action of heat stabile enterotoxin of *E. coli*. Nature (London) 271:755, 1978.

20. Azis KMS: Diarrhea toxin obtained from a waterbloom-producing species, *Microcystis aeruginosa* Kutzing. Science 183:1206, 1974.

21. Gamble JL, Fahey KR, Appleton J, MacLachlan E: Congenital alkalosis with diarrhea. J Ped 26:509, 1945.

22. Darrow DC: Congenital alkalosis with diarrhea. J Pediatr 26:519, 1945.

23. Holmberg C, Perheentupa J, Louniala K: Colonic electrolyte transport in health and in congenital chloride diarrhea. J Clin Invest 56:302, 1975.

24. Said SI, Faloona GR: Elevated plasma and tissue levels of vasoactive intestinal polypeptide in the watery diarrhea syndrome due to pancreatic, bronchogenic and other tumors. N Engl J Med 293:155, 1975.

25. Gardner JD: Pathogenesis of secretory diarrhea. *In* Field M, Fordtran JS, Schultz SG (eds): Secretory Diarrhea. Williams & Wilkins, Baltimore, 1980.

26. Sunshine P, Kretchmer, N: Studies of small intestine during development. III. Infantile diarrhea associated with intolerance to disaccharides. Pediatrics 34:38, 1964.

27. Clark JT, Quillian W, Schwachman H: Chronic diarrhea and failure to thrive due to intestinal disaccharidase insufficiency. Pediatrics 34:807, 1964.

28. Lifshitz F, Coello-Ramirez P, Guiterez-Topete G: Monosaccharide intolerance and hypoglycemia in infants with diarrhea. J Pediatr 77:595, 1970.

29. Tripp JH, Muller DPR, Harries JT: Mucosal (NA$^+$-K$^+$)-ATPase and adenylate cyclase activities in children with toddler diarrhea and the postenteritic syndrome. Pediatr Res 14:1382, 1980.

30. Binder HJ: Pathophysiology of bile acid and fatty acid induced diarrhea. *In* Field M, Fortran JS, Schultz SG (eds): Secretory Diarrhea. Williams & Wilkins, Baltimore, 1980.

31. Cline WS, Lorenzsohn V, Benz L, et al: The effects of sodium ricinolate on small intestine function and structure. J Clin Invest 58:380, 1976.

32. Avery GB, Villavicencis O, Lilly JR, Randolph JG: Intractable diarrhea in early infancy. Pediatrics 41:712, 1968.

33. Rossi TM, Lebenthal E, Nord KS, Fazili RR: Extent and duration of small intestine mucosal injury in intractable diarrhea of infancy. Pediatrics 66:730, 1980.

34. Daum F, Cohen MI, McNamera H, Finberg L: Intestinal osmolality and carbohydrate absorption in rats treated with polymerized glucose. Pediatr Res 12:24, 1978.

35. Klish WJ, Udall JN, Colvin RT, Nichols BL: The effect of intestinal solute load on water secretion in infants with acquired monosaccharide intolerance. Pediatr Res 14:1343, 1980.

36. Islam MR, Greenough WB III, Rahaman MM, et al: Lobon-gur (common salt and brown sugar) oral rehydration solution in the diarrhoea of adults. Dacca, Bangladesh International Centre for Diarrhoeal Disease Research. Bangladesh, April 1980 (Scientific Report No. 361, p. 17).

37. Collyns W: Malignant cholera: bleeding, cold salt and water in gallons, mercurial frictions, etc. Lancet 1:113, 1832.

38. Rance TF: Treatment of the malignant cholera in the parish of St. Luke, Middlesex. Lancet 2:110, 1832.

39. Phillips RA: Water and electrolyte losses in cholera. Fed Proc 23:705, 1964.

40. Hirschhorn N, Kinzie JL, Sachar DB, et al: Decrease in net stool output in cholera during intestinal perfusion with glucose-containing solution. N Engl J Med 279:176, 1968.

41. Nalin DR, Levine MM, Mata L, et al: Oral rehydration and maintenance of children with rotavirus and bacterial diarrhoeas. Bull WHO 57:453, 1979.

42. Finberg L, Mahalanabis D, Nalin D: Oral therapy for dehydration in acute diarrhoeal diseases with special reference to the global Diarrhoeal Diseases Control Programme. WHO/BAC/DDC79:1, 1979, p. 6 (unofficial document).

43. Levine MM, Hughes TP, Black RE, et al: Variability of sodium and sucrose levels of simple sugar/salt oral rehydration solutions prepared under optimal and field conditions. J Pediatr 97:324, 1980.

Chapter 21

MALNUTRITION: MARASMUS AND KWASHIORKOR

Severe undernutrition involving either calorie or protein insufficiency, and sometimes both, causes serious morbidity and mortality to many of the world's infants. These states may be lumped into a single category, protein-calorie malnutrition, or split into two categories: (1) energy lack with adequate protein (marasmus), and (2) protein insufficiency with relatively normal calorie intake (kwashiorkor). When undernourished or malnourished infants become ill, the accompanying disturbance in water and electrolyte metabolism usually dominates the pathophysiology of the process and frequently determines the outcome of the illness.

Most intercurrent illnesses are infectious. Many infections are enteric, particularly since a high incidence of malnutrition occurs where poverty and poor hygiene exist. Enteric infections give rise to the symptoms of diarrhea and vomiting, each of which may produce profound effects. Diarrhea causes loss of water and electrolyte; vomiting may do this as well but, more important, it prevents intake of water and salts. The blocking of water intake gives rise to the most rapidly dangerous circumstance.

Enteric infections, because of these consequences, are the principal killer of malnourished infants. In fact, the combination of malnutrition and enteric infection is the leading cause of worldwide mortality in infancy beyond the neonatal period — this despite the fact that in "developed" countries there is very little such mortality. Nonenteric infections in malnourished infants also disturb water and electrolyte homeostasis and therefore will be briefly mentioned in this section as well.

Clearly, prevention of this causally linked chain of events by adequate nutrition (e.g., successful breast-feeding) and by effective sanitation is the ultimate goal of pediatric practice. In the meantime, clinicians must deal with physiologic disturbances, understanding both the normal and the pathophysiologic mechanisms in order to bring about correction.

WATER CONTENT, DISTRIBUTION, AND TURNOVER

Body water content, distribution, and turnover all vary with age and to some extent with nutritional status. In malnourished states, the tissues are not equally or proportionately affected. Adipose tissue is absent. Muscle tissue is sacrificed before visceral organs, so composition may change radically. Individual body tissues also deviate considerably from the average overall proportion of water. Compact bone has little associated water; most viscera, on the other hand, have more water than muscle, and so on.

Muscle tissue makes up most (60 per cent) of the lean body mass (LBM) in well-nourished individuals, so it usually dominates the assessment of cell water and solute. Since muscle tissue has less water, the proportion of body water in marasmic patients is higher than in well-nourished individuals, approaching 75 per cent or more of the LBM. In kwashiorkor, where low plasma protein levels lead to low plasma volume but expansion of interstitial fluid (edema), the water content of the body may easily exceed 80 per cent of the LBM. These differing water contents are very important for an overall grasp of the changes in physiology imposed by poor nutrition.

Perhaps even more important are the distributional changes affecting body fluids. As mentioned earlier, each of the compartments and subcompartments has a discrete and important physiologic function. As usual, we are concerned with ICF, ECF generally, and the blood plasma. The ICF in healthy infants makes up about 45 per cent of the LBM (50 per cent in older children and adults). The ECF is about 25 per cent of the LBM in infants. About 6 per cent of LBM is plasma, about 15 per cent interstitial fluid, and about 4 per cent the slower equilibrating extensions of the ECF. When body composition is distributed by under- or malnutrition, changes may occur in distribution as well as in content. Lack of calories leads to disturbed cell protein content and, in some way not well understood, to a lower osmolality. Thus, in marasmus osmolality is frequently in the range of 245 to 265 mOsm/kg. As already indicated, the presence of fewer muscle cells leads to higher total body water (TBW). Fewer cells generally means that most of the excess will be in the ECF.

When kwashiorkor (protein deficiency) is present, plasma albumin levels drop and edema results. The amount of edema and the plasma volume are regulated by a balance among blood pressure, oncotic pressure, and tissue back pressure. The last is determined by elasticity, which is, in turn, dynamic. In any event, plasma volume is low and vulnerable to further decreases, thus impairing the vital functions of gas exchange and renal regulation of ECF composition. Under the stress of disease, further distortion may occur and require the clinician to pinpoint therapeutic efforts and also to calculate what is needed rather than what may have been lost. Hypo-osmolality characterizes kwashiorkor, and the regulatory systems of ADH, aldosterone-renin-angiotensin, and others adapt to maintain the status quo. This will be further described in the succeeding section.

ELECTROLYTE CONTENT AND DISTRIBUTION

As noted in earlier chapters, sodium and chloride ions have a special role in mammalian physiology. These ions, restricted for the most part to the ECF, thus determine by their content the partitioning of body water into its two main compartments. We have previously made the point that malnourished infants characteristically have lower body fluid osmolality than do normal infants. The mechanism is not fully understood, although most would agree that the type and quantity of muscle protein synthesis and the sufficiency of energy for the Na-K-ATPase pump are two probable factors. Studies of malnourished patients' fluids and tissues have shown low concentration of sodium in the ECF coupled with a rather high rate of entry and retention of sodium in the muscle cell water.[1]

A reduction in protein (nonpermeable solute), a lack of energy for active transport, or both could bring about this result. At the observed levels, the usual regulatory systems that help maintain homeostasis continue to operate, defending the distorted but adaptive steady state. Increasing sodium intake results only in increased excretion. If excretory capacity is exceeded, water retention and edema result. Administering potassium to replace cell water sodium also results only in excretion, not in "correction" of the hyponatremia.[2]

A consequence of this adaptive steady state, for the clinician, is that hyper- and hyponatremia must be redefined for these patients. Since 1955,[3] hypernatremia has been defined by a concentration of sodium in *serum* of greater than 150 mEq/l. In fact, any rapid elevation of the ECF sodium concentration that creates a gradient greater than 12 mEq/l (a final concentration greater than 5 mEq/l in ECF) produces the same physiologic consequence no matter what the initial level. If the patient is well adapted, a sharp sudden rise in ECF osmolality subjects him to possible CNS damage, particularly when sodium salts (extracellular obligates) are the source of the gradient. Conversely, a sharp drop in sodium concentration as a result, for example, of drinking 30 to 40 ml/kg of plain water within an hour, will cause swelling of cells generally and of the brain particularly.

These cell changes occur in both marasmus and kwashiorkor; however, in kwashiorkor the situation is further complicated by expanded ECF and low plasma volume. Restoration of plasma volume by rapid protein administration may lead to relative hypervolemia and provoke pulmonary edema.

A further risk is loss of mineral, especially potassium, through the sharply augmented urine output.

Potassium deficiency in severely malnourished individuals has been noted by many workers.[1, 2] The primacy of the findings in pathogenesis has been doubted,[2] but the need to supply large amounts of potassium during recovery has been emphasized by the same workers.[4]

Hydrogen ion and bicarbonate (CO_2) show no characteristic deviations because of malnutrition per se. However, renal capacity to excrete hydrogen ions and to reabsorb bicarbonate is reduced.[5] Ammonia production, however, has been observed to be normal, possibly because of increased levels of glutamine in malnourished subjects.[6] Offsetting of the renal incapacity for acid excretion is effected by the reduced release (and dietary presence) of sulfate and phosphate from protein metabolism.

Magnesium, the cation closest to potassium in concentration in ICF, frequently becomes deficient in malnourished infants.[7] Specific symptoms are not often manifest until refeeding is begun, and then only if insufficient magnesium is provided.

Bone mineral deposition is deficient in malnourished infants to various degrees, depending on the degree of calorie and protein deficits and the mineral content of the diet. Suffice it to say that regardless of calcium and vitamin D intake, if bone matrix formation is deficient, mineralization also will be inadequate. Bone matrix formation is, of course, dependent on adequate calorie and protein intake. Osteoporosis is, therefore, the rule in deficiency of energy and protein. Although one usually thinks of rickets as dependent on growth to be manifest, this is not the case when either calcium or phosphate intake is also very low and there is, simultaneously, inadequate vitamin from either sunlight or diet. Under these extreme conditions, rickets may accompany marasmus.

When severe malnutrition is complicated by intercurrent infection or other insult, levels of phosphorus in plasma may fall below 1 mg/dl. Patients with such a condition rarely survive, probably because such a low phosphate pool interferes with energy processes. There have been survivors following intravenous phosphate administration, but such cases are anecdotal and thus far the benefit of this therapy is uncon-firmed by controlled studies in either animals or patients.

Trace mineral deficiencies may also be present in malnutrition. The role of these deficiencies in water and electrolyte disturbances is not known to be important. However, protein synthesis, upon which the plasma level of albumin is dependent, does depend in part on adequate amounts of iron and copper in the body and perhaps on zinc and manganese as well.

EFFECTS OF DISEASE

Infection intercurrent with malnutrition initiates a series of events resulting in a catabolic spiral that often is ultimately fatal. Water and electrolyte changes are a usual part of these events. During adaptation to severe undernutrition, the rates of both protein synthesis and catabolism are diminished. Catabolic processes are slowed even more than synthetic processes, resulting in a slower-than-normal turnover.[8] Infection (e.g., measles) markedly increases catabolism but not, of course, synthesis. With the resultant increased turnover, plasma albumin levels fall; marasmus will convert to kwashiorkor or kwashiorkor edema will be exacerbated. These events place stress on water and electrolyte balance, disturbing the integrity and physiologic function of the body water compartments. The result may be catastrophic.

If the infection is an enteric one, the symptoms of diarrhea and vomiting will cause *losses* of water and salts and deficient *intake* of water, salts, and calories and, further, will aggravate malabsorption, making even more rapid a downward spiral. The inflammatory diarrheas (e.g., rotavirus) worsen intestinal absorption, while the secretory diarrheas (e.g., cholera, toxigenic *E. coli*) produce higher stool losses of water and sodium but less malabsorption. Knowledge of etiology is good, therefore, not only for prevention and, when available, specific therapy but also for the planning of physiologic supportive therapy, which is more often the crucial factor in therapeutic success or failure.

Loss of plasma volume, either from shifts in body fluid compartments or from general depletion of water and sodium, produces the most dangerous clinical condition — progressive circulatory failure and shock. Five assessment points have been defined: Volume considerations are primary in the assessment of problems of hydration; plasma volume is the most apt to require emergency attention. As usual, next in order of consideration is the distribution of water in the body space compartments, which is mostly a matter of sodium metabolism. After these two assessments, disturbances in hydrogen ion, in cell potassium and magnesium, and, finally, in the skeletal mineral calcium and in phosphate should be evaluated. All these points of assessment are more complex in severely malnourished patients than in others.

Chronic diarrhea will produce chronic mineral deficiencies that are difficult to correct and therefore important to recognize early. The intracellular ions, potassium and magnesium, are especially vulnerable to marked deficiency in chronic diarrheal states.

EFFECTS OF TREATMENT

Against the background sketchily outlined here for the special problems of malnourished patients, the knowledge of parenteral fluid therapy gained over the past 70 years may be readily applied. Parenteral therapy is required for patients with circulatory failure, for those with CNS damage (however temporary), and for those who for any other reason cannot take water, salts, and calories by mouth.

The view apparently held by some that all patients with dehydrating diarrhea require a period of no oral intake has never been supported by data and, indeed, has never been tenable. For example, clinicians have long known that breast-feeding, despite lactose content, may and usually should be sustained in the presence of diarrhea. This has less relevance to the treatment of malnourished infants, however, since breast-fed infants are not usually malnourished. Abstinence from cow's milk feedings has long been recommended because such feedings increase stool losses. We now know that lactose as well as protein is an offender and that the high renal solute load exacerbates the danger. "Resting the bowel" has never had a scientific or empirical basis; removing *milk* has been supported empirically, although it has also been

recurrently challenged by some investigators.

By 1945, specific glucose-electrolyte solutions were being offered as rational therapy for patients either following initial parenteral hydration or prior to the development of dehydration during enteritis. In subsequent years, our understanding of the coupling of glucose and sodium in intestinal absorption has made the physiological use of such solutions even more rational than was first realized. There remains controversy over the optimal concentration of glucose and electrolytes. Part of this problem arises from a secondary perceived need for a single solution that can be used in developing regions of the world. To develop an optimal approach, it is necessary to first go back to basic physiologic considerations and then to see that practical matters concerning distribution, storage, availability, and education must modify the approach to achieve the greatest good for the greatest number of people.

The principles of an oral hydration regimen are identical to those of parenteral therapy, modified only by the special features of the two routes of entry. In a dehydrated patient there is a deficit that must be replaced. When plasma volume is severely compromised, probably only an intravenously administered emergency phase will succeed in preventing fatality. Let us consider here only those situations in which such a phase is not required.

In most dehydrated infants, most of the deficit is from the ECF. In patients with the high-volume stool output of secretory diarrhea, this is almost always so. Replacing such a deficit calls for the administration of a solution with a relatively high sodium content. Sodium concentrations of 75 to 150 mEq/l have been used successfully in parenteral schemes. Lesser concentrations have also been tried but with less overall success. For many years, we have used and recommended 75 mEq/l for parenteral deficit replacement in infants for whom there are not sufficient data to individualize the therapy. The solution for oral usage currently recommended by the WHO (ORS) contains 90 mEq/l of sodium. The current composition of ORS is modified from a recommendation devised for adult patients with cholera (120 mEq/l of sodium). Either 75 or 90 mEq/l is theoretically quite satisfactory as a deficit replacement solution for infants. An oral solution should also contain glucose to facilitate sodium uptake and to combat ketosis. The ORS concentration is 111 mmol/l. To replace losses, potassium is needed in an amount sufficient to deliver about 3 mEq/kg per day. Concentrations between 15 and 30 mEq/l are suitable. The anions should provide chloride and base in a ratio of from 3:1 to 4:1.

Deficit replacement, except when the dehydration is hypernatremic, should be rapid — over 6 to 8 hours if possible. After this, less sodium and relatively more water is needed. Where ORS is the only solution available, some method must be developed to achieve a second solution with lower solute content. Breast milk is suitable but, as pointed out earlier, is not usually available for infants who are already malnourished. Plain water, one part for every two of ORS, will dilute the sodium appropriately but the potassium perhaps a bit too much. Nonetheless, if economic and social factors necessitate a single solution, this regimen making use of plain water is probably the wisest.

In sites with better facilities and larger staffs, there is no reason to limit the armamentarium to a single solution. In the United States, Canada, and western Europe, infant diets high in solute help make hypernatremic dehydration a common occurrence. About one third of these cases are severe. Since not all will be detected clinically, even the initial rehydration solution, whether parenteral or oral, should be safe. After deficit replacement, a lower sodium level is even more clearly needed. A second solution, containing about 50 mEq/l of sodium and 20 mEq/l of potassium (plus chloride, base, and glucose) should be available. This solution is also useful for early replacement of milk at the outset of disease, before dehydration occurs.

Much energy is currently being wasted on polemics concerning oral rehydration because of the belief of some that there is a single preparation for all circumstances. There is every reason to believe this to be a false premise. Moreover, there are techniques, as illustrated earlier, that enable one to adapt to circumstances. Each region should develop the therapeutic approaches best suited to its resources. The ideal approach would be individualized treatment for each patient. In practice, only groups of patients need be identified for special handling.

Malnutrition, poverty, and limited medical or public health resources are usually found together. The lower prevalence of hypernatremia among malnourished infants makes the higher-solute solution more widely acceptable in that milieu. The second solution will usually be plain water. For temperate-zone urban populations with relatively good economic and medical resources, oral therapy may be carried out with an armamentarium similar to that used in parenteral therapy. This comprises at least two preparations.

The electrolyte problems of malnutrition represent a frontier for clinicians. The current wave of excitement about oral hydration may well stimulate research into mechanisms that will further elucidate unsolved problems in the field. The importance of this cannot be doubted if we realize that of all the children dying of the combination of malnutrition and diarrhea, half will have "electrolyte imbalance" assigned as the proximate cause of death.[9]

REFERENCES

1. Metcoff J, Frenk S, Yoshida T, et al: Cell composition and metabolism in kwashiorkor (severe protein-calorie malnutrition in children). Medicine 45:365, 1966.
2. Nichols BL, Alvarado M, Hazelwood CF, et al: Clinical significance of muscle potassium depletion in protein-calorie malnutrition. J Pediatr 80:319, 1972.
3. Finberg L, Harrison HE: Hypernatremia in infants. Pediatrics 16:1, 1955.
4. Nichols BL, Alvarado M, Rodriguez SJ, et al: Therapeutic implications of electrolyte, water and nitrogen losses during recovery from protein-calorie malnutrition. J Pediatr 84:759, 1974.
5. Alleyne GAO: The effect of severe protein-calorie malnutrition on the renal function of Jamaican children. Pediatrics 39:400, 1967.
6. Klahr S, Alleyne GAO: Effects of chronic protein-calorie malnutrition on the kidney. Kidney Int 3:129, 1973.
7. Linder GC, Hansen JDL, Karabus CD: The metabolism of magnesium and other inorganic cations and of nitrogen in acute kwashiorkor. Pediatrics 31:552, 1963.
8. Viteri EF, Arroyave G: Protein-calorie malnutrition. In Goodhart RS, Shils ME (eds.): Nutrition in Health and Disease. Lea & Febiger, Philadelphia, 1973, p. 604.
9. Galvan RR, Calderon JM: Deaths among children with third-degree malnutrition: influence of the clinical type of the condition. Am J Clin Nutr 16:351, 1965.

Chapter 22

THERAPY OF HYDRATION
PROBLEMS IN RENAL DISORDERS

The purpose of this brief chapter is to review special problems of water and electrolyte management during acute and chronic renal disease. No attempt will be made here to discuss kidney disease in depth. Earlier in this work the physiologic role of the kidney in water regulation has been briefly reviewed. There are a number of excellent texts on kidney disease in children[1] and in general[2] that the reader should consult for deeper understanding of those diseases. Comments on specific problems that need to be met in children who present with acute glomerular nephritis and other causes of acute renal failure or the nephrotic syndrome and some remarks on the special handling of children who have chronic renal failure follow.

ACUTE GLOMERULAR NEPHRITIS AND ACUTE RENAL FAILURE

Probably the most common cause of oliguria and anuria in children is acute glomerular nephritis. This illness is most often caused by the beta-hemolytic streptococcus, group A, and generally is manifest from ages 3 through 15 years. Presentation of the patient may include any or all of the following clinical signs: peripheral edema, oliguria, azotemia, albuminuria, hematuria, and hypertension. Our concern will be with edema, the genesis of which is primarily oliguria or temporary anuria for days or even weeks. Occasionally, the patient with acute nephritis will have such profuse early albuminuria that he or she will become nephrotic, a syndrome discussed in the next section. This state is usually transient and can be identified; therefore, it is not further discussed in this section.

The oliguria of acute nephritis is produced by generalized glomerular damage with marked reduced filtration. The result of this is retention of salt, water, and other excretory products, causing expansion of the extracellular fluid. This problem of expanded plasma volume is the most serious early hazard for patients with nephritis, because hypervolemia may lead to pulmonary edema associated with cardiac dilatation and death.

The important part of the management of such patients is the anticipation of plasma volume expansion and the prevention of its occurrence. This is done rather simply by restriction of fluid intake to the amount that is estimated to be lost through the skin, lungs, and stool. If there is some, though meager, urine formation, this volume may be added to the patient's intake on the following day.

In addition to restriction of fluid volume, sodium and potassium salts should be withheld whenever the oliguria is severe — sodium because it adds specifically to the extracellular increase and potassium because rising levels of potassium in the plasma are toxic to the myocardium. Additional control of excess potassium may be achieved by several clinical means. The use of oral potassium-binding exchange resins is one way to remove small amounts of potassium in the stool. For more acute, threatening circumstances, the simultaneous administration of insulin and glucose will move potassium into cells and bind some of it with glycogen (see Chapter 7).

The patient's water intake should be

estimated by the principles outlined in Chapters 4 and 15. Carbohydrate calories in the form of glucose or sucrose should be added to minimize cell breakdown, and the patient should be maintained in this way until the oliguria subsides. Some patients never have a significant oliguric phase. In many it lasts for only a few days, and uncommonly there may be total anuria for two weeks and even more. For whatever length of time the oliguria persists, the management indicated here should be employed, with no water allowed for urine formation except what was observed on the previous day.

In modern hospitals dialytic procedures are available for the management of anuria. The decision as to when to introduce dialysis will depend on the circumstances and resources. Either peritoneal dialysis or hemodialysis may be used. However, as indicated previously, it is possible to maintain patients without dialysis for periods of up to two weeks. This is not necessarily the optimal way to do it, but the fact that the option exists is reassuring, at least under some circumstances.

The hypervolemic state inhibits release of antidiuretic hormone (ADH). As has been pointed out in previous chapters, this is an important signal to the pituitary-hypothalamic system. On the other hand, this effect may sometimes be counteracted by a drop in sodium concentration during periods of high water intake. As with the increased blood volume — indeed, because of it — the low ADH in this disorder stands in contrast to that of the nephrotic syndrome discussed below.

Acute renal failure may also be produced by renal vascular damage to the medulla or by direct toxic reaction to tubules by substances like bromate and borates. Drugs and toxins also may sometimes crystallize in the tubules, causing obstructive uropathy; myoglobinuria and sulfonamide excess are examples. Probably the most common cause of acute renal failure in children is posthypovolemic shock. The entity known as the hemolytic-uremic syndrome may also have a prolonged anuric phase. Rarely, Henoch-Schönlein (anaphylactoid) purpura may produce a nephropathy with oliguria or anuria. Regardless of the cause, the dangers to the child are similar to those of the renal failure induced by acute glomerular nephritis. The same management plan is indicated, consisting of reduced water intake; no sodium or potassium salts or, indeed, other mineral ions; and the provision of carbohydrate to offset some of the catabolic events. Careful management can, again, usually sustain such patients for as long as 12 to 14 days, if necessary. More detailed discussions of acute renal failure should be consulted for greater detail.[3]

THE NEPHROTIC SYNDROME

In the nephrotic syndrome, loss of protein in the urine causes the protein concentration of the plasma to fall below the level necessary to sustain the hydrostatic-oncotic balance. Many complex factors are involved in sustaining the plasma volume under the threat of depletion. Nonetheless, a useful simplification is that the breaking point occurs when the plasma albumin is at a level of 2.4 mg/dl. At this level of albumin, more water and salt escape to the interstitial fluid than are returned with each pass of the circulation. Edema — i.e., increased interstitial fluid — presents and rapidly increases. Distended tissue eventually encounters resistance as the limits of elasticity are approached, and a temporary new balance is struck from back pressure. If the hypoalbuminemia persists, tissues, particularly the skin, give a little more each hour and the edema progresses until maximal anasarca ensues. When the limits of elasticity have been reached, the skin or other tissue finally is literally torn. The body cavities, particularly the abdomen and thorax, become reservoirs of fluid as well. It should be pointed out that the hypoalbuminemia of malnutrition and protein-losing enteropathy produces a somewhat similar clinical picture, although the pathogenesis is obviously different.

The protein loss that occurs in nephrotic states results from a permeability defect of the glomerulus that can be caused by a variety of things. The most common cause is still not understood, and the disorder is therefore often referred to as the idiopathic nephrotic syndrome of childhood. An immunologic pathogenesis is suspected. The pathophysiology is better understood. The protein leak in this empirically described illness is variable in both extent and duration. In addition, there are spontaneous and sometimes frequent remissions and relapses. Regardless of the etiology and the extent of lesion, patients with this syndrome, in contradistinction to oliguric, hypervolemic patients with acute nephritis, are hypovolemic. In fact, this hypovolemia may lead to considerable initial diagnostic confusion with nephritis, because the secondarily reduced renal blood flow may lead to both hematuria and, by compensatory mechanisms, hypertension. The clinician must sort out these differences and decide which are primary and which are secondary.

In nephrotic patients the hypovolemia will stimulate ADH release, which, of course, tends to cut back water excretion. The task of the physician responsible for a patient's hydration is to help maintain an adequate plasma volume, an appropriate sodium concentration, and sufficient urine output so that renal failure is not added to the patient's problems. So long as the patient is putting out urine, he or she may be maintained with reasonable, though not excessive, water intake and normal (though, again, not excessive) amounts of dietary salts and potassium. Severe restriction of these three elements is not only unnecessary but, indeed, even unwise.

Modern treatment of most kinds of nephrotic syndrome, including the idiopathic, usually seals the glomerular leak in the course of a week or so, the usual therapeutic agent being a synthetic steroid of the glucocorticoid type. Generally, the administration of intravenous albumin is not very effective, because the amount administered simply pours into the urine. Potent diuretics also are not often useful, because they increase salt and water output at the cost of creating hypovolemia and mineral depletion.

There are some times when diuretics are useful. One such time is when edema progresses, causing marked stretching of the abdomen, vulva, or scrotum to the point of rupture, offering an invitation to infection. Maneuvers that can bring temporary relief include the simultaneous administration of an infusion of albumin coupled with the use of a potent diuretic like furosemide to relieve a little of the edema without worsening the hypovolemia. Such maneuvers may buy at least a few days' time until the glomerular losses are reduced or ended.

Because of the many different homeostatic mechanisms that are operative, the albumin level in plasma of approximately 2.4 gm/dl may be seen in patients presenting no edema, maximal edema, or any intermediate degree. Levels appreciably below 2.4 gm/dl are invariably associated with edematous states. Patients with levels above this will at least be free of the hypoalbuminemic type of edema.

CHRONIC RENAL FAILURE

Chronic renal disease is characterized by the retention of such excretory products as urea, phosphate, sulfate, hydrogen ion, and potassium. The challenge in fluid and electrolyte therapy is to minimize the hazard. With respect to potassium, a fairly safe clinical rule is that so long as the urine volume is within the normal range, ordinary amounts of dietary potassium are tolerable, even though the renal clearance is extremely low and azotemia is present.

When oliguria supervenes, potassium restriction becomes necessary. Even without oliguria, when there is phosphate ($H_2PO_4^-$) and sulfate (HSO_4^-) retention, these anions should be reduced in the diet. Phosphate and sulfate are found primarily in association with protein. Protein requirements for a patient with chronic renal disease are minimal, since growth is usually arrested, and it is therefore wise to reduce protein intake to a level as low as is compatible with cell repair. When high quality protein or proteins are chosen, this can mean that as little as 6 or 7 per cent of calories may be protein. This not only will reduce the acidic anion load but also will be reflected in lessened azotemia. The urea itself is probably not harmful, but it acts as a useful marker for the clinician. Some vegetables contain fairly substantial amounts of phosphate, which means minimizing them in the diet as well. Phosphate ion, in addition to contributing an acid load, interacts with calcium to produce disturbances in calcium homeostasis. This, too, is countered by reducing diet phosphate. The role of vitamin D metabolites, important in this regard, is somewhat beyond the scope of this work; Chapter 8 provides background information.

The pathophysiology of chronic renal disease has recently been reviewed.[1]

REFERENCES

1. Edelmann CM (ed): Pediatric Kidney Disease. Little, Brown, Boston, 1978.

2. Strauss MB, Welt LG (eds): Diseases of the Kidney. 2nd Ed. Little, Brown, Boston, 1971.

3. Franklin SS, Maxwell MH: Acute Renal Failure. *In* Maxwell MH, Kleeman CR (eds): Clinical Disorders of Fluid and Electrolyte Metabolism. McGraw-Hill Book Co., New York, 1979.

4. Bricker NS, Fine LG: The pathophysiology of chronic renal failure. *In* Maxwell MH, Kleeman, CR (eds): Clinical Disorders of Fluid and Electrolyte Metabolism. McGraw-Hill Book Co., New York, 1979.

Chapter 23

PROBLEMS OF THE CENTRAL NERVOUS SYSTEM: ANATOMIC AND PHYSIOLOGIC REVIEW

The special anatomy and physiology of the central nervous system requires particular emphasis in the context of problems of water and minerals. In earlier chapters dealing with the problems of hypernatremia and hyponatremia (Chapter 11 and 14) and in discussions of antidiuretic hormone (ADH) production, we have covered a number of the problems of interest. These will not be reviewed again here; however, a few disease states bear discussion after a consideration of their unique anatomic and physiologic features.

ANATOMY

It has been known since 1822 that intravenously injected substances that enter virtually all tissues of the body sometimes do not enter the brain.[1] A number of factors are involved in this; most relate to the particular anatomic properties of the brain capillaries and the membranes that bound the cerebral spinal fluid. Figure 23–1 illustrates this morphology. The structures involved in creating the blood-brain and blood-CSF barriers include the endothelium of brain capillaries, the astrocytic processes, the thick basement membrane of the brain capillaries, and the thick cell wall. The brain capillary basement membranes function as an epithelial sheet. Brain capillaries, unlike others in the body, are made of a single layer of endothelial cells consisting of a dense cytoplasm with a few vesicles. They are connected to each other with tight junctions that act to form a continuous layer. The basement membrane surrounding the cells is then covered by glial cells whose astrocytic processes make up 85 per cent of the capillary surface. This structure also charac-

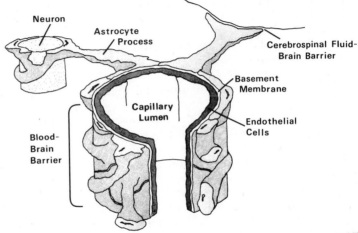

Figure 23–1. Diagrammatic rendition of the blood-brain barrier. The principal components are astrocytic foot processes, endothelial cells with tight junctions, and a thick capillary basement membrane. The cerebrospinal fluid–brain barrier consists primarily of choroid plexus and ependyma.[4] (From Arieff AL, and Schmidt RW: Fluid and electrolyte disorders and the central nervous system. In Maxwell MH, and Kleeman CR (eds): Clinical Disorders of Fluid and Electrolyte Metabolism. 3rd Ed., New York, McGraw-Hill Book Co., 1980, page 1415. Used with permission.)

terizes the intracerebral arterioles and venules. Together with the thick neuronal cell walls, this tissue constitutes most of the blood-brain barrier. The thick lipid cell wall excludes small molecules that pass out of cerebral capillaries but are not soluble in lipid.

The extracellular space of the brain, as elsewhere, is considered a fluid compartment outside the cells. In reality, this may not be an anatomic space within the brain but rather a physiologic one measured by injected markers that have a distribution we regard as extracellular. To some extent, astroglial water may contribute to this space. In the brain, unlike other body tissues, the sodium space is not larger than the chloride space. For greater detail, the interested reader is referred to several excellent discussions of the anatomy and physiology of the brain.[2-6]

The osmotically active solute of the brain differs somewhat from that of other tissues. Arieff and coworkers state that the approximate concentration (in millimoles per kilogram of wet weight) in the cerebral cortex of mammalian species is as follows:

Na$^+$	50–60	mmol/kg
K$^+$	85–100	mmol/kg
Chloride	35–45	mmol/kg
Bicarbonate	10–12	mmol/kg
Ca^{2+}	1–2.8	mmol/kg
Mg^{2+}	5–6	mmol/kg

From this it is obvious that the sum of the inorganic cations far exceeds that of the inorganic anions. Clearly, most of the anions, then, are organic and include polyionic organic phosphates, lipids, and proteins. The work of Thurston and coworkers has made clear that taurine, glutamate, and aspartate may assume particular importance as organic anions[8] (see Chapter 11). It is of interest that, following the induction of severe hypoglycemia, about half the increase in brain solute is due to the presence of particles not determined by the usual analysis.[9]

The entry of drugs into the nervous system is subject to the same physical and chemical laws that regulate the entry of other molecules. Lipid solubility and the degree of ionization are of especial importance in this transport system. The cerebrospinal fluid (CSF), which is a portion of the extracellular fluid of the brain, differs in composition from plasma in several ways.

There is very little protein present in the CSF, so the usual clinical electrolyte measurements of this fluid show virtually no unmeasured anion. Sodium and chloride concentrations corrected for water volume and Donnan distribution seem to derive directly from the plasma. Because of these factors, chloride concentration in CSF as measured is 15 to 20 mEq/l higher than in the plasma. Concentrations of potassium and calcium, however, do not follow the plasma concentrations precisely, and make clear that the CSF is not simply a filtrate of plasma but results at least in part as a secretion. There is variation even among mammalian species for the normal potassium and calcium concentrations. In humans, the potassium concentration in the CSF is usually a little under 3 mEq/l. Calcium is also slightly lower in CSF. Magnesium in the CSF is slightly higher than in plasma.

The acid-base characteristics of the CSF are of particular concern. The CSF pH may be controlled independently of plasma pH because the capillary endothelium is much more permeable to ionized CO_2 than to bicarbonate. In general, the CSF pH is 0.1 unit less than the plasma pH. Therefore, weak acids tend to be excluded from the CSF and weak bases tend to be concentrated there. Whenever there is a clinical circumstance that causes a rapid change in the bicarbonate level in plasma, the effect on CSF pH is, paradoxically, the reverse of that on plasma pH. For example, after the rapid administration of bicarbonate, the plasma pH rises. Because the equilibrium reaction converts some of the bicarbonate to CO_2 and because CO_2 diffuses much more rapidly into the CSF than does the bicarbonate, the pH of the CSF falls.[10] A very important clinical circumstance that may give rise to this problem is the rapid treatment of any kind of acidemia. The discrepancy between the fluids becomes even more pronounced if there is, for any reason, difficulty in exhaling CO_2.

Against this background, it is now desirable to discuss a few clinical situations involving the central nervous system that are not covered elsewhere in this work.

TRAUMA: HYPOXIA

When trauma to the brain or a prolonged period of hypoxia has occurred, brain cells become damaged. This damage leads to an accumulation of small molecules in the cells, some of which molecules are not readily diffusible. This, in turn, draws water into the cells to the maximal extent that the cells are distensible within their mechanical limitations. Such cellular swelling is also seen after poisoning by lead, tin and a number of other substances. This swelling may become extensive enough to close off by pressure some small vessels, leading to further cell damage and infarction.

To some extent this swelling may be controlled by therapeutic maneuvers with intravenous water and hypertonic solute. Hypertonic solutions of mannitol, a substance that is confined to the extracellular space, have been particularly useful in reducing brain swelling. Mannitol molecules are promptly excreted in the urine because they are not reabsorbed. Thus, the agent and the excess water carried by it osmotically may be thought of as arriving in the urine, when renal function permits. The important thing, however, is that the hypertonic mannitol has first, by establishing an osmol gradient, withdrawn cell water — in particular, cell water of the brain. Hypertonic solutions of glucose initially act similarly. Glucose, however, will eventually diffuse into cells and will be metabolized. Thus, a rebound phenomenon occurs. Corticosteroids, through an unknown mechanism, reduce cerebral swelling, but there is approximately a 24-hour time-lag between administration of the drug and observable effect.

INFECTIONS OF THE MENINGES

During bacterial meningitis, there is, of course, altered permeability from the blood to the brain and the CSF. In addition, the irritation of the brain is a stimulus to the production of ADH. Finally, in bacterial infections of almost any kind, a water load develops from cell destruction that is resistant to excretion.[11, 12] Whether this is mediated by ADH is still unclear. All these factors tend to produce a hyponatremic state during bacterial meningitis. They also make the patient vulnerable to a sudden increase in intracranial pressure following the administration of a rapid infusion of hypotonic solutions. For this purpose, a 5 per cent solution of glucose is hypotonic because of the active transport of glucose across brain

capillaries. Since the meningitis has already increased the intracranial pressure, such water loads are dangerous to the point of being lethal. Thus, deficit repair during meningitis, particularly when it must be rapid, should always be effected with solutions that have a sodium concentration close to that of extracellular fluid. Maintenance water should always be delivered slowly, whether by vein or by mouth.

TUBERCULOUS MENINGITIS

In chronic tuberculous meningitis, a special and rather unusual situation exists: hyponatremia and hypochloremia affect the CSF as well as body fluids generally. This is the basis for the former diagnostic use of chloride concentration in the spinal fluid in days before sodium analyses were readily available. Although patients will display the usual fluctuations during the periods of dehydration and rehydration, at a steady state they will almost invariably show hyponatremia and hypochloremia.

When patients with tuberculous meningitis were analyzed some years ago by a variety of studies including tissue analysis, interesting results were obtained that are not yet fully explainable.[13] Despite the hyponatremia of these patients, who had usual salt intakes, there was no decrease in total body sodium or muscle tissue sodium. Although there was some increase in body water in these undernourished patients, the increase was not sufficient to account for the dilution. It was discovered that there was, instead, a marked deficiency of muscle cell potassium with considerable entry of sodium into the muscle cells.

If sodium chloride is given patients with tuberculous meningitis, the plasma and CSF values can be brought to normal but the patients are edematous and demonstrably sicker. When large amounts of potassium are given, the ion simply spills into the urine unless given so fast that toxicity occurs. On the other hand, when these patients begin to recover, potassium from the diet is retained in cells, sodium returns to the ECF, volume adjusts, and a normal electrolyte pattern returns. Although this phenomenon has been ascribed by some authors to changes in ADH secretion, we tend to believe that ADH is not significantly involved in the genesis of these events. They remain unexplained and perhaps represent a clue to cerebral components of body composition that are not yet appreciated.

REFERENCES

1. Crone C: General properties of the blood-brain barrier with special emphasis on glucose. In Cserr HF, Fenstermacher JO, Fencl V (eds): Fluid Environment of the Brain. Academic Press, New York, 1975, pp. 33–46.
2. Davson H: Physiology of the Cerebrospinal Fluid. Little Brown, Boston, 1967.
3. Rapoport SI: Blood-Brain Barrier in Physiology and Medicine. Raven Books, Abelard-Schuman Ltd, New York, 1976.
4. Arieff AI, Schmidt RW: Fluid and electrolyte disorders and the central nervous sytem. In Maxwell MH, Kleeman CR (eds): Clinical Disorders of Fluid and Electrolyte Metabolism, 3rd Ed, McGraw-Hill, New York, 1979.
5. Katzman R, Pappius HM: Brain Electrolyte and Fluid Metabolism. Williams & Wilkins, Baltimore, 1973.
6. Goldstein GW: Pathogenesis of brain edema and hemorrhage: role of the brain capillary. J Pediatr 64:357, 1979.
7. Arieff AI, Kerian A, Massry SG, DeLima J: Intracellular pH of the brain: alterations in acute respiratory acidosis and alkalosis. Am J Physiol 230:804, 1976.
8. Thurston JH, Haurart RE, Dirgo JA: Taurine: a role in osmotic regulation of mammalian brain and possible clinical significance. Life Sci 26:1561, 1980.
9. Arieff AI, Guisado R, Lazarowicz VC: The pathophysiology of hyperosmolar states. In Andreoli TE, Grantham JJ, Rector FC (eds): Disturbances in Body Fluid Osmolality. American Physiological Society. Williams & Wilkins, Baltimore, 1977.
10. Posner JB, Plum F: Spinal fluid pH and neurologic symptoms in systemic acidosis. N Engl J Med 277:605, 1967.
11. Gonzalez C, Finberg L, Bluestein D: Electrolyte concentrations during acute infections in infants and children. Am J Dis Child 107:476, 1964.
12. Finberg L, Gonzalez C: Experimental studies on the hyponatremia of acute infections. Metabolism 14:693, 1965.
13. Harrison HE, Finberg L, Fleischman E: Disturbances of ionic equilibrium of extracellular and intracellular electrolytes in patients with tuberculous meningitis. J Clin Invest 31:300, 1952.

Chapter 24

DISORDERS OF THE ADRENAL GLAND AS CAUSES OF ELECTROLYTE DISTURBANCES: DIAGNOSIS AND TREATMENT

ADRENOCORTICAL INSUFFICIENCY IN INFANCY

Following birth the function of the fetal adrenal glands changes dramatically from the production of steroids, such as dehydroepiandrosterone sulfate (DHEAS), which serve as precursors for placental estrogen synthesis, to a major role in the maintenance of fluid and electrolyte balance. The adrenal gland of the human fetus is 10 to 20 times larger than the adult gland relative to body weight.[1] Eighty per cent of the adrenal is occupied by the fetal zone, which involutes rapidly and disappears completely by approximately the sixth month of life. As the fetal cortex involutes, it is replaced by adult-type cells, resulting in three distinctive zones: the zona glomerulosa (mineralocorticoids), zona fasciculata (glucocorticoids), and zona reticularis (adrenal androgens).

The clinical manifestations of abnormal adrenal function in the newborn period result in most instances from inadequate secretion of glucocorticoids, mineralocorticoids, or both. For a list of clinical signs of adrenal insufficiency in infancy and childhood, see Table 24–1.[2]

As a consequence of enzyme defects in steroidogenesis affecting the adrenal as well as the gonad, production of glucocorticoids, mineralocorticoids, and sex steroids may be increased or decreased.

Virilization of the external genitalia in females or undervirilization in male infants may result. Despite little variation in the

Table 24–1. Clinical Manifestations of Adrenal Insufficiency in Infancy and Childhood

CORTISOL DEFICIENCY
  Hypoglycemia
  Vasomotor collapse
  Hyperpigmentation (ACTH excess)
  Apneic spells
  Seizure

ALDOSTERONE DEFICIENCY
  Vomiting
  Poor feeding
  Hyponatremia
  Urinary salt wasting
  Hyperkalemia
  Metabolic acidosis
  Failure to thrive
  Volume depletion
  Hypotension
  Dehydration
  Cyanosis
  Shock

ANDROGEN EXCESS OR DEFICIENCY
  Ambiguous genitalia

phenotype, ambiguity of the external genitalia at birth may have many causes.[3] Precise diagnosis is essential for appropriate therapy, both short-term and long-term, and for proper genetic counseling.

Causes of adrenal insufficiency in the neonatal period and childhood are listed in Table 24–2. These causes include primary and secondary adrenocortical insufficiency. Primary adrenocortical insufficiency is due to failure of the gland to secrete adequate amounts of hormone, even with maximal stimulation. Secondary adrenocortical in-

171

Table 24–2.   Causes of Adrenal Insufficiency in Infancy and Childhood

---

Congenital adrenal hypoplasia secondary to ACTH
    deficiency:
        Autosomal recessive
        X-linked
Adrenal hemorrhage
Congenital adrenal unresponsiveness to ACTH
Addison disease
Isolated hypoaldosteronism
Schilder disease
Isolated deficiency of aldosterone synthesis due to
        18-hydroxylase deficiency
        18-hydroxysteroid dehydrogenase deficiency
Pseudohypoaldosteronism—End organ unresponsive-
    ness to aldosterone
Congenital adrenal hyperplasia
Deficiency of enzymes prior to pregnenolone 20, 22-
    desmolase deficiency
3β-Hydroxysteroid dehydrogenase deficiency
17-Hydroxylase deficiency
21-Hydroxylase deficiency
11β-Hydroxylase deficiency

---

sufficiency occurs because of insufficient stimulation of the adrenal gland by the trophic hormones ACTH (adenocorticotropic hormone) and angiotensin. Since the primary effect of ACTH is control of cortisol synthesis and secretion, glucocorticoid insufficiency characterizes ACTH insufficiency, and patients with anterior hypopituitarism usually do not have disturbances of mineral metabolism or require mineralocorticoid hormone replacement.

Clinically, disorders of adrenal function are most critical in the newborn period and in infancy. They may produce abnormalities of fluid and electrolyte balance, vomiting, hypoglycemia, vasomotor collapse, or ambiguous genitalia in males and females, representing inborn defects of steroidogenesis that may be expressed in the adrenal as well as the gonad.

The glucocorticoids exert an effect on electrolyte metabolism via their effects on the kidney. The effect on the glomerular filtration rate (GFR) is evidenced by the low GFR in adrenally insufficient patients. GFR rises in both normal and adrenally insufficient subjects after administration of glucocorticoids in pharmacologic doses. Glucocorticoids also exert another important effect, augmenting renal water excretion. Thus, patients with adrenal insufficiency are unable to dilute urine sufficiently to excrete a water load normally, and the extracellular fluid therefore becomes diluted.

Excretion of a dilute urine also requires maintenance of impermeability to water in the collecting duct, so that water cannot readily diffuse back into the circulation. The impermeability to water depends upon the absence of antidiuretic hormone (ADH), and glucocorticoids appear to inhibit secretion of ADH. Lack of glucocorticoids also increases the water permeability in distal renal tubular cells.

Among the adrenal steroids, aldosterone has the strongest sodium-conserving action. As with cortisol, the primary determinant of the plasma level of aldosterone is the secretion rate. The secretion of aldosterone is controlled by ACTH, the renin-angiotensin system, and serum potassium concentration, but the most important of these is the renin-angiotensin system (see also Chapter 7). The role of ACTH in the control of aldosterone secretion is probably only a permissive one.

CONGENITAL ADRENAL HYPOPLASIA

Congenital adrenal hypoplasia of the adrenal glands may occur in combination with congenital hypoplasia or aplasia of the pituitary. Congenital adrenal hypoplasia is often associated with anencephaly. Isolated and familial forms have been described.[4, 5]

Infants may present with vomiting, convulsions, cyanosis, apneic spells, and hypoglycemia.[6] Until recently, most patients died in early infancy. A clue to the antenatal existence of this condition may be extremely low maternal levels and excretion of estrogens, particularly estriol, reflecting lack of DHEAS as a precursor substance provided by the fetal adrenal gland. This clue is particularly useful in mothers with a previous history of sudden, unexplained death of a newborn infant.[2]

Characteristically, plasma levels and urinary excretion of all steroidal hormones are low or undetectable. Since gonadal function is normal, genitalia are normally formed. The differential diagnosis includes adrenal insufficiency, adrenal hemorrhage, or congenital adrenal hyperplasia due to 20, 22-desmolase deficiency—a block in the earliest steps in steroid biosynthesis. Therapy consisting of replacement of glucocorticoids and mineralocorticoids may be life-saving.

ADRENAL HEMORRHAGE

Adrenal hemorrhage can occur in the newborn period and be associated with adrenal insufficiency. The etiology of this condition is unknown, but birth trauma to the large and rapidly involuting newborn adrenal is the most widely accepted theory. The onset is usually between the second and seventh day of life.[7] The clinical findings may be severe (see Table 24–1). There may be unexplained jaundice and a palpable abdominal mass. Calcification of the adrenal gland may be visible within three or four weeks and persists for life.[8] Treatment, after correction of shock and rehydration, is with replacement of gluco- and mineralocorticoids and is commonly lifelong, although resolution and spontaneous recovery may occur.

HEREDITARY ADRENOCORTICAL UNRESPONSIVENESS TO ACTH

This syndrome is characterized by recurrent vomiting episodes and hypoglycemia, often manifesting as seizures, and hyperpigmentation of the skin and buccal mucosa. In the absence of electrolyte disturbances, this constellation suggests glucocorticoid deficiency and overproduction of ACTH with its inherent melanocyte-stimulating hormone activity. Plasma cortisol, urinary 17-hydroxycorticoids, and 17-ketosteroids are low, yet aldosterone levels or production rates are low and increase promptly in response to a low sodium diet.[9, 10] Antibodies to adrenal tissue are not present in affected patients.[10] ACTH levels are high and adrenal steroids do not respond to administered ACTH.[11]

Treatment consists of appropriate replacement with glucocorticoids; supplemental salt and mineralocorticoid administration are not necessary, since mineralocorticoid responsiveness to angiotensin II is conserved.

A variant of this syndrome, associated with achalasia of the cardia and disturbed autonomic function, including deficient lacrimation, has recently been described.[11a]

ADDISON DISEASE

Primary atrophy is considered the leading cause of idiopathic Addison disease.[12] Autoantibodies against select or all layers of the adrenal, which are frequently present, suggest strongly that it is an autoimmune disorder. Antibodies against other tissues (e.g., gonads, pancreas) are often found in Addison disease as well.[13] Addison disease may occur in association with other endocrinopathies, particularly idiopathic hypoparathyroidism, chronic lymphocytic thyroiditis, diabetes mellitus, hyperthyroidism, and pernicious anemia. Chronic mucocutaneous candidiasis is frequently associated with Addison disease and may even antecede it.[14]

The clinical manifestations of cortisol and aldosterone deficiency are described in Table 24–1. There is little, if any, rise in plasma cortisol after ACTH infusion. A failure to respond to ACTH stimulation can be considered diagnostic. Glucocorticoid *and* mineralocorticoid therapy is necessary. For maintenance steroid dosages, see Table 24–5.

A defect in water excretion has been demonstrated in both primary and secondary adrenal insufficiency. It is this defect in water metabolism and the tendency to lose sodium in the urine that account for the frequently observed hyponatremia in these patients.

SELECTIVE DEFICIENCY OF ALDOSTERONE SECRETION

Selective deficiency of aldosterone secretion without alterations in cortisol production results in persistent hyperkalemia, renal salt wasting, and postural hypotension. The hyperkalemia may be associated with profound muscle weakness and cardiac arrhythmias. Etiologies include specific deficiencies of the enzymes involved in aldosterone biosynthesis (see Fig. 24–1 and Table 24–2), selective destruction of the zona glomerulosa, or a deficiency in renin production. In the disorders of aldosterone biosynthesis and in those situations in which the zona glomerulosa alone appears to fail, plasma renin activity is usually elevated. By contrast, in those disorders in which alterations in the function of the renin angiotensin system are observed, plasma renin activity is generally unmeasurably low.[15]

The clinical manifestations of isolated hypoaldosteronism are promptly reversed

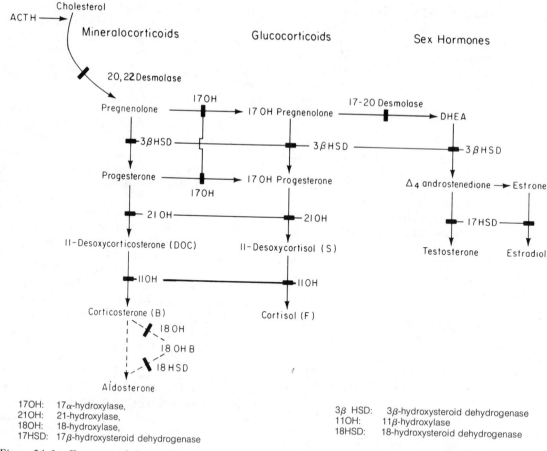

Figure 24–1. Enzymatic deficiencies in the biosynthetic and metabolic pathways of mineralocorticoids, glucocorticoids, and sex hormones.

by the administration of exogenous mineralocorticoids, such as 9α-fluorocortisol.

PSEUDOHYPOALDOSTERONISM

Pseudohypoaldosteronism is a renal tubular disorder characterized by excessive urinary sodium loss. This disorder is manifested by repeated episodes of dehydration, hyponatremia, and hyperkalemia during infancy. Pseudohypoaldosteronism is due to an end-organ defect in the distal renal tubule, with profound failure of response to endogenous aldosterone. Aldosterone secretion and urinary excretion are usually elevated and the plasma renin activity is high. Other adrenal hormones are normal. The sodium concentration in sweat is elevated.

None of the sodium-conserving organs in which there is sodium transport dependent on mineralocorticoids (kidney, salivary and sweat glands, colon) respond to mineralocorticoid therapy.[16] The only avenue of therapy is, therefore, oral sodium chloride supplement.

ADRENAL HYPERFUNCTIONING STATES

Hypercortisolism

Cushing disease refers only to endogenous secretion of excessive glucocorticoids secondary to excess secretion of pituitary ACTH by a pituitary adenoma. *Cushing syndrome* may be due to either adrenal cortical tumor or hyperplasia, but an adrenal tumor is more likely if features of both hypercortisolemia and virilization are present. The term *Cushing syndrome* accordingly applies to patients suffering from either excessive endogenous or excessive exogenous glucocorticoids. The typical clinical manifestations of Cushing syndrome include facial rounding and a plethoric appearance, truncal obesity, buffalo hump, weakness and fatigue, thinning of the skin, striae, hyperpigmentation in the skin folds, ecchymosis due to increased capillary fragility, hypertension, and growth failure. The exact clinical picture in any child is determined by the severity and duration of the hypercortisolism, the presence or absence of associated mineralocorticoid, and androgen or estrogen excess. Thus, the protein-wasting action of cortisol is often masked in children with adrenal carcinoma by the anabolic effect of androgens.[17, 18]

Abnormal electrolyte findings in patients with Cushing syndrome result to a large extent from the effects of cortisol. Serum potassium may be decreased, and as a result a hypokalemic alkalosis may be present. Sex steroids and aldosterone may also be elevated. Elevated glucocorticoids, nonsuppressible by standard doses of exogenous glucocorticoid (dexamethasone), establish the diagnosis.[19]

It is important to start the patient on parenteral glucocorticoids both before and immediately after surgery to avoid a crisis of adrenal insufficiency.

Hyperaldosteronism

Causes of hyperaldosteronism are listed in Table 24–3. The separation into primary and secondary hyperaldosteronism is based on whether the stimulus for increased secretion of aldosterone comes from the adrenal gland itself or from an extra-adrenal source. If the stimulus is intra-adrenal, there is a decreased level of circulating plasma renin activity. In secondary aldosteronism, there is an excess of circulating plasma renin activity.[15]

Primary hyperaldosteronism is a rare but potentially curable cause of hypertension. As outlined in Chapter 7, the principal action of aldosterone is on the distal tubule of the kidney to enhance the reabsorption of sodium. At this site, obligatory exchange of potassium or hydrogen ions for reabsorbed sodium takes place. Accordingly, autonomous pathologic excess aldosterone production leads to potassium depletion and development of a metabolic alkalosis. It is

Table 24–3. Causes of Hyperaldosteronism*

A. Primary Hyperaldosteronism
  1. Adrenocortical hyperplasia
     a. Glucocorticoid suppressible
     b. Glucocorticoid nonsuppressible
  2. Adrenocortical adenoma

B. Secondary Hyperaldosteronism
  1. Physiologic
     a. Decreased plasma volume (upright posture, dehydration, hemorrhage)
     b. Electrolyte imbalance (K^+ loading, Na^+ depletion)
  2. Pathologic
     a. With edema (nephrotic syndrome, congestive heart failure, severe hypoproteinemia, cirrhosis)
     b. Without edema (congenital or acquired renovascular disease)
  3. Bartter syndrome
  4. Renal tubular insensitivity to aldosterone (pseudohypoaldosterone)
  5. Cystic fibrosis

*Adapted from New MI, Peterson RE: Disorders of aldosterone secretion in childhood. Pediatr Clin North Am 13:43, 1966.

important to identify this condition before surgery, because the blood pressure response to adrenalectomy may be highly variable. In patients with a solitary adenoma, adrenalectomy can be performed with a high probability of cure of hypertension and correction of the electrolyte abnormalities. In patients with bilateral adrenal hyperplasia, bilateral adrenalectomy frequently fails to reduce the blood pressure, although the hyperkalemic alkalosis is corrected.[15]

Hypokalemia (< 3.5 mEq/l) is the most consistent biochemical finding. Metabolic alkalosis is also present. An alkaline and isotonic urine is produced with markedly increased bicarbonate and ammonia excretion. Serum calcium and magnesium levels are almost always normal. Carbohydrate intolerance may be present and is a reflection of chronic potassium depletion acting on both insulin secretion and its peripheral action.[20]

Primary hyperaldosteronism is suspected in a hypertensive, hypokalemic patient who shows renal potassium loss on a normal sodium and potassium intake. The final diagnosis of primary hyperaldosteronism requires documentation of aldosterone excess as measured by plasma aldosterone or a metabolite of aldosterone in the urine. In addition, depressed plasma renin activity has to be documented.[21] To document inappropriately high aldosterone, measurements are made on a high sodium intake. It should be noted that sodium loading will intensify potassium depletion.[22]

Causes of secondary hyperaldosteronism are listed in Table 24–3. Plasma renin activity is high in secondary hyperaldosteronism.

In general, secondary hyperaldosteronism is associated with one of the following:[15]

1. Depletion of extracellular fluid volume, such as sodium depletion or severe water deprivation

2. Reduction of plasma volume (hypoproteinemia)

3. Sequestration of blood on the venous side of the circulation (cirrhosis)

BARTTER SYNDROME (see also Chapter 28)

Bartter syndrome is a special cause of secondary hyperaldosteronism. This syndrome commonly occurs in late infancy or early childhood and is characterized by hypokalemia, hypochloremia, alkalosis, normal blood pressure, hyperaldosteronism, and hyperplasia of the juxtaglomerular apparatus,[23] with elevated plasma renin activity.[23] Other features include growth retardation and muscle weakness. Plasma renin activity and the aldosterone response to infused angiotensin are diminished.[23]

The precise pathogenesis of Bartter syndrome is unknown, but impaired reabsorption of sodium in the ascending limb of the loop of Henle seems likely.[24] Erythrocyte sodium transport is abnormal in Bartter syndrome. If this alteration could be related to the pathophysiology of Bartter syndrome, it would lend support to the assumption that there is a genetically determined defect of membrane ion transport.[24]

There is considerable evidence that renal prostaglandin (Pg) has a role in the pathogenesis of Bartter syndrome. PgA is elevated in plasma, and the urinary excretion of PgE_2 and $F_2\alpha$ is also elevated.[25, 26] Increased production of prostaglandins is probably secondary to potassium depletion.[27] It is highly probable that the short-term clinical improvement with indomethacin[25] depends upon inhibition of prostaglandin synthetase. Similar effects have been

found for ibuprofen and aspirin.[28, 29] It is too early to assess the long-term effects and safety of blockers of prostaglandin synthetase.

Bartter syndrome may be mimicked by gastrointestinal causes, such as covert vomiting, by abuse of potent diuretics or laxatives, or by a dietary deficiency of chloride. Urine screens will pick up thiazides or furosemide. Urinary chloride determination will be diagnostic if induced vomiting is suspected: During a high chloride intake the patient with Bartter syndrome will show urinary chloride wasting whereas the patient with metabolic mimicry of Bartter syndrome (vomiting or familial chloride diarrhea) will show chloride sparing.[30] This syndrome of pseudo-Bartter is probably more common than true Bartter syndrome.[31]

CONGENITAL ADRENAL HYPERPLASIA

Congenital adrenal hyperplasia (CAH) is an inborn error of metabolism transmitted by an autosomal recessive gene. The clinical manifestations can be correlated with the different defects of cortisol synthesis. A simplified scheme of adrenal steroidogenesis is depicted in Fig. 24–1. The various forms of CAH are associated with specific enzyme defects, and the salient clinical and laboratory features are presented in Table 24–4.

The pathophysiology of these enzyme defects and their diagnosis can best be understood in the context of the following features:

1. Site and severity of the enzyme defect

2. Overproduction of precursors

3. Impact of androgens on virilization, and differentiation of external genitalia and somatic growth

4. Impact of impaired glucocorticoid biosynthesis on glucose homeostasis and the ability to withstand stress

5. Impact of mineralocorticoid deficiency on fluid and electrolyte homeostasis[2, 3]

Only a brief outline will be presented here. Detailed reviews are available in standard texts.[32, 32a] We emphasize here diagnosis and treatment, particularly treatment in time of stress.

Table 24–4. Clinical and Biochemical Features in Adrenal Insufficiency

	SALT-WASTING	HYPER-TENSION	AMBIGUOUS GENITALIA		SERUM					URINE	
			Virilized Female	Incomplete Male	Cortisol	Aldosterone	Renin	17OHP	DHEA	17OHCS	17KS
Hypoplasia	Severe	—	No	No	Decrease	Decrease	Increase	Decrease	Decrease	Decrease	Decrease
Hemorrhage	Moderate-Severe	—	No	No	Decrease	Decrease	Increase	Decrease	Decrease	Decrease	Decrease
20,22-Desmolase deficiency	Severe	—	No	Yes	Decrease	Decrease	Increase	Decrease	Decrease	Decrease	Decrease
3β-HSD Deficiency	Severe	—	Yes	Yes	Decrease	Decrease	Increase	Decrease	Increase	Decrease	Increase
17-Hydroxylase deficiency	None	+	No	Yes	Decrease	Normal—Decrease	Decrease	Normal—Sl. Increase	Decrease	Decrease	Decrease
21-Hydroxylase deficiency simple virilizer	None	—	Yes	No	Decrease	Normal	Normal—Sl. Increase	Increase	Increase	Decrease	Increase
salt waster	Moderate-Severe	—	Yes	No	Decrease	Decrease	Increase	Increase	Increase	Decrease	Increase
11-Hydroxylase deficiency	None	+	Yes	No	Decrease	Decrease	Decrease	Normal—Sl. Increase	Increase	Increase	Increase
Aldosterone synthesis block	Severe	—	No	No	Normal	Decrease	Increase	Normal	Normal	Normal	Normal
Pseudohypoaldosteronism	Severe	—	No	No	Normal	Increase	—	Normal	Normal	Normal	Normal
Unresponsiveness to ACTH	None	—	No	No	Decrease	Normal—Low	Increase	Normal	Normal	Decrease	Decrease

Abbreviations: 17OHP, 17-hydroxyprogesterone; DHEA, Dehydroepiandrosterone; 17OHCS, 17-hydroxycorticosteroids; 17KS, 17-ketosteroids. (Adapted from Sperling MA: Newborn adaptation: adrenocortical hormones and ACTH. In Tulchinsky D: Maternal-Fetal Endocrinology. W. B. Saunders Co., Philadelphia, 1980, p 387.)

Cholesterol Desmolase Deficiency

This defect results in impaired synthesis of all three classes of adrenal steroids and in severe salt wasting. The male with this defect has ambiguous genitalia. This suggests that the defect is also present in the testis. The biosynthetic defect involves the side-chain cleavage converting cholesterol to pregnenolone. Early recognition and proper treatment should permit survival of these infants, as in Addison disease of infancy.[33]

3β-Hydroxysteroid Dehydrogenase (3β-HSD) Deficiency

This defect also results in decreased synthesis of all three classes of steroids. There is impaired secretion of aldosterone, cortisol, and testosterone, which leads to male pseudohermaphroditism and life-threatening salt-wasting in infancy. The female with this defect shows only minimal clitoral enlargement, probably owing to the extremely high amounts of DHEA, a weak androgen.[34]

Congenital adrenal hyperplasia due to 3β-HSD deficiency must be suspected in a newborn infant with salt-wasting who has ambiguous genitalia. Urinary or plasma DHEA measurement will be diagnostic.

Since stress in the immediate postnatal period may elevate DHEA levels in infants with normal adrenal function, DHEA reference values for newborn infants should be consulted before the diagnosis of 3β-HSD is contemplated.[35] Treatment consists of glucocorticoids and fluodrocortisone (9α-fluorocortisol, Florinef).

17α-Hydroxylase Deficiency

Glucocorticoids and sex steroids are secreted in diminished amounts as a result of this defect. The decrease in cortisol production results in increased ACTH secretion, which leads to compensatory increases in the production of corticosterone (a weak glucocorticoid) and desoxycorticosterone (DOC; a mineralocorticoid). Hypertension, hypokalemia, and alkalosis are frequently present and are probably due to increased desoxycorticosterone production. Increased DOC levels will lead to sodium retention, and this in turn causes depressed aldosterone secretion. Lifelong therapy with glucocorticoids is mandatory.[36]

21-Hydroxylase Deficiency

Impairment of 21-hydroxylation is the most common enzymatic deficiency observed in CAH and accounts for approximately 95 per cent of CAH cases. The deficiency results in decreased cortisol synthesis; this in turn increases ACTH secretion. Consequent to the increased ACTH secretion is overproduction of cortisol precursors (17-hydroxyprogesterone) and androgens, the biosynthesis of which do not require 21-hydroxylase.

The salt-wasting form of this disease is life-threatening. It must be recognized within the first few weeks of life. Symptoms may not appear until the fifth to twelfth day of life. While the genital ambiguity in females with CAH immediately triggers diagnostic studies, first-born males with normal genitalia may go undetected and are therefore at increased risk for rapid virilization, salt-wasting crisis, or both, depending on the severity of the enzyme defect. An early sign is an increase in serum potassium levels. Such infants have a poor appetite and lose more weight than is physiologic. This is due to an excessive sodium loss, which results in severe water loss and marked dehydration.[32] There is also apathy, vomiting, diarrhea, and abdominal pain. As sodium depletion approaches 50 per cent of the total exchangeable sodium, small additional losses rapidly lead to severe, symptomatic hyponatremia. The inability to secrete aldosterone combined with the overproduction of steroids, possibly promoting a salt-losing tendency (e.g., progesterone) results in acute adrenal crisis.

There is no direct correlation between the degree of virilization of the external genitalia and the severity of the enzyme deficiency.

In light of recent advances demonstrating a close genetic linkage between HLA-genotype and both simple virilizing and salt-wasting forms of 21-hydroxylase deficiency, it is now clear that the forms represent different degrees of severity of a single enzyme deficiency. The close genetic linkage between the HLA-B locus and the gene for 21-hydroxylase indicates that the latter gene is on chromosome number 6. Prenatal diagnosis of CAH due to 21-hydroxylase deficiency has become possible by measurement of 17-hydroxyprogesterone in amniotic fluid. In addition, HLA typing of

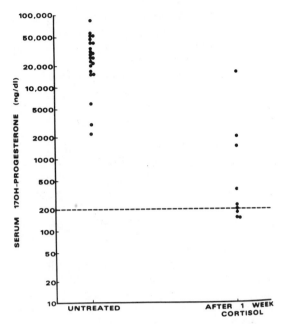

Figure 24–2. Serum 17OH-progesterone levels in infants with congenital adrenal hyperplasia (CAH) before and after one week of cortisol therapy. The staggered line indicates the upper limit of normal. (From Hughes, IA, and Winter JSD: The application of a serum 17OH-progesterone radioimmunoassay to the diagnosis and management of congenital adrenal hyperplasia. J. Pediat. 88:766, 1976. Used with permission.)

amniotic cells can establish the diagnosis in a pregnancy at risk (previous affected child). Prenatal diagnosis of CAH will help the family and the physician prepare for the infant with CAH.[37] Among siblings, males and females are equally affected. In the United States the incidence of 21-hydroxylase deficiency has been reported as 1:11,000 to 1:40,000.[38]

Both salt-wasters and simple virilizers have elevated plasma levels of 17-hydroxyprogesterone (Fig. 24–2) as well as of various androgens. Measurement of 17-hydroxyprogesterone by a micromethod using eluates of filter paper impregnated with blood permits the rapid screening of newborn infants for this defect.[38] Screening of newborn infants for this form of congenital adrenal hyperplasia is potentially life-saving, since the first newborn male with salt-wasting disease may go unrecognized until he presents in crisis. Plasma renin activity is markedly elevated in salt wasters. Plasma renin activity may be moderately elevated even in simple virilizers.[39]

11-Hydroxylase Deficiency

A defect in 11-hydroxylation results in the hypertensive form of CAH. The hypertension and lack of salt-wasting are attributed to excessive DOC production.[32]

TREATMENT IN 21-HYDROXYLASE DEFICIENCY AND 11-HYDROXYLASE DEFICIENCY

In the newborn period clinical features suggesting adrenal insufficiency are, predominantly, electrolyte imbalance, dehydration, and hypoglycemia with or without genital ambiguity. Accompanying vomiting may easily lead to the wrong diagnosis — that is, pyloric stenosis. The electrolyte pattern should aid in establishing the diagnosis firmly. Thus, in pyloric stenosis there is hypochloremic alkalosis as a result of the loss of gastric juice containing hydrochloric acid; serum potassium is normal to low; and serum sodium is usually normal. In mineralocorticoid deficiency states, serum sodium is low, potassium is elevated, and chloride is normal. There may be a metabolic acidosis.

When genital ambiguity is present, congenital enzyme defects have to be ruled out. Rapid determination of the genetic sex is necessary and should precede sex assignment. Treatment of the electrolyte and volume disturbance with balanced saline solutions *and* DOCA (desoxycorticosterone acetate), 1 mg IM daily, should begin during the work-up. Because the dehydration is primarily extracellular, isotonic saline is appropriate. Administration of DOCA will not interfere with the measurement of 17-ketosteroids, pregnanetriol, or 17-hydroxyprogesterone.

If infusion of isotonic saline does not correct the metabolic acidosis, sodium lactate may be added to the solution. Serum electrolytes, hematocrit, and body weight have to be monitored carefully during the acute phase, since too much salt, DOCA or fluids may lead to edema, hypertension, hypernatremia, and hypokalemia.

The sex of assignment should be guided by the anatomy of the external and internal genitalia, the possibility that puberty will conform to the sex of assignment, and the capacity for sexual activity and fertility.[3]

Table 24–5. Treatment of Congenital Adrenal Hypoplasia During Maintenance and Stress[*]

	MAINTENANCE (mg/day)	STRESS (mg/day)
Cortisol Replacement		
PO cortisol	25 per m²	75 per m²
IM cortisol	12.5 per m²	37.5 per m²
IV cortisol sodium succinate (Solu-Cortef)	–	50–100
Aldosterone Replacement		
PO 9α-fluorocortisol	0.05–0.1	0.05–0.1
IM DOCA	–	1–3

[*]Adapted from Migeon CJ: Diagnosis and treatment of adrenalcortical disorders. In DeGroot LJ (ed): Endocrinology, Vol. 2. Grune and Stratton, New York, 1979.

After the diagnostic workup is completed, in the immediate postnatal period, IM hydrocortisone, 25 mg/m² every 24 hours, and DOCA 1 to 2 mg IM daily, should be used. Within two to three weeks of age, oral therapy with 9 α-fluorocortisol may be initiated (Table 24–5). There is no longer any need for subcutaneous DOCA pellets in infants. However, mineralocorticoid replacement does not obviate the need for additional salt, 1 gm per each 10 kg of body weight. The aim of treatment in simple viriliz-

ing CAH is suppression of the excessive androgen production and cessation of virilization with concurrent maintenance of normal growth and development. Since the physiologic secretion of cortisol is 12.1 ± 2.9 mg/m² in 24 hours, the daily IM injection of 12.5 mg of cortisol to a child with a body surface of 1 m² will represent adequate replacement therapy.[32] Since this is impractical, different modes of administration have been developed (see Table 24–5). Because of its short half-life in plasma (90 min) and because of partial inactivation of the hormone by gastric acidity, the maintenance daily dose of oral cortisol must be approximately twice the physiologic production (see Table 24–5).

The suggested oral replacement dose of hydrocortisone is therefore 20 to 25 mg/m²/day.[40] The proper distribution of this dose into three daily doses remains controversial, some recommending a larger dose at night to suppress the nighttime ACTH surge, others giving the larger part of the dose in the morning.[40] Prednisolone or prednisone (5 and 6 mg/m²/day, respectively) may also be successfully used. Both drugs have a longer half-life in plasma (200 min) (Table 24–6). The dose may not be so easily adjustable to the individual needs

Table 24–6. Characteristics of Commonly Used Glucocorticoids and Mineralocorticoids[*]

DURATION OF ACTION	BIOLOGIC HALF-LIFE (hrs)	PLASMA HALF-LIFE (min)	GLUCO-CORTICOID ACTIVITY[†]	EQUIVALENT GLUCOCORTICOID DOSE (mg)	MINERALO-CORTICOID ACTIVITY[‡]
GLUCOCORTICOIDS					
SHORT-ACTING					
Cortisol	8–12	90	1	20	1
Cortisone	24–36	30	0.7	25	0.7
Prednisolone	12–36	200	4	5	0.7
6 α-Methyl prednisolone	12–36	200	5	4	0.5
INTERMEDIATE-ACTING					
Triamcinolone	36–48	200	5	4	nil
LONG-ACTING					
Dexamethasone	36–54	300	30	0.75	2
MINERALOCORTICOIDS					
Aldosterone			0.1	–	400
9α-Fluorocortisol			10	–	400

[*]Table compiled from Fass B: Glucocorticoid therapy for non-endocrine disorders. Pediatr Clin North Am 26:251, 1979, and Liddle GW: The adrenal cortex. In Williams RH (ed); Textbook of Endocrinology. W. B. Saunders Co., Philadelphia, 1974.

[†]Relative values. Cortisol is assigned a value of 1.

[‡]Relative values. Aldosterone is assigned a value of 400.

of the child, especially in infancy. Other, more potent synthetic compounds such as dexamethasone are not recommended.[41, 42]

In both the simple virilizing *and* salt-wasting form, 9α-fluorocortisol, 0.05 to 0.1 mg/day, is added to the therapy to suppress renin to the normal range if renin is elevated. Normalization of plasma renin activity provides a smoother control.[39] Sodium repletion also normalizes ACTH levels (Fig. 24–3). Blood pressure determinations must be taken frequently in these patients.

Since the half-life of 9α-fluorocortisol is about 16 hours, it does not need to be administered more than once a day. It should be noted that there is no need for adjustment of the replacement of mineralo-corticoid therapy in relation to body size. This is probably related to the fact that the secretion rate of aldosterone in children after two weeks of age is not significantly different from that of older children and adults.[32]

Efficacy of therapy is evidenced by orderly growth and maturation, including normal bone age progression. Laboratory evidence for adequate therapy includes the normalization of plasma androgens and 17-hydroxyprogesterone to concentrations of less than 200 μg/dl[43] (see also Fig. 24–2).

The tendency toward sodium loss appears to be less marked after the first two or three years of life; it does not, however, disappear. The reasons for this change are not known.

The infant's family should keep a syringe with 100 mg hydrocortisone for emergency IM injection. Affected children should carry on their persons an identification card or tag so that IM hydrocortisone therapy can be initiated promptly in emergency situations. Adrenal crisis may thus be averted.

Physiologically, the adrenal gland responds to stress with a marked increase in secretion of cortisol. Patients with CAH and patients treated with steroids for more than two weeks are unable to do so. Additional steroid is necessary. If this is not done, adrenal insufficiency with postural hypotension, shock and hypoglycemia may ensue. In moderate stress the dose should be doubled, and during major infections it should be tripled, particularly in salt-wasters (see Table 24–5). Quick return to maintenance levels — as soon as possible — is necessary to avoid problems of over-treatment leading to poor growth and iatrogenic Cushing syndrome.

In 11-hydroxylase deficiency, mineralo-corticoid therapy or added salt is not necessary.

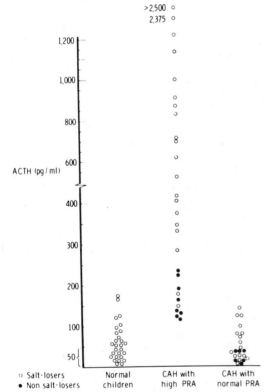

Figure 24–3. ACTH levels in normal children and in seven patients with congenital adrenal hyperplasia treated with constant replacement doses of glucocorticoids equivalent to 25 mg/m²/day of hydrocortisone. Samples were drawn between 0800 and 0900 h. Levels of plasma renin activity (PRA) were high during the ad lib., normal and low sodium diets. Normal PRA levels were achieved by sodium repletion with a high sodium diet or additional 9α-fluorocortisol or both. (From Rösler A, Levine LS, Schneider B, et al: The interrelationship of sodium balance, plasma renin activity and ACTH of congenital adrenal hyperplasia. J Clin Endocrinol Metab 45:500, 1977. Copyright © 1977. The Endocrine Society. Used with permission.)

Preparation of Patients for Surgery

Whenever possible, the patient should be hospitalized one day prior to surgery to evaluate carefully his electrolyte status. Three times maintenance levels of IM cortisol should be given the night before surgery. This is continued on the day of surgery and also for the next two to three days. Thereafter the dose can be reduced quickly,

Table 24–7.   Treatment of Adrenal Insufficiency During Surgery

	IM CORTISOL (mg/m²/day)	IV SOLU-CORTEF (mg/day)	IM DOCA (mg/day)
Day prior to surgery	37.5–50		(Florinef PO 0.05–0.1 mg/day)
Pre-anesthesia	37.5–50		
During surgery		50–100, Continuous infusion	1–3
Day after surgery:			
1	37.5–50		1
2	37.5–50		1
3	37.5–50		1
4	37.5–50		1
5	Resume replacement therapy°		

°If there is any intercurrent complication, continue the "stress" coverage.

and regular replacement doses can be resumed by the fifth day. With intercurrent complications it may be necessary to continue this "stress therapy" longer. Fluorocortisol doses generally do not have to be increased; it is, however, advisable to give 1 mg of DOCA IM on the day of surgery when no oral therapy can be given (Table 24–7).

At the time of emergency, such as surgery, IM cortisol therapy is started simultaneously with immediate administration of 50 mg of hydrocortisone. This is followed by a continuous infusion of 50 to 100 gm of hydrocortisone added to intravenous fluid given during surgery. Normal (0.9 per cent) or 0.45 per cent saline with 20 mEq/l potassium added should be used as intravenous fluid (see Table 24–7). Patients with chronic adrenal insufficiency (Addison disease) are treated with glucocorticoids and mineralocorticoids in the same dose range as patients with CAH.

Withdrawal of Steroid Therapy

As a general rule, patients who have received glucocorticoids for a week or less do not require a period of decreasing dosage. Patients who have received such therapy for more than a week may have suppression of adrenocorticol function.[44]

The suppression is far less on alternate-day dosage regimens. The cortisol response to insulin-induced hypoglycemia of patients on alternate-day therapy is comparable to that of controls, which indicates that the ability of their hypothalamic pituitary adrenal (HPA) axis to respond to stress is intact.[45, 46] Patients on alternate-day therapy

were found to have fewer steroid side-effects — i.e., no hypertension, minimal changes in fat distribution, and most important in children, a normal growth rate.[47]

The biologic half life of steroids (see Table 24–6) is another factor determining the length and the degree of ACTH suppression after glucocorticoid therapy.

Recovery of function after steroids have been stopped is highly variable. In a study of asthmatic children who had been treated with a high dosage of prednisone for between six months and five years, all had achieved normal morning cortisol levels and a normal response to hypoglycemia two to four weeks after stopping the medication.[48]

Studies in adults show a considerably wider range in the length of time required for recovery.[49] Recovery may last as long as 12 months.[50] Recovery of function of the adrenal cortex lags behind that of the pituitary. Early in recovery, acute stress from, for example, hypoglycemia will raise ACTH while the adrenal cortex remains unresponsive.[51]

Recovery of adrenal function can be tested by an ACTH test, a morning plasma cortisol determination, or both. If the plasma cortisol concentration is greater than 10 μg/dl or the ACTH response of cortisol is greater than 30 μg/dl, normal adrenal function can be assumed.[52] A recent study comparing ACTH test results with cortisol levels during and after surgery shows an excellent correlation between the two.[53] Response to insulin-induced hypoglycemia is also a good indicator of the recovery of functional integrity of the HPA axis.[54] The metyrapone test is very informative yet more time-consuming than the tests discussed earlier.

Since it is difficult to determine, without proper testing, whether recovery of the HPA axis has indeed occurred, it is prudent to treat with glucocorticoids during the acute event any patient who experiences medical or surgical illness within one year after cessation of corticosteroid therapy[55] (see Table 24–6 for doses).

Cortisone acetate administered intramuscularly is poorly absorbed and produces low blood levels of circulating cortisol. Hydrocortisone hemisuccinate should be used instead for acute coverage.[56]

Steroid withdrawal in a patient who is disease-free should rapidly proceed to maintenance level (25 mg/m²/day of hydrocortisone). Thereafter, one halves the dose over two to four weeks or switches to alternate-day therapy with maintenance doses.[44] The morning cortisol levels will indicate how to proceed further. In patients with suspected hypothalamic or pituitary disease, one proceeds in the same fashion. If the morning cortisol is too low, it is advisable to continue treatment for another month and to repeat the test. If the morning cortisol is finally in the normal range, the stress response of plasma cortisol to insulin-induced hypoglycemia should be tested after all steroids have been discontinued for several days.[52] In patients with a history of seizure disorders, the plasma cortisol response during a glucogen stimulation test may be the preferred test to evaluate integrity of the HPA axis.[60]

ACUTE ADRENAL INSUFFICIENCY

Acute adrenal insufficiency is the result of combined cortisol deficiency, aldosterone deficiency and often some precipitating stress. Extracellular volume depletion may lead to dehydration, hypotension and possibly shock. Hypoglycemia may complicate this picture further. It can usually be assumed that a patient in acute adrenal insufficiency is depleted of 20 per cent of his or her extracellular fluid volume. It is important to remember that, in contrast to the sodium wasting, there is potassium retention. Thus, supplementary potassium is contraindicated unless hypokalemia develops later, as a consequence of excessive treatment with adrenal steroids.

The keys to therapy include appropriate steroid hormone replacement and careful fluid and electrolyte replacement. One must not depend upon sodium-retaining steroids to replenish sodium stores once they have become depleted.

The following steps should be taken:

1. Initially, an isotonic balanced sodium (150 to 160 mEq/l) solution with either 5 or 10 per cent glucose is administered at a rate of 100 to 120 ml/kg of body weight for the first 24 hours for children less than 20 kg, and 75 ml/kg for children over 20 kg. Twenty to 25 per cent of the total calculated replacement fluid may be given in the first two hours. After the first day, maintenance therapy may be continued as a balanced sodium (75 mEq/l) salt solution. When intravenous therapy has been discontinued, and when the child takes fluid by mouth, additional sodium chloride, 1 gm for each 10 kg of body weight, should be given.

2. A soluble hydrocortisone product, hemisuccinate or phosphate, should be given immediately intravenously, 1.5 to 2 mg/kg of body weight, followed by 1 to 2 mg/kg every six hours. Intramuscular steroids are slowly absorbed and therefore are not used in the acute phase.[61] Intramuscular hydrocortisone, 2 mg/kg per day, is given in the recovery phase. Plasma levels are maintained for 24 hours or longer with this drug.

3. Desoxycorticosterone acetate (DOCA), 1 to 3 mg, is given intramuscularly at once. The dose can be repeated in the first 24 hours. Once the acute crisis is over, 1 to 2 mg per day of DOCA usually suffice. This compound helps restore electrolyte balance and diminishes salt requirements. Patients who have a DOCA pellet implanted may need less sodium and less DOCA intramuscularly. Overtreatment may lead to hypertension, edema, hypernatremia, hypokalemia and cardiac failure. Serum electrolytes should therefore be determined twice daily until a stable state is achieved.

4. If shock persists, pressor agents may be necessary for circulatory support.

REFERENCES

1. Lanman JT: The adrenal gland in the human fetus. An interpretation of its physiology and unusual developmental pattern. Pediatrics 27:140, 1961.

2. Sperling MA: Newborn adaptation: adrenocortical hormones and ACTH. In Tulchinsky D, Ryan KJ (eds): Maternal-Fetal Endocrinology. W.B. Saunders, Philadelphia, 1980, p 387.

3. Saenger P, Levine LS, Pang S, et al: Sexual ambiguity at birth. In Bailey J, Hafez ESE (eds): Diagnostic Andrology. Martinus Nijhoff Publishing Co., The Hague, Netherlands, 1980, p. 31.

4. Weiss L, Mellinger RC: Congenital adrenal hypoplasia: an x-linked disease. J Med Genet 7:27, 1970.

5. Sperling MA, Wolfsen AR, Fisher DA: Congenital adrenal hypoplasia: an isolated defect of organogenesis. J Pediatr 82:44, 1973.

6. Pakravan P, Kenny FM, Depp R, et al: Familial congenital absence of adrenal glands: evaluation of glucocorticoid, mineralocorticoid, and estrogen metabolism in the perinatal period. J Pediatr 84:74, 1974.

7. Black J, Williams DI: Natural history of adrenal hemorrhage in the newborn. Arch Dis Child 48:173, 1973.

8. Kuhn J, Jewett T, Munschauer R: The clinical and radiographic features of massive neonatal adrenal hemorrhage. Radiology 99:647, 1971.

9. Kelch RP, Kaplan SL, Biglieri EG, et al: Hereditary adrenocortical unresponsiveness to adrenocorticotropic hormone. J Pediatr 81:726, 1972.

10. Migeon CJ, Kenny FM, Kowarski A, et al: The syndrome of congenital adrenocortical unresponsiveness to ACTH: report of six cases. Pediatr Res 2:501, 1968.

11. Spark RF, Etzkorn JR: Absent aldosterone response to ACTH in familial glucocorticoid deficiency. N Engl J Med 297:917, 1977.

11a. Allgrove J, Clayden GS, Grant DB, et al: Familial glucocorticoid deficiency with achalasia of the cardia and deficient tear production. Lancet 1:1284, 1978.

12. Irvine WJ, Stewart AG, Scarth L: A clinical and immunological study of adrenocortical insufficiency (Addison's disease). Clin Exp Immunol 2:31, 1967.

13. Newfeld M, Blizzard RM: Polyglandular autoimmune disease. Pediatr Ann 9:43, 1980.

14. Craig JM, Schiff LH, Boone JE: Chronic moniliasis associated with Addison's disease. Am J Dis Child 89:669, 1955.

15. Melby JC: Diagnosis and treatment of hyperaldosteronism and hypoaldosteronism. In De Groot LJ (ed): Endocrinology, Vol 2. Grune and Stratton, New York, 1979, p 1225.

16. Oberfield SE, Levine LS, Carey RM, et al: Pseudohypoaldosteronism: multiple target organ unresponsiveness to mineralocorticoid hormones. J Clin Endocrinol Metab 48:228, 1979.

17. Gilbert MG, Cleveland WW: Cushing's syndrome in infancy. Pediatrics 46:217, 1970.

18. Streeten DHP, Faas FH, Elders MJ, et al: Hypercortisolism in childhood: shortcomings of conventional diagnostic criteria. Pediatrics 56:797, 1975.

19. Winter JSD: Cushing's syndrome in childhood. In Gardner LI (ed): Endocrine and Genetic Diseases of Childhood and Adolescence. W.B. Saunders Co., Philadelphia, 1975, p 500.

20. Conn JW: Hypertension, the potassium ion and impaired carbohydrate tolerance. N Engl J Med 273:1137, 1965.

21. Horton R: Aldosterone: review of its physiology and diagnostic aspects of primary aldosteronism. Metabolism 27:1525, 1973.

22. Conn JW, Rovner DR, Cohen EL, et al: Normokalemic primary aldosteronism. JAMA 195:21, 1966.

23. Bartter FC, Pronove P, Gill JR, et al: Hyperplasia of the juxtaglomerular complex with hyperaldosteronism and hypokalemic alkalosis: a new syndrome. Am J Med 33:811, 1962.

24. Gardner JD, Simopoulos AP, Lapey A, et al: Altered membrane sodium transport in Bartter's syndrome. J Clin Invest 51:1565, 1972.

25. Gill JP, Frölich JC, Bowden RE, et al: Bartter's syndrome: a disorder characterized by high urinary prostaglandins and a dependence of hyper-reninemia on prostaglandin synthesis. Am J Med 61:43, 1976.

26. Fichman MP, Telfer N, Zia P, et al: Role of prostaglandins in the pathogenesis of Bartter's syndrome. Am J Med 60:785, 1976.

27. Galvez OG, Roberts BW, Bay WH, Ferris TF: Hemodynamic changes with hypokalemia. Clin Res 24:559A, 1976.

28. Vinci JM, Gill JR Jr, Bowden RE, et al: The kallikrein-kinin system in Bartter's syndrome and its response to prostaglandin synthetase inhibition. J Clin Invest 61:1671, 1978.

29. Norby L, Lentz R, Flamenbaum W, et al: Prostaglandins and aspirin therapy in Bartter's syndrome. Lancet 2:604, 1976.

30. Veldhuis JD, Bardin CW, Demers LM: Metabolic mimicry of Bartter's syndrome by covert vomiting. Am J Med 66:361, 1979.

31. Higgins JT Jr, Mulrow PJ: Fluid and electrolyte disorders of endocrine disease. In Maxwell MH, Kleeman CR (eds): Clinical Disorders of Fluid and Electrolyte Metabolism, 3rd ed. McGraw-Hill, New York, 1980, p. 1291.

32. Migeon CJ: Diagnosis and treatment of adrenocortical disorders. In De Groot LJ (ed): Endocrinology, Vol 2. Grune and Stratton, New York, 1979, p 1203.

32a. New MI, Dupont B, Pang S, et al: An update of congenital adrenal hyperplasia. Recent Prog Horm Res 37:105, 1981.

33. Kirkland RT, Kirkland JL, Johnson C, et al: Congenital lipoid adrenal hyperplasia in an eight-year-old phenotypic female. J Clin Endocrinol Metab 36:488, 1973.

34. Bongiovanni AM: The adrenogenital syndrome with deficiency of 3β-hydroxysteroid dehydrogenase. J Clin Invest 41:2086, 1962.

35. Levine LS, Lieber E, Pang S, New MI: Male pseudohermaphroditism due to 17-ketosteroid reductase deficiency diagnosed in the newborn period. Pediatr Res 14:480, 1980 (abstract).

36. New MI: Male pseudohermaphroditism due to 17α-hydroxylase deficiency. J Clin Invest 49:1930, 1970.

37. Pollack M, Levine LS, Pang S, et al: Prenatal

diagnosis of congenital adrenal hyperplasia (21-hydroxylase deficiency) by HLA typing. Lancet 1:1107, 1979.

38. Pang S, Hotchkiss J, Drash A, et al: Microfilter paper method for 17α-hydroxyprogesterone radioimmunoassay: its application for rapid screening for congenital adrenal hyperplasia. J Clin Endocrinol Metab 45:1003, 1977.

39. Rösler A, Levine LS, Schneider B, et al: The inter-relationship of sodium balance, plasma renin activity and ACTH in congenital adrenal hyperplasia. J Clin Endocrinol Metab 45:500, 1977.

40. Brook CGD, Zachmann M, Prader A, et al: Experience with long-term therapy in congenital adrenal hyperplasia. J Pediatr 85:12, 1974.

41. Laron Z, Pertzelan A: The comparative effect of 6α-fluoroprednisolone, 6α-methylprednisolone and hydrocortisone on linear growth of children with congenital adrenal hyperplasia and Addison's disease. J Pediatr 73:774, 1968.

42. Stempfel RS, Sheikholislam BM, Lebovitz HE, et al: Pituitary growth hormone suppression with low dosage, long-acting corticoid administration. J Pediatr 73:767, 1968.

43. Hughes IA, Winter JSD: The application of a serum 17OH progesterone radioimmunoassay to the diagnosis and management of congenital adrenal hyperplasia. J Pediatr 88:766, 1976.

44. Migeon CJ, Weldon VV, Guild HG: Iatrogenic adrenal cortical suppression. In Heald FP, Hung W (eds): Adolescent Endocrinology. Appleton-Century-Crofts, New York, 1970.

45. Ackerman GL, Nolan CM: Adrenocortical responsiveness after alternate-day corticosteroid therapy. N Engl J Med 278:405, 1968.

46. Sadeghi-Nejad A, Senior B: Adrenal function, growth and insulin in patients treated with corticoids on alternate days. Pediatrics 43:277, 1969.

47. McEnery PT, Gonzalez LL, Martin LW, et al: Growth and development of children with renal transplants: use of alternate-day steroid therapy. J Pediatr 83:806, 1973.

48. Morris HG, Jorgensen JR: Recovery of endogenous pituitary-adrenal function in corticosteroid-treated children. J Pediatr 79:480, 1971.

49. Graber AL, Ney RL, Nicholson WE, et al: Natural history of pituitary-adrenal recovery following long-term suppression with corticosteroids. J Clin Endocrinol Metab 25:11, 1965.

50. Melby JC: Systemic corticosteroid therapy: Pharmacology and endocrinologic considerations. Ann Intern Med 81:505, 1974.

51. Byyny RC: Withdrawal from glucocorticoid therapy. N Engl J Med 295:30, 1976.

52. Chamberlin P, Meyer WJ: Management of pituitary-adrenal suppression secondary to corticosteroid therapy. Pediatrics 67:245, 1981.

53. Kehlet H, Binder C: Value of an ACTH test in assessing hypothalamic-pituitary-adrenocortical function in glucocorticoid-treated patients. Br Med J 2:147, 1973.

54. Kehlet H, Blichert-Toft M, Lindholm J, et al: Short ACTH test in assessing hypothalamic-pituitary-adrenocortical function. Br Med J 1:249, 1976.

55. Aceto T, Blizzard RM, Migeon CJ: Adrenocortical insufficiency in infants and children. Pediatr Clin North Am 9:177, 1962.

56. Fariss BL, Hane S, Shinsako J, et al: Comparison of absorption of cortisone acetate and hydrocortisone hemisuccinate. J Clin Endocrinol Metab 47:1137, 1978.

57. Fass B: Glucocorticoid therapy for non-endocrine disorders: withdrawal and "coverage." Pediatr Clin North Am 26:251, 1979.

58. New MI, Peterson RE: Disorders of aldosterone secretion in childhood. Pediatr Clin North Am 13:43, 1966.

59. Liddle GW: The adrenal cortex. In Williams RH (ed): Textbook of Endocrinology. W.B. Saunders Co., Philadelphia, 1974, p 246.

60. Frasier SD: A review of growth hormone stimulation tests in children. Pediatrics 5:929, 1974.

61. Bongiovanni AM: Acute adrenal insufficiency. In Smith CA (ed): The Critically Ill Child: Diagnosis and Management, 2nd Ed. W.B. Saunders Co., Philadelphia, 1977, p 46.

Chapter 25

HEART FAILURE

Heart failure can be "forward" or "backward," left-sided or right-sided, acute or chronic, and high-output or low-output. But the phrase "heart failure" usually implies congestive heart failure, which is the type in which water and electrolytes are most important. Heart failure can be due to diseases affecting the heart tissue itself, such as myocarditis; to arrhythmias; and to impaired coronary artery circulation as well as to physiologic abnormalities such as hypoxia, acidemia, and hypoglycemia, and derangements of sodium, potassium, calcium, and magnesium metabolism. It can be caused by an increased pressure load, as with pulmonary or systemic hypertension or with obstructing lesions of the heart or vessels as in aortic stenosis, coarctation of the aorta, or pulmonary stenosis.

Asymmetric circulatory volume loads, as with shunting of blood through a ventricular septal defect or patent ductus arteriosus, cause heart failure, as do such regurgitant valvular lesions as aortic or mitral insufficiency. Heart failure can also be caused by shunts, such as those with arteriovenous fistula, vasodilator drugs, and liver disease. Excessive administration of blood, plasma, or other fluids, particularly when renal function is impaired, also produces congestive heart failure, even with an otherwise intact cardiovascular system. Such "heart failure," as well as that resulting from thyrotoxicosis, glomerular insufficiency (see Chapter 22), marked anemia, and beriberi, threatens the patient with pulmonary edema even though the cardiac muscle may be pumping maximally. Management should, therefore, generally be directed toward the underlying condition and not toward the heart.

The physiology and pathophysiology of heart failure and edema have been discussed elsewhere (Chapters 5 and 13). Congestive heart failure, through a variety of mechanisms, produces increased extracellular fluid volume. The increased blood volume and increased venous pressure that are important factors in producing symptomatic edema may also be, paradoxically, important compensatory mechanisms that augment cardiac output by increasing ventricular filling and stroke volume. Lowering of the blood volume and venous pressure may, therefore, have a deleterious effect on cardiac output.[1]

Increased venous pressure and increased blood volume are not, in themselves, indications for reducing venous pressure or blood volume but should be considered guides to the extent of disease, much as the sign of fever is a guide in infections. As with fever, after a certain point these manifestations of disease may become pathogenetic in themselves, producing further damage or symptoms that may then require therapy. It is usually far better to treat the cause of the illness, when possible, rather than signs and symptoms. Initial efforts, when time is available, should be directed at finding the etiology of the heart failure and providing specific treatment.

Congestive heart failure that produces limitation of function and retarded growth and development requires nonspecific therapy, regardless of etiology. As left atrial pressure rises in heart failure, the pressure in the pulmonary capillaries and larger pulmonary vessels rises also. Distended pulmonary vessels can constrict large airways where they pass in close proximity. Since small airways travel in the same connective tissue sheath as the pulmonary vessels, as the vessels distend they can compress the adjacent airways.

Increased capillary pressure will cause increased flow of fluid across pulmonary capillaries into the lung interstitium, which may also compress small airways, and the fluid may eventually enter the alveoli as frank pulmonary edema.[2] This compression of intrathoracic airways produces airway obstruction similar in many ways to bronchial asthma, increasing the work of breathing and producing greater demands for increased cardiac output for transport of oxygen, energy substrate, and carbon dioxide, which will worsen heart failure. Airway obstruction is also likely to produce decreased pleural and interstitial pressure. The resulting increase in transcapillary pressure will tend to increase the flow of fluid from the capillary and thus tend to produce pulmonary edema.[3]

The accumulation of fluid in the interstitium of the lung, in addition to producing airway obstruction, will decrease pulmonary compliance, further increasing the work of breathing. As fluid accumulates in the interstitium, the interstitial pressure tends to rise, decreasing further flow from the capillary. Fluid in the interstitium of the lung is removed by the lymphatic system, and lymphatic integrity is important in ameliorating the effect of raised capillary pressure. If the lymphatics are diseased, obstructed, already overburdened, or entering into a high pressure venous drainage system, then pulmonary edema will tend to occur with lesser degrees of congestive heart failure and will be more severe.

Since the airway obstruction and decreased compliance will not be symmetric, a ventilation perfusion imbalance will occur and produce hypoxia, which, if it is severe enough, will result in metabolic acidosis with acidemia. This will accentuate the previous problems by further impairing muscle function and increasing cardiac demands. Pulmonary edema fluid in the alveoli and airways will further impede gas exchange by interfering with ventilation and diffusion and also by producing right-to-left shunting of blood, worsening the hypoxia. If unrelieved, hypoventilation will ensue, followed shortly by death.

It is apparent that the effects of cardiac failure on the respiratory system are important; they may be manifested by tachypnea, chest-wall retractions, wheezing, rales, dyspnea, and finally, perhaps, bloody foam coming from the mouth or endotracheal tube. Pulmonary edema may be confirmed by the characteristic x-ray changes of the lung, which may be accompanied by pleural fluid and cardiomegaly.

The respiratory distress will make eating and drinking difficult, since a portion of the airway is required for eating and drinking. Breathing has the higher priority when the patient has to choose between it and eating or drinking. In addition, vascular congestion and decreased blood flow to the gastrointestinal tract further impair its function.

Whereas left-sided heart failure produces major effects in the pediatric patient, right-sided congestive failure is less of a problem. With only right-sided failure, systemic venous pressure is increased, distending peripheral veins, raising systemic capillary pressure, and producing generalized edema, which is worse in dependent portions of the body, as well as hepatomegaly, splenomegaly, and possibly ascites. Such effects, although not so dramatic as those of left-sided failure, may produced disabling symptoms and disturbance of organ function. Unfortunately, pediatric patients, particularly infants, rarely present with only one-sided heart failure; usually both sides fail together.

Regardless of the etiology, certain basic principles and methods are applicable to the therapy of almost all types of heart failure.

1. Rest. Decreased work will lead to decreased transport requirements and decreased demand for cardiac output and may, in itself, reverse heart failure. This can be accomplished for the patient as appropriate by such measures as bed rest, reassurance, placement of the patient in a neutral thermal environment, relief of respiratory distress, and sedation.

2. Oxygen Delivery. Except in patients with right-to-left shunting, oxygen administration will almost always raise the arterial PO_2 to normal levels. Oxygen can be administered by tent, mask, nasal prongs, incubator, or head box as required and as desired but should not be thought of as optimal. Usually, a patient resistant to one means of administration will find another quite acceptable. This will improve oxygen delivery to tissues, decrease requirements for cardiac output, and decrease anaerobic metabolism.

One of the main control points determining cardiac output is the oxygen demand of the tissues.[4] As oxygen requirements increase, cardiac output increases, and vice versa. In animals, isovolumetric changes in hematocrit also bring inverse changes in cardiac output, so that raising oxygen-carrying capacity by raising hematocrit reduces cardiac output and lowering hematocrit increases it.[5] As a clinical example, heart failure may occur in patients with severe anemia with the resulting requirement for high cardiac output, even though their cardiovascular systems are otherwise entirely normal. As another example, one physiologic adaptation to chronic hypoxemia is increased hematocrit. No such adaptation occurs physiologically in patients with heart failure who do not also have hypoxemia. A useful maneuver in patients with severe intractable heart failure and normal or low hematocrits is to raise the hematocrit slowly without raising blood volume, by giving over a few days a series of small transfusions of packed red blood cells (5 ml/kg over several hours), in order to decrease requirements for blood flow for oxygen supply to tissues. In this way, cardiac output may be decreased without lowering tissue oxygen consumption, and the heart failure may be relieved.

3. Digitalis. Digitalis dosage should be appropriate for the age and weight of the patient and should be modified by the patient's response, signs of toxicity, and serum levels. Hypercalcemia and hypokalemia will increase digitalis toxicity.

4. Diuretics[6,7] **(Table 25–1).** The diuretics most often used are furosemide, chlorothiazide, hydrochlorothiazide, and spironolactone; mercurials and acetazolamide are mainly of historical interest.

Furosemide can be given intravenously, intramuscularly, or orally at dosages from 0.25 to 6 mg per kg, up to two or three times daily, but preferably the lesser amount less often. Furosemide is a "loop diuretic," so called because it works by blocking Cl^- reabsorption at the thick portion of the ascending loop of Henle. It is extremely effective in producing diuresis and is so potent that it may decrease extracellular fluid volume to the point of causing prerenal azotemia and even shock. In addition to increasing water loss, it induces potassium, chloride, calcium, and magnesium diuresis, retention of uric acid, which may result in hyperuricemia, and occasionally produces hyperglycemia. Potassium loss may be exaggerated further by the increased levels of aldosterone in heart failure, but without diuretics the drop in potassium is usually self-limited and of no great magnitude, particularly if the intakes of sodium and chloride are restricted.[8]

An effective therapeutic response to furosemide is the brisk diuresis of more than 2 to 3 per cent of the body weight in a three- to four-hour period, with relief of edema, respiratory distress, tachypnea, tachycardia,

Table 25–1.   Urinary Electrolyte Composition During Diuresis*

	VOLUME (ml/min)	pH	Na⁺	K⁺ (mEq/l)	Cl⁻	HCO₃⁻
Control	1	6	50	15	60	1
Mannitol	10	6.5	90	15	110	4
Mercurial	7	6	150	8	160	1
Acetazolamide	3	8.2	70	60	15	120
Benzothiadiazides (thiazides)	3	7.4	150	25	150	25
Ethacrynic acid	8	6	140	10	155	1
Furosemide	8	6	140	10	155	1
Triamterene	3	7.2	130	5	120	15
Amiloride	2	7.2	130	5	110	15
Aminophylline	3	6	150	15	160	1

*Data are representative of results that would be observed in man or dog during normal hydration and acid-base balance. Such findings are readily reproducible during the peak of diuresis and following a single maximally effective dose. However, a significant range of urinary values may be anticipated; a single value is given here solely to facilitate comparison of one drug to another. Excretion rates are obtainable as the product of urinary volume and composition. (From Goodman LS, Gilman A (eds): The Pharmacological Basis of Therapeutics, 6th Ed. Macmillan Publishing Co., New York, 1980. Copyright © 1980, Macmillan Publishing Co., Inc. Used with permission.)

and the other signs of heart failure for which it was given. If this response has not been obtained, a higher dosage may be given, but with lack of a substantial diuresis the diagnosis of congestive cardiac failure should be reconsidered. Ethacrynic acid acts similarly to furosemide and has similar potency, although it has been used less often in young children.

Chlorothiazide and hydrochlorothiazide, which act at the distal convoluted tubule, are used in the treatment of hypertension but have less current use in the treatment of heart failure. They may produce hyperuricemia, hypercalcemia, hyperglycemia, hypokalemia, hyponatremia, metabolic alkalosis, and renal damage, and these complications should be looked for. Acetazolamide, a carbonic anhydrase inhibitor that acts mainly on the proximal convoluted tubule, producing a diuresis of water, sodium, potassium, and bicarbonate, is also little used except for alkalinization of the urine, as in the treatment of salicylate or other poisonings.

Dietary intake can usually supply enough of the electrolytes lost in the urine except, occasionally, potassium. Extra potassium can be given by supplementation of the diet with oral or intravenous KCl, or losses can be lessened by concurrent administration of spironolactone or triamterene. Spironolactone is a weak diuretic, but it acts as an aldosterone antagonist at the terminal distal portion of the tubule of the nephron. By inhibiting potassium-sodium exchange at this site, it decreases potassium loss in the urine. Triamterene, which has had little trial in children, works directly at this site. The serum potassium levels of patients treated with spironolactone or triamterene should be measured frequently since severe hyperkalemia may develop. A possible detrimental effect of spironolactone may be the increase in calcium excretion that it produces. Good dietary sources of extra potassium are orange, grape, and apple *juices*, which contain from 24 to 65 mEq/l of K^+ with small amounts of sodium (ranging from 0.1 to 2.5 mEq/l), but not fruit *punches*, fruit *drinks*, or carbonated beverages, which have much lower concentrations of potassium.

In addition to producing hypokalemia, with its significant impairment of gastrointestinal, cardiac, and general muscle functions, deficit of body potassium results in metabolic alkalosis, which may add its effects to the pathophysiology. Therefore, potassium deficit from diuretics requires prevention and treatment. Since most potassium is intracellular, the serum level of potassium may not correlate with total body potassium, particularly since the serum levels of K^+ are influenced by the blood pH and are usually lower in alkalemia and higher in acidemia regardless of the total body stores. A clue to a developing deficit in total body potassium is the development of metabolic alkalosis, which is manifest by a rising level of total CO_2, bicarbonate, and base excess. If this occurs, even if serum potassium levels seem normal, potassium chloride supplementation is usually advisable.

Care must be taken not to administer too high a concentration of K^+ too quickly intravenously, particularly in a patient with renal impairment, or else cardiac arrest may follow. This risk can be reduced by keeping concentrations of potassium in intravenous fluids below 40 mEq/l at the usual maintenance IV rate, by not giving intravenous potassium to an anuric patient, or by administering potassium orally, usually 2 to 3 mEq/kg/day and up to 9 mEq/kg/day when there is a deficit. Potassium chloride should be used if metabolic alkalosis is also present, and potassium acetate, bicarbonate, gluconate or citrate with a metabolic acidosis. Serum potassium levels should be checked to avoid potentially lethal hyperkalemia. Potassium should not be given as an enteric-coated tablet, which may cause local intestinal damage.

With excessive dietary NaCl restriction and excessive diuretic administration, hyponatremia may be produced; this should be looked for by periodic determination of Na^+ in serum and avoided or treated by increasing Na^+ intake or decreasing the diuretics.

Mercurial diuretics, which act at the same site as furosemide — that is, in the thick ascending limb of the loop of Henle — have fallen into disfavor since they are nephrotoxic and not so effective as furosemide (see Fig. 13–1, page 110).

5. Theophylline. A drug that has had its periods of favor and disfavor in the past but that now requires another look is theophylline. A lot has been learned about the pharmacology of theophylline in recent years; it has returned to popularity in the

Table 25-2.   Content of Infant Feedings

FEEDING	% OF CALORIES P	Fat	CHO	CAL/ML.	NA (mEq/l)	(mEq/100 cal)	CL (mEq/l)	mEq/100 cal	K (mEq/l)	(mEq/100 cal)	CA (mg/l)	(mg/100 cal)	P (mg/l)	(mg/100 cal)	RENAL SOLUTE (mOsm/100 cal)
Human milk	8	51	41	0.67	6	0.9	10	1.4	12	1.8	340	51	150	22	12
Whole cow's milk	22	49	29	0.67	22	3.3	30	4.5	37	5.5	1200	180	930	139	33
Skim cow's milk	40	5	55	0.34	22	6.6	30	9.0	37	11	1200	360	930	278	66
Evaporated cow milk: H_2O (1:1) + 5 g CHO/dl	17	37	46	0.9	22	2.4	30	3.3	37	4.1	1200	133	930	103	24
EM:H_2O (1:1) + 10 g CHO/dl	11	33	56	1.1	22	2	30	2.7	37	3.4	1200	109	930	85	20
Infant formula°	10	50	40	0.67	8	1.2	12	1.8	15	2.4	520	78	400	60	16
Infant formula + 5 g CHO/dl	8	42	50	0.87	8	0.9	12	1.4	15	1.7	520	60	400	46	12
Pregestimil† – protein hydrolysate, no lactose	13	36	51	0.67	13	1.9	16	2.4	18	2.7	600	90	400	60	19
PM 60-40† – low mineral milk	9	47	44	0.67	7	1	13	2	15	2.2	400	60	200	30	14

°Representative of the major commercial infant formulas.

†Commercial preparations; product composition as of 1981.

The infant feedings above illustrate the problem of trying to reduce sodium and other renal solute while maintaining adequate protein intake. The practical minimum of protein, when from high-quality animal sources, is about 8 per cent of total daily calories (12 to 15 per cent from vegetable sources). With the ideal or reference protein (chicken egg albumin), the percentage of protein calories theoretically could be as low as 5 to 6 per cent. Human milk with excellent biologic protein is highly satisfactory at 8 per cent of calories. With cow's milk or other good animal protein, it is wise to use a slightly higher minimum, e.g., 10 per cent of calories, because digestion and absorption may be relatively inefficient and biologic value slightly lower. The usual modifier for feedings is carbohydrate, which produces no renal solute. Renal solute comes from protein, primarily as urea, and from minerals, primarily sodium salts. Note that when the sodium load is reduced by carbohydrate dilution, so is the phosphorus load, which may also be important (Chapter 33) in other conditions. Note also that skim milk, when a major portion of the diet, is a particularly poor feeding, providing maximal stress to water balance.

treatment of asthma and should be re-evaluated for the treatment of heart failure. It increases cardiac output by inotropic effect, it is a diuretic, and it directly decreases pulmonary vascular resistance. This should make it particularly effective in heart failure secondary to pulmonary hypertension, but good clinical trials are needed.

6. Water and Salt Restriction. Although most patients in cardiac failure can manage to excrete a water load, those in severe failure may not be able to do so. Water intake in such patients should, therefore, be limited to maintenance requirements. This can be accomplished by giving a more concentrated feeding while decreasing obligatory renal solute per calorie — that is, by adding carbohydrate or fat to the infant formula. If this is done, care should be taken, when reducing the electrolyte and protein per calorie, not to drop the proportion of the total calories from animal protein to below about 8 per cent (Table 25–2), lest protein malnutrition occur. Since cow milk has an extremely high protein content, it is a good foundation to which carbohydrate and fat can be added. If carbohydrate or fat is added to a standard infant formula, which is designed to be similar to human milk, the proportion of calories from protein can easily be too low. Care should also be taken to avoid increasing excessively the osmolality of the feeding, since vomiting, diarrhea, and possibly necrotizing enterocolitis (in small infants) may be produced.

The usual infant diet is relatively low in sodium, since the amount of sodium in most milks is less than 30 mEq/l. The use of a diuretic can eliminate the excess dietary salt, if any, in the urine without posing extreme restrictions on diet, but salt should not be added to feedings, and commercial soups, which are very high in sodium, should be avoided.

Adequacy of sodium restriction should be assessed by evaluating relief of symptoms and signs of congestive heart failure on the one hand, and hyponatremia and hypovolemia on the other. In the unusual case in which the amount of salt in the usual milk feeding is thought to be excessive, commercially available milk products with lower sodium concentrations and lower renal solute loads can be used (see Table 25–2). In patients with hypervolemic states, simple restriction of salt and water may correct the hypervolemia while attention is directed to removing the underlying cause.

7. Relief of Edema. If systemic or pulmonary edema persists, Starling's Law of the capillary can be applied and tissue pressure increased in order to decrease edema. This can be effected by having the patient wear elastic stockings or elevate the limb for lower extremity edema, by placing the patient in a sitting position to decrease pulmonary venous pressure, or by raising alveolar pressure. Any such maneuver that will increase mean alveolar pressure — such as intermittent positive pressure breathing (IPPB) with high inspiratory pressure and long inspiratory time, a pressure mask, or continuous positive airway pressure — will tend to decrease or reverse pulmonary edema.

On the other hand, the weaning of patients from respirators is frequently complicated by the development of acute pulmonary edema as the mean alveolar pressure is reduced. This phenomenon is surprisingly easy to misdiagnose and accounts for the difficulty in breathing spontaneously that some cardiac patients have after being on a respirator.

8. Other Methods. Rotating tourniquets are rarely used in children, owing to the relatively small size of children's extremities, and phlebotomy rarely proves necessary. Vasodilation with such drugs as sodium nitroprusside or hydralazine requires further evaluation.

In summary, the presence of heart failure and its therapy produces vulnerability to electrolyte disturbances, which in turn may exacerbate the heart failure. These may be anticipated and prevented or corrected by application of physiologic principles.

REFERENCES

1. Kaloyanides GJ: Pathogenesis and treatment of edema with special reference to the use of diuretics. In Maxwell MH, Kleeman CR: Clinical Disorders of Fluid and Electrolyte Metabolism. McGraw-Hill, New York, 1980, Chapter 13, p 647.
2. Robin ED, Cross CE, Zelis R: Pulmonary edema. N Engl J Med 288:239, 1973.
3. Oswalt CE, Gates GA, Holmstrom FMG: Pulmona-

ry edema as a complication of acute airway obstruction. JAMA 238:1833, 1977.

4. Sullivan SF: Oxygen transport. Anesthesiology 37:140, 1972.

5. Replogle RL, Merrill EW: Experimental polycythemia and hemodilution. J Thorac Cardiovasc Surg 60:582, 1970.

6. Mudge GH: Diuretics and other agents employed in the mobilization of edema fluid. In Goodman LS, Gilman A: The Pharmacological Basis of Therapeutics. Macmillan Publishing Co., New York, Chapter 39, p 817, 1975.

7. Bailie MD, Linshaw MA, Stygles VG: Diuretic pharmacology in infants and children. Pediatr Clin North Am 28:217, 1981.

8. Morgan DB, Davidson C: Hypokalaemia and diuretics: an analysis of publications. Br Med J 109:905, 1980.

Chapter 26

PROBLEMS IN LIVER FAILURE

Cirrhosis in children most often follows infantile biliary disease including external biliary atresia, infantile hepatitis, and progressive biliary dysplasia. A few patients with cystic fibrosis, Wilson disease, galactosemia, alpha$_1$-antitrypsin deficiency, and other disorders also develop cirrhosis each year. In addition, acute hepatitis and toxic causes exist. What follows in this brief chapter is a consideration of some of the problems of cirrhosis in its late stages.

When chronic liver disease produces cirrhosis, portal hypertension results and ascites frequently follows. The ascites may be aggravated by a reduction in plasma albumin as a result of inadequate albumin manufacture by the liver. The ascitic fluid forms from transudation in the sinusoidal bed of the liver. The protein level in ascitic fluid of this variety may reach levels of 3.0 gm/dl, which is higher than usual for transudates though it is usually less.

Loss of plasma water and electrolyte to the abdomen reduces plasma volume, which stimulates mechanisms for volume protection so that renal conservation of sodium and water follows. Measures of plasma volume in ascites have usually been high.[1] One explanation for this is that the "effective" plasma volume is low but the value for plasma volume measured by dilution is high because some of the marker used in measurement is diluted in an expanded portal venous bed. Alternatively, it has been suggested that sodium retention occurs first in the sequence of events, followed by plasma volume expansion and overflow ascites.[2] Renin and aldosterone levels are high in cirrhosis, probably not because of slow degradation but because of increased adrenal output.[3] There may be a disturbance of internal renal blood flow, but its mechanism, if any, remains obscure.

Edema other than ascites also appears in cirrhosis. Low oncotic pressure and pressure on lower extremity vessels are two factors that contribute to edema; pressure on lower extremity vessels adds to dependent edema only. These explanations do not cover all instances of edema, however, and some mechanisms have not yet been elucidated. Cirrhotic patients usually show hyponatremia. If effective plasma volume is low, antidiuretic hormone (ADH) production with water retention can be expected. Slow degradation of ADH by the liver may be another pathway to hyponatremia.

Hyperventilation commonly occurs in chronic liver disease.[4, 5] This leads to alkalosis with compensatory reduction of ECF bicarbonate. The relationship of these events to ammonia levels in plasma and brain has not been worked out clearly. Certainly an alkalemia would shift NH_3 to the brain and precipitate or aggravate encephalopathy. Attempts to treat the respiratory alkalemia in order to reverse encephalopathy have not been effective, however.[6]

Many of the problems in patients with liver disease and edema may be aggravated or even initiated by diuretic therapy. In particular, large potassium losses lead to metabolic alkalosis as a result of the replacement of potassium by hydrogen in cells and of contraction of the ECF. This problem may be offset by providing potassium supplements during diuretic therapy, by using spironolactone as part of the diuretic therapy, or by providing lysine or arginine HCl supplements. Most experience with

193

these approaches has been in adults, since far fewer pediatric patients with cirrhosis are seen or have been studied.

REFERENCES

1. Lieberman FL, Reynolds TB: Plasma volume in cirrhosis of the liver: its relation to portal hypertension, ascites, and renal failure. J Clin Invest 46:1297, 1967.
2. Lieberman FL, Denison EK, Reynolds TB: The relationship of plasma volume, portal hypertension, ascites formation, and renal sodium retention in cirrhosis: the overflow theory of ascites. Ann NY Acad Sci 170:202, 1970.
3. Rossoff L Jr, Zia P, Reynolds TB, Horton R: Studies of renin and aldosterone in cirrhotic patients with ascites. Gastroenterology 69:698, 1975.
4. Vanomee P, Poppell JW, Glichsman AS, et al: Respiratory alkalosis in hepatic coma. Arch Intern Med 97:762, 1956.
5. Prytze H, Thomsen AC: Acid-base status in stable, terminal, and portocanal shunted patients. Scand J Gastroenterol 11:249, 1976.
6. Posner JB, Plum F: The toxic effects of carbon dioxide and acetazolamide in acute hepatic encephalopathy. J Clin Invest 39:1246, 1960.

Chapter 27

DIABETES MELLITUS

The pathophysiologic mechanisms that underlie diabetes are still not fully understood, and detailed discussion of the various possible defects of metabolism in this state are outside the scope of this book. In childhood diabetes, once the disease is well established, there is a total lack of endogenous insulin. When diabetes is not controlled, serious disturbances of hydration, hydrogen ion metabolism, and osmolality may occur.

Correction of these disturbances by supportive means is often life-saving. Although control of the underlying process by the use of insulin remains the fundamental therapy, in the first 12 to 24 hours following an episode of severe ketoacidosis or hyperosmolar coma, supportive fluid and electrolyte management takes priority in the urgent matters of immediate restoration. Even if no insulin is available, the patient's most serious physiologic disturbances can be reversed. Insulin, of course, is recommended for correction of the underlying biochemical disturbance. We do recommend that the insulin not be given very rapidly, since rapid administration will lead to further water, hydrogen ion, and electrolyte changes, some of which are potentially lethal. Specifically, if insulin is given intravenously, it should be by continuous low-dose administration, not by bolus infusions.[1, 2, 3]

The following simplified schema is useful in interpreting the abnormalities of water and electrolyte balance associated with uncontrolled diabetes mellitus. Two processes are apparently present in untreated diabetes; both are abolished when exogenous insulin is administered:

1. A decrease in the cellular utilization of glucose in the formation of glycogen stores, and its incorporation in anaerobic glycolysis.

2. An increase in the rate of gluconeogenesis from amino acids, and increased lipolysis resulting in the release of depot fat.

The effects of these processes may be summarized as follows:

1. Elevation of the blood glucose derived both from the gastrointestinal tract and from release from live cells.

2. Rise in plasma fatty acids with increased hepatic ketone body formation.

3. Decrease in the formation of acetyl-COA in muscle because of slowing of anaerobic glycolysis. This, in turn, depresses Krebs cycle activity, resulting in a fall in the production of succinyl-CoA. Thus, breakdown of acetoacetic acid is blocked, causing this metabolite and beta-hydroxybutyric acid (the reduced form) to accumulate in plasma.

The rise in blood glucose leads to an increase in plasma osmolality owing to the block preventing the entry of glucose into cells. The hyperosmolar state is complicated by osmotic diuresis, which is the inevitable consequence of the filtration of glucose at a rate that exceeds the tubular maximum. Thus, glycosuria occurs, with polyuria and loss of solute, particularly potassium, in the urine. In severe cases, dehydration sets in with marked depletion of extracellular water. In situations of extreme hyperglycemia, the hypertonicity of the extracellular fluids may be huge, with a correspondingly large depletion of intracellular water.

Gluconeogenesis leads to protein breakdown, release of potassium into the blood, and loss of potassium in the urine; thus, intracellular potassium depletion is almost always present. The serum potassium will not reflect this, because in states of dehydration, renal function is impaired. Thus, hyperkalemia may be present initially, but the serum level may fall precipitously with treatment of the dehydration and acidosis plus the administration of insulin.

The rise in the blood level of acetoacetic acid leads to a rise in the hydrogen ion concentration of the blood. Initially, the pH is maintained by stimulation of respiration with a fall in PCO_2. With decreased renal filtration and increasing acidosis, the blood pH will eventually drop, leading to acidemia.

The management of diabetic ketoacidemia in childhood involves two therapeutic approaches. The first is the correction of the underlying metabolic deficiency—that is, the insulin deficiency. This deficiency is relatively easy to manage in children, since severe insulin resistance is rarely seen in this age group. On the contrary, even children with severe acidemia are usually remarkably insulin-sensitive and rarely require huge or repeated doses of insulin.

The management of the water and electrolyte disturbances here does not differ fundamentally from that in any state of dehydration. It is necessary to ensure that the blood volume has been re-established, that the deficit is replaced, and that enough fluid is given to control ongoing water losses and establish normal maintenance. Diabetic dehydration differs from other forms in that usually severe polyuria is present despite water loss. This is, of course, because the high blood glucose level continues to exert its effect as an osmotic diuretic. It is apparent, therefore, that the use of hypertonic glucose as a volume expander is contraindicated.

Occasionally, the degree of dehydration is so severe that shock is present. At this stage urinary suppression may occur, but it should be emphasized that this is extremely rare. In either situation, therapy should commence with a solution that is approximately isotonic. Plasma should be used when shock is present, but saline-lactate or saline-bicarbonate solution, 20 to 60 ml/kg depending on the degree of shock and dehydration, with a sodium concentration of 130 mEq/l, is often adequate. The fluid should be given as rapidly as possible.

The rest of the estimated deficit should be given as a solution of 2 to 5 per cent dextrose containing sodium in a concentration of about 70 mEq/l within the next two to three hours.

Thereafter, continued therapy will depend on the condition of the patient and on his or her response to insulin and fluid therapy. In the average patient, urine output will have begun to decrease as the expected fall in the blood glucose level occurs. In general, it is advisable to stop intravenous fluid therapy as soon as possible and shift to oral intake. The management of the acidemia or acidosis requires no special measures. The use of hypertonic sodium bicarbonate to correct calculated deficits carries with it the risk of increasing the hyperosmolality already present and may increase intracerebral acidemia as well.[4] The presence of hyponatremia should not be used as a signal for the enthusiastic administration of normal saline or $\frac{1}{6}$ molar lactate over and above the amount that has been used to correct the deficit in the blood volume. As discussed in earlier chapters, factitial hyponatremia results either from excess lipid in the serum or, more commonly, because hyperglycemia is accounting for osmotic space in the ECF. When the glucose level falls and the accompanying water is redistributed, sodium levels will be restored.

Potassium administration should commence as soon as it is clear that no renal shutdown is present. It should be recalled that, regardless of the initial potassium value, a significant deficiency is present. When the acidosis has been treated and insulin administered, potassium will begin to re-enter the cells. Thus, the hyperkalemia that was present initially may, in a few hours, be changed to hypokalemia. When possible, a serum potassium level should be obtained after about three hours of therapy. A normal or low value indicates that potassium should be added to the intravenous fluids in concentrations ranging from 20 to 40 mEq/l, depending on the serum level. If the initial potassium level is normal or low, potassium may be given as soon as the patient passes urine.

Nonketotic hyperosmolar coma is seen less often in children than in adults. The absence of ketosis may result from the effect of increased osmolality on lipolysis; sodium salts and glucose may differ in this regard.[5] In animal experiments, hypertonic sodium concentrations inhibited epinephrine-induced lipolysis and hypertonic glucose had a variable effect.[5] Nevertheless, the CNS pathophysiology is similar to that of hypernatremic dehydration, since in the absence of insulin, glucose becomes a relative extracellular obligate, much as are sodium and chloride. The possibility of hemorrhage if the condition develops rapidly and the changes in symptoms correlated with idiogenic osmol formation are the same as in hypernatremic dehydration.[6] Accordingly, the same therapeutic caution exists— namely, slow restoration of normal osmolality with a low-sodium, high-potassium infusion.

Hypophosphatemia may occur in diabetic ketoacidosis. It has been suggested that this disturbance may impair glucose metabolism, reflecting decreased tissue sensibility in insulin.[7] This provides a rationale for phosphate infusion, the value of which has not yet been confirmed by clinical studies.

REFERENCES

1. Veeser TE, Glines MH, Niederman LG, Monteleone JA: Low-dose intravenous insulin therapy for diabetic ketoacidosis in children. Am J Dis Child 131:308, 1977.
2. Edwards GA, Kohaut EC, Wehring B, Hill, LL: Effectiveness of low-dose continuous intravenous insulin infusion in diabetic ketoacidosis. J. Pediatr 91:701, 1977.
3. Waldhäusl W, Kleinberger G, Korn A, et al: Severe hyperglycemia: effects of rehydration on endocrine derangements and blood glucose concentration. Diabetes 28:577, 1979.
4. Ohman JL Jr, Marliss EB, Aoki TT, et al: The cerebrospinal fluid in diabetic ketoacidosis. N Engl J Med 284:283, 1971.
5. Turpin BP, Duckworth WC, Solomon SS: Simulated hyperglycemic hyperosmolar syndrome. Impaired insulin and epinephrine effects upon lipolysis in the isolated rat fat cell. J Clin Invest 63:403, 1979.
6. Arieff AI, Guisado R, Lazarowitz VC: The pathophysiology of hyperosmolar states. In Andreoli TE, Grantham JJ, Rector FC Jr (eds): Disturbances in Body Fluid Osmolality. The American Physiological Society, Williams & Wilkins, Baltimore, 1977, pp 227–250.
7. DeFronzo RA, Lang R: Hypophosphatemia and glucose intolerance: evidence for tissue insensitivity to insulin. N Engl J Med 303:1259, 1980.

Chapter 28

METABOLIC DISORDERS AFFECTING WATER AND ELECTROLYTES

In addition to diabetes mellitus, there are a number of diseases, endocrine or metabolic in character, genetic or acquired, in which the pathogenesis involves water and electrolyte metabolism. Ten of them are discussed here, with emphasis on diagnostic features, clinical characteristics, links to electrolyte physiology, and, when known, treatment. The first four involve water intake and excretion; the others involve electrolyte or other solute changes as the primary disturbance.

DIABETES INSIPIDUS

Diabetes insipidus is caused by a deficient production and release of antidiuretic hormone (ADH; arginine vasopressin —see Chapter 4). In a small number of patients, diabetes insipidus occurs as a genetic disease. Both autosomal dominant and X-linked recessive modes of inheritance have been described. Most patients have had an acquired destructive lesion in the region of the hypothalamus. Histiocytosis, encephalitis, sarcoidosis, tuberculosis, leukemia, head trauma, and postneurosurgical states constitute most of the underlying diseases, although there are others. A partial deficiency may also occur.

The symptoms are polyuria and polydipsia. The patients do well as long as they are able to drink enough to replace the obligatory high volume of urine. The urine osmolality will range between 50 and 200 mOsm/kg (specific gravity 1.001 to 1.005) and cannot rise above an osmolality of 300 mOsm/kg after water deprivation.

Differential diagnosis includes compulsive water drinking, nephrogenic diabetes insipidus, and absence of the thirst center. Only the first of these is likely to cause uncertainty if a proper concentration study is carried out. Partial defects may be harder to define. When intake falls behind urine output, as is particularly likely during intercurrent illness, hypernatremia results. Usually this increasing osmolality is slow enough that the more dangerous aspects of hypernatremia—cerebrovascular bleeding problems—do not occur. Similarly, when treatment is being given with electrolyte-free water (by infusion or orally), the renal losses are so great that the development of gradients producing cerebral swelling (Chapter 17) is unlikely.

Management of patients with diabetes insipidus may be accomplished by replacement therapy. The natural vasopressin product from animals (Pitressin) may be used. The half-life of an aqueous preparation of injected vasopressin is about 20 minutes, making it unsatisfactory for therapy. As a nasal spray or snuff, vasopressin preparations are too irritating for most patients. An oily preparation is effective but must be injected. Recently, the synthetic 1-desamino-8-D-arginine vasopressin (DDAVP) has been successful with intranasal administration.

NEPHROGENIC DIABETES INSIPIDUS

Nephrogenic diabetes insipidus may also be either inherited or acquired. Most affected children come from families with an X-linked recessive trait in which the renal tubule cells do not respond to ADH.[1] In older individuals, either drugs or systemic disease may produce a similar phenotype. In the genetic variety, male infants present very early with polyuria and polydipsia.

The clinical picture is just like diabetes insipidus, except that exogenous ADH has no effect: the physiologic problem is hypernatremic dehydration; the severity of the condition and the patient's water replacement needs are the same as those discussed in the previous section. The principal therapy for these children is the prevention of episodes of dehydration. Diuretics such as chlorothiazide reduce free water clearance and may have limited therapeutic usefulness.[2]

ABSENT THIRST CENTER

The absence of a thirst center may result from trauma or may occur especially as a complication of surgical removal of a craniopharyngioma. It is also seen in diseases of the CNS as a solitary defect or in combination with other central disturbances such as defective temperature regulation, obesity, and breathing irregularity (Ondine's curse).[3, 4] In postsurgical patients, diabetes insipidus may also be present, complicating management of each condition greatly. Again, hypernatremic dehydration is the hazard. Here, when the lesion is unaccompanied by diabetes insipidus, rapid water loading may precipitate water intoxication. Management of the condition consists of ensuring, through training or supervision, that the patient drinks water regularly and copiously.

TRUE SYNDROME OF INAPPROPRIATE ADH SECRETION

Excess ADH unrelated to physiologic stimuli to the hypothalamic-pituitary complex occurs from secretion of ADH or something very similar, with the same activity, from an ectopic focus, usually a malignant neoplasm. It is rarely seen in children. The tumors include oat cell carcinoma of the lung, adenocarcinoma of the intestine, and lymphomas.[5] Affected patients develop hyponatremia and are vulnerable to water intoxication from excessive water loads.

FANCONI SYNDROME

Fanconi syndrome has come to designate a disorder of the proximal renal tubules manifesting a defect in reabsorption of phosphate, amino acids, and glucose. In addition, problems in conservation of water, sodium, potassium, and bicarbonate ion may be present. The syndrome has many causes. It appears as a part of the genetic disorder cystinosis, the form in which it was originally described by Fanconi as well as by deToni and Debre. It may also be seen as an independent (idiopathic) disorder or in Lowe syndrome, tyrosinemia, sometimes galactosemia, Wilson disease, and glycogen storage disease. Finally, heavy metal (e.g., lead) poisoning and degraded tetracycline also cause the syndrome.

Diagnosis requires analysis of the urine under controlled circumstances. The low phosphorus level in plasma may lead to rickets, and detection of either the phosphorus level or the rickets may alert the clinician to the diagnosis. Management consists of treatment of the underlying condition, if any, and symptomatic replacement of missing mineral. Correction of acidemia, if present, and administration of vitamin D for the control of rickets may be needed.

BARTTER SYNDROME

Patients with Bartter syndrome have an inability to reabsorb chloride in the thick segment of the loop of Henle.[6] They are characterized by hypochloremic, hypokalemic metabolic alkalosis; hyper-reninemia; aldosteronism; and excessive renal production of prostaglandin E_2. In early infancy, hyponatremia also is usually present. Affected infants have normal blood pressure and hypertrophy of the renal juxtaglomerular apparatus. Dietary chloride deficiency mimics this picture closely. Management includes potassium chloride supplements for all ages plus sodium for small infants. Prostaglandin inhibitors have also been useful to some extent, as have potassium-sparing diuretics in older children.

PSEUDOHYPOALDOSTERONISM

Described first in 1958, pseudohypoaldosteronism remains quite rare.[7] It is thought to represent the inability of the renal tubule to respond to aldosterone. Hyponatremia, hypochloremia, and mild hyperkalemia occur, but adrenal function remains normal, which distinguishes this condition from salt-losing of adrenal origin. Treatment is by replacement of sodium chloride to restore normovolemia. Preliminary data indicate lesser severity of the disturbance with increasing age.

PSEUDOHYPERALDOSTERONISM

This rare autosomal dominant condition, also known as Liddle syndrome, is characterized by hypokalemic alkalosis and hypertension with negligible aldosterone secretion.[8] The electrolyte excretion is not affected by either an aldosterone antagonist or an inhibitor of aldosterone synthesis. Potassium chloride supplements plus triamterene have proved helpful.

PERIODIC PARALYSIS

Two varieties of periodic paralysis are seen, involving familial recurrent paralysis and changes in potassium levels in the plasma. One variety, which usually starts late in childhood, is precipitated by high carbohydrate intake and characterized by low potassium levels. Potassium administration is helpful during attacks. The other variety starts earlier in life. The paralytic episodes usually start during rest after exercise and last up to a few hours. The level of potassium is elevated and potassium loads may stimulate attacks. The more severely affected children develop mild permanent weakness.

GALACTOSEMIA

Galactosemia results from a deficiency of either galactose-1-phosphate uridylyltransferase or galactokinase. The transferase deficiency, which has several variants, is the more severe illness. When patients with disorders arising from either cause ingest galactose, a variety of toxic events occur. Here we are interested only in one of them, which is usually not the most prominent — namely, the swelling of brain cells, which produces the syndrome of pseudotumor cerebri.[9, 10]

An alternative pathway of galactose metabolism occurs with reduction of galactose to galactitol. This alcohol or polyol is found in brain cells; it does not diffuse out of them readily, which leads to swelling from osmotic forces. A pseudotumor may result and be the presenting symptom. Treatment is removal of galactose from the diet.

REFERENCES

1. Waring AJ, Kajdi L, Tappan V: A congenital defect of water metabolism. Am J Dis Child 69:323, 1945.
2. Crawford JD, Kennedy GC: Chlorothiazide in diabetes insipidus. Nature (London) 183:891, 1959.
3. Conely SB, Brocklebank JT, Taylor IT, Robson AM: Recurrent hypernatremia: a proposed mechanism in a patient with absence of thirst and abnormal excretion of water. J Pediatr 89:898, 1976.
4. Travis LB, Dodge WF, Waggener JD, Koshemsant C: Defective thirst mechanism secondary to a hypothalamic lesion: studies in a child with adipsia, polyphagia, obesity, and persistent hyperosmolality. J Pediatr 70:915, 1967.
5. Friedman AL, Segar WE: Antidiuretic hormone excess. Pediatrics 94:521, 1979.
6. Gill JR Jr, Bartter FC: Evidence for a prostaglandin-independent defect in the loop of Henle as a proximal cause of Bartter's syndrome. Am J Med 65:766, 1978.
7. Cheek DB, Perry JW: A salt-wasting syndrome in infancy. Arch Dis Child 33:252, 1958.
8. Liddle GW, Bledsoe T, Coppage WS Jr: A familial renal disorder simulating primary aldosterone secretion. In Banlieu EE, Robel P (eds): Aldosterone. Blackwell Scientific Publications, Oxford, 1963.
9. Huttenlocher PR, Hillman RE, Hsia YE: Pseudotumor cerebri in galactosemia. J Pediatr 76:902, 1970.
10. Litman N, Kanter A, Finberg L: Galactokinase deficiency presenting as pseudotumor cerebri. J Pediatr 86:410, 1975.

Chapter 29

ELECTROLYTE PROBLEMS IN POISONINGS: SALICYLATES AND PHOSPHATES

Accidental poisoning and drug reactions are an important part of clinical pediatrics. A number of poisonings produce problems in water and mineral balance. Most toxins injure an organ system directly or through a metabolic pathway. A few representative poisons are listed in Table 29–1 along with an indication of the systems involved and the location in this book of relevant information. Additional information may be found in pediatric texts and in specialized books on poisons.[1]

Two drugs that may be toxic in overdosage are discussed here because of the relatively high frequency of poisonings and the unusual and complex metabolic nature of their toxicity. They are salicylates (usually aspirin) and sodium phosphate salts used either as hypertonic enema preparations or as laxatives.

SALICYLATE (ORTHOHYDROXYBENZOATE) POISONING

Aspirin (acetylsalicylic acid) poisoning has long been the most common poisoning of children. Accidental single dose ingestion by toddlers, suicide attempts by adolescents, and inadvertent overdosage in therapy produce the clinical events. Diagnosis is

Table 29–1.   Common Poisons and Their Effects on Fluid and Electrolyte Metabolism

POISON	SYSTEM(S) INVOLVED	WATER/MINERAL ASPECT	CHAPTER
Acetaminophen[6]	Hepatic	Minimal except when secondary to liver failure	26
Bromate salts	Renal	Anuria	22
Carbon tetrachloride	Renal Hepatic	Edema Na and K retention	22, 26
Lead	CNS Renal	Cerebral swelling Fanconi syndrome	23, 28
Mercury	Renal Gastrointestinal CNS	Anuria	22
Salicylate	CNS Renal Cell metabolism Glucose homeostasis	H^+ ion changes Dehydration	29
Sodium phosphate hypertonic oral or rectal	Calcium homeostasis CNS	Tetany Hypernatremia	29

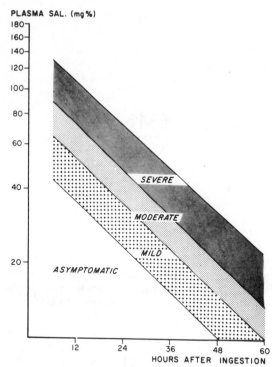

PLASMA SAL. (mg%)

Figure 29–1. Relationship of plasma salicylate concentration to severity of intoxication. (Adapted by Winters RW (ed), The Body Fluids in Pediatrics, Little Brown, Boston, 1973, from Done AK, Pediatr 26:800, 1960, by permission.)

made on the basis of the patient's history and confirmed by measuring the level of salicylate in serum. There are a number of elegant studies of the pharmacokinetics of salicylate and of possible genetic differences among individuals in the metabolism of this drug.[2, 3] Judgment concerning the level has to take into account the time of the ingestion. A. K. Done has prepared a nomogram useful for this purpose, which is shown in Figure 29–1.[4]

Once the diagnosis of salicylate poisoning has been made, the therapist will have to consider a number of important variables before beginning treatment. Most important among these are whether the poisoning resulted over a short period of time, such as from a large dose ingested accidentally or with suicidal intent, and the age of the patient. A lesser matter concerns the type of salicylate preparation. Most commonly the offender is aspirin; less commonly, oil of wintergreen (methylsalicylate) is ingested. Because oil of wintergreen is liquid, a very large dose may be easily swallowed. A level teaspoonful of the fluid equals 5 gm of

methylsalicylate. Thus, dosage rather than any special property of the agent probably accounts for the high incidence of severe salicylate poisonings.

Salicylate preparations are efficiently and rapidly absorbed from the duodenum. On entering the blood the salicylate ion binds loosely to plasma albumin but then rapidly diffuses throughout the body water, resulting in a decrease in blood level of salicylate prior to significant excretion. If the salicylate is swallowed when the stomach is empty, peak blood levels are reached in 75 to 90 minutes. About two hours later a plateau is reached, and then the level decreases gradually owing to excretion. After a large dose, complete excretion takes days if no assistance is given.

The major pathway of excretion is through the urine, in which the drug appears as the free salicylate ion and as two soluble conjugates formed in the liver, a glycuronide and salicyluric acid (a glycine conjugate). About 90 per cent of the ingested dose eventually appears in the urine. Because the action of the liver takes place slowly, large doses of salicylate cannot be cleared rapidly by hepatic action. The excretion of free salicylate by the kidney, like that of any ion of a weak acid, is enhanced by an alkaline pH in the renal tubular fluid. In the case of salicylate, a change of urine pH from 6.5 to 7.5 (a tenfold decrease in hydrogen ion) produces almost a tenfold increase in salicylate owing to inhibition of renal tubular reabsorption of the ionized form. Thus, whereas the free form is about 20 per cent of the total salicylate in an acid urine, it constitutes 80 to 95 per cent of an alkaline urine at pH values above 7.5.

The toxicity of large doses of salicylate affects the central nervous system and energy metabolism. Salicylate irritates the brain in general and stimulates the respiratory center in particular, causing primary hyperventilation. The molecular basis for this is not known, but the effect seems to be a direct one, resulting in early overbreathing with consequent reduction in the blood P_{CO_2}. The brain irritation may result in coma or convulsions, findings usually manifest in severe toxicity.

The predominant effects on metabolism are as follows: First, there is an inhibition of two Krebs-cycle enzymes, alpha-keto-glutaric dehydrogenase and succinic dehydrogenase, leading to gluconeogenesis and ketosis. Second, uncoupling of oxidative phosphorylation causes a hypermetabolic state manifested by fever and increased oxygen consumption. Some of these effects tend to cancel each other physiologically, while others act together to augment the damage.

A particularly complicated situation arises with hydrogen ion metabolism and the acid-base status. The primary depression of PCO_2 characterizes all poisoned patients. However, in the very young, from toddlers to children 5 years of age (the most frequent victims of accidental ingestion), this phenomenon does not result, as might be expected, in a respiratory alkalemia and alkaluria. The reason derives from the rapidly developing metabolic events wherein keto-acid production results in a sharp reduction of bicarbonate ion. This at first "compensates" and then ultimately, within a few hours, swamps the direct ventilatory effect on hydrogen ion level, resulting in acidemia. The acidemia, in turn, completes a vicious circle, because the renal excretion of salicylate is inhibited by the resultant acid urine. Fever and diaphoresis from the hypermetabolic state join with the hyperventilation to increase water losses, a circumstance worsened by nausea, which limits water intake. These conditions predispose to a hypernatremic type of dehydration with a metabolic acidemia plus an independently low PCO_2.

The effects of salicylate on carbohydrate metabolism may be reflected in disturbances in blood glucose levels: early hyperglycemic, and later hypoglycemic levels sometimes are seen. In animals, ample liver storage of glycogen protects against salicylate poisoning. Clinical observations make it seem likely that this is true of humans as well. In addition, over a period of a few days, salicylate depresses prothrombin production. Aspirin, but not other salicylates, seriously interferes with platelet adherence, and, large doses of salicylate damage renal tubules. There are many other actions of salicylate, but for the purposes of this discussion, these are the pertinent ones.

Acute Poisonings

Young children are frequently brought to physicians after having ingested large doses of salicylate over a short period of time. A dose exceeding 200 mg/kg invariably produces toxicity if absorbed; doses of less than 100 mg/kg in a previously healthy child are not dangerous. The effects of intermediate amounts cannot be safely predicted. Correlation of these doses with blood levels shows that plateau, or steady-state, levels exceeding 30 mg/dl are invariably associated with symptoms. Peak levels (at 90 minutes) may reach as high as 50 mg/dl without symptoms, however. If the child is seen within the first two hours after ingestion (up to 6 hours for oil of wintergreen), either emesis should be induced or gastric lavage carried out to remove any residual drug from the stomach.

Following this step, the goals of therapy are twofold: (1) to correct the progressive physiologic disturbances of water balance, acid-base status, and carbohydrate metabolism, and (2) to hasten the removal of salicylate. These aims may be accomplished simultaneously by appropriate techniques that can hydrate, cause hydrogen ion removal, and remove the salicylate through the urine or, if necessary, by dialysis. Our experience with more than 600 consecutive hospitalized patients following single large ingestions, who were seen within 24 hours of poisoning, indicates that the renal route of excretion is satisfactory in the regimen described in the following paragraphs; dialysis has not proved necessary for this group of patients, all of whom survived apparently undamaged.

The following five steps are recommended for therapy:

1. Adequate hydration with an excess of water to provide a high volume of urine.

2. Ample provision of glucose (as a 5 per cent solution) to provide excess substrate for Krebs cycle activity and to replenish liver glycogen.

3. Provision of sufficient base to correct acidosis. Some of the base should be provided as the potassium salt as soon as urine formation has been observed.

4. Provision of excess base to alkalinize the urine, in conjunction with administration of carbonic anhydrase inhibitor.

5. Administration of the carbonic anhydrase inhibitor, acetazolamide, 5 mg/kg of body weight, subcutaneously immediately and repeated two more times at five-hour intervals. This drug is given as a facilitator of base excretion only in conjunction with

systemic alkalinization to obtain an alkaline urine without the risk of excess sodium administration. Similarly, this drug reduces risks from overvigorous implementation of Step 4.

The first four steps are implemented with individual variation depending on the state of hydration of the patient. If marked dehydration is present, emergency rehydration with replacement of deficit may be necessary. When hydration is not severely disturbed, an immediate, rapidly running, intravenous solution of $1/6$ molar sodium lactate, bicarbonate, succinate, or acetate (the lactate is as satisfactory as the others) in 5 per cent glucose should be started. The sodium concentration of such a solution is 167 mEq/l, which would be excessive if it were not possible to facilitate sodium excretion by simultaneous administration of acetazolamide.

As soon as urine is obtainable, the pH should be checked at regular intervals until it reaches 7.5 or higher. This usually takes less than an hour, frequently as few as 20 minutes. At this point, the sodium concentration of the intravenous solution should be reduced to about 40 to 50 mEq/l, and 20 mEq of potassium ion per liter should be added. The anions should be about half base (lactate, bicarbonate, or acetate) and half chloride. The potassium ion is important because potassium levels in serum are low in salicylate poisoning and because the acetazolamide enhances potassium loss as well as sodium loss. The rate of the infusion should be adjusted to provide water at about two to three times the ordinary maintenance allowance; e.g., at a rate of about 300 ml/kg/day in a 2-year-old child.

In patients with milder poisoning and in those who present very early following ingestion and before marked acidosis, the initial intravenous base concentration may be held to the lower (50 mEq/l) concentration of the sodium salt. The acetazolamide should be given promptly and potassium added when urine formation is demonstrable.

Acetazolamide without base administration would not be safe, because acidosis would be worsened. A further problem might result from a worsening of the acidemia produced by administration of acetazolamide unopposed by base; the CSF would, at least initially, be more alkaline and the salicylate would migrate preferentially to the brain.[5]

Acetazolamide has been associated with the occurrence of convulsions. We have seen this symptom a number of times prior to therapy and only rarely afterward, leaving open the question of causal relationship. We have not, in any event, seen lasting harm from these convulsions.

Attempts to alkalinize the urine by administration of sodium bicarbonate or other bases without the acetazolamide are not advised, because of the risks of severe hypernatremia or of rapidly decreasing cerebrospinal fluid pH through CO_2 diffusion, which occurs much faster than bicarbonate ion movement into the CSF.

If no urine is formed after the initial hydration, indicating serious oliguria, either peritoneal or extracorporeal dialysis should be instituted, with application of the same principles but without dependence on the renal mechanisms to remove the salicylate. The peritoneal route, while providing a satisfactory method for correcting the physiologic disturbances, does not provide a very efficient means of salicylate removal. The addition of albumin to the dialysate helps. Extracorporeal dialysis, on the other hand, is highly efficient in both physiologic correction and removal of toxin. The hazards include anticoagulation, the inherent risks of blood transfusion, and possible blood volume or blood pressure disturbances. In our experience, only patients neglected for three days or more and those suffering chronic salicylism with renal damage (as well as, obviously, patients with independent severe kidney disease) have required dialysis.

We do not recommend the use of tromethamine or exchange transfusion for acute salicylate poisoning, because of hazards involved and the inefficient removal of the drug.

In older patients with large short-term ingestions, usually adolescents attempting suicide, management is similar except that much less base is necessary initially, because there may be a primary respiratory alkalemia with alkaline urine and there is thus considerable delay in the onset of metabolic acidosis. The rest of the management proceeds in the same way, with acetazolamide being given promptly.

Chronic Toxicity

The term *chronic toxicity* applies to patients who have had doses of salicylate over a period of days or weeks, usually in a high therapeutic dosage range. However, in this type of poisoning the patient may be very sick or even die with levels that are well below 30 mg/dl. Indeed, there is little correlation between illness and salicylate level in these patients, in whom iatrogenesis is all too often the basis of the problem. In this group, the effects of salicylate on prothrombin production, platelets, and renal tubules are more important than in acute poisoning. Vitamin K as the K_1 oxide, 5 to 10 mg intravenously, should be administered quickly (not exceeding 1 mg/min). Fresh blood transfusion is in order if bleeding is observed. The previously discussed mode of therapy may be carried out unless oliguria becomes apparent, in which case dialysis, either peritoneal or extracorporeal, is indicated.

SODIUM PHOSPHATE POISONING

Children have been poisoned by receiving a high dosage of hypertonic sodium phosphate/bicarbonate salts either as an enema or from overdosage of a laxative preparation.[7, 8] The resulting disturbance may include hypernatremia, hyperphosphatemia, hypocalcemia, alkalemia, and dehydration. The hypocalcemia results directly from the hyperphosphatemia. The disturbance presents difficulties in treatment. Although intravenous calcium is indicated, there is considerable concern about the possibility that calcium salts will precipitate in the kidney or other tissue. We have given low-dose, continuous calcium infusion without harm: 10 ml of 10 per cent calcium gluconate per 500 ml of solution. The hypernatremia should be managed as in Chapter 17. Modification for alkalemia and hypocalcemia is clearly required. A maximal rate

of fluid intake consistent with the degree of hypernatremia should be sought.

Finally, it should be pointed out that even water and salt are potential poisons and substances that may figure in child abuse. Salt and sodium bicarbonate have been used as murder weapons on children, with death or permanent brain damage resulting. Forced water drinking as a form of child abuse has also been reported,[9, 10, 11] as has withholding of water, producing hypernatremic dehydration.[12]

REFERENCES

1. Gosselin RE, Hodge HC, Smith RP, Gleason MN: Clinical Toxicology of Commercial Products. Williams & Wilkins, Baltimore, 1976.
2. Levy G, Tsuchiga T: Salicylate accumulation genetics in man. N Engl J Med 287:430, 1972.
3. Furst DE, Gupta N, Paulus HE: Salicylate metabolism in twins. J Clin Invest 60:32, 1977.
4. Done AK: Salicylate intoxication. Significance of measurement of salicylate in blood in cases of acute ingestion. Pediatrics 26:800, 1960.
5. Hill JB: Experimental salicylate poisoning. Pediatrics 47:658, 1971.
6. Koch-Wesser J: Acetaminophen. N Engl J Med 295:1297, 1976.
7. Davis RF, Eichner JM, Bleyer WA, et al: Hypocalcemia, hyperphosphatemia, and dehydration following a single hypertonic phosphate enema. J Pediatr 90:484, 1977.
8. Levitt M, Gessert C, Finberg L: Inorganic phosphate (laxative) poisoning resulting in tetany in an infant. J Pediatr 82:479, 1973.
9. Dugan S, Holliday MA: Water intoxication in two infants following the voluntary ingestion of excessive fluids. Pediatrics 39:418, 1967.
10. Nickman SL, Buckler JMH, Weiner LB: Further experiences with water intoxication. Pediatrics 41:149, 1968.
11. Partridge JC, Payne ML, Leisgang JJ, et al: Water intoxication secondary to feeding mismanagement. AM J Dis Child 135:38, 1981.
12. Pickel S, Anderson C, Holliday MA: Thirsting and hypernatremic dehydration. Pediatrics 45:54, 1970.

Chapter 30

ASTHMA

Asthma is a potentially fatal, extremely common acute and chronic illness of variable severity and unknown etiology. It is characterized by reversible episodes of bronchial narrowing from bronchospasm, exess mucus, and vascular congestion and may be precipitated by allergens, emotional factors, inhaled irritants, cold inspired air,[1] and viral infections. Management employs allergen and irritant avoidance, psychotherapy, immunotherapy, bronchodilation and steroids.

Attention to water, gas, and mineral metabolism is important in the management of asthma, since dehydration increases the viscosity of airway secretions, decreases their clearance, and makes airway obstruction worse. Dehydration also will impair circulatory efficiency, leading to tissue starvation, hypoxia, and acidosis. These, in turn, will weaken muscle function, including that of the respiratory muscles, and will decrease CNS function and respiratory drive. Overhydration may lead to hyponatremia and to pulmonary and cerebral edema. Administration of an aerosol may induce bronchospasm, while inhalation of dry air or oxygen will increase the degree of inspissation of secretions.

Asthma increases the work of breathing, so that there are increased requirements for water, oxygen, and calories with increased carbon dioxide production. Owing to the bronchospasm, hypoxia is common. With mild disease, hyperventilation occurs, increasing water loss in the expired air; it is accompanied by respiratory alkalosis and alkalemia. Both respiratory acidosis and metabolic acidosis may then supervene, progressing in severity as the disease worsens; these may serve as important markers for worsening disease and as guides to therapy. The administered drugs and the disease itself may produce cardiac arrhythmia, altered circulatory dynamics, and conflicting effects on salt and water excretion. Steroid and antidiuretic hormone levels are increased.[2]

WATER REQUIREMENTS

Asthma increases water requirements by three main mechanisms. During an attack, the work of breathing is increased, which raises the rate of metabolism and increases water requirements proportionately. The hyperventilation characteristic of the less severe attacks, which are the most common, causes increased water loss in the expired air. (With severe asthma and hypoventilation, this source of water loss will decrease.) Theophylline, a commonly used medication, is a diuretic as well as a bronchodilator.

These increases in water requirements are partially offset by the endogenous production of water as hydrogen-containing energy substrates are oxidized. In addition, increased levels of steroids, from both endogenous and exogenous sources, decrease the output of salt and water in the urine. Urine volume is further diminished by increased ADH levels stimulated by decreased stretch of the atrial receptors.[2]

The oxygen cost of normal breathing at rest has been estimated to be from 1 to 5 per cent of total oxygen consumption. Oxygen consumption is directly related to caloric expenditure, so that for every liter of oxygen consumed, roughly 5 cal is expended.[3] For every calorie expended, roughly 1 ml of water is required. It follows, therefore, that calorie requirements and water requirements for normal breathing at rest are also less than 5 per cent of the total.

Increased respiratory work increases oxygen consumption.[4] It has been estimated that the oxygen cost of breathing can rise to as much as 50 per cent of the total oxygen requirement in patients with very severe respiratory distress, with proportional increases in calorie and water requirements. This increased water requirement does not include the additional increase in insensible water losses in the expired air from hyperventilation, which may be three times the amount lost at rest, going from about 15 per cent of total maintenance water requirements to about 35 per cent.

From these considerations we estimate that an extreme degree of respiratory distress will increase water requirements from two to three times the basal water requirements. For a 1-year-old infant weighing 10 kg, this will be from 100 to 150 ml/kg per day (50 ml/kg basal requirement times 2 or 3); for a 4-year-old child weighing 20 kg, this will be from 90 to 135 ml/kg per day; and for a 70-kg adult, it will be from 40 to 60 ml/kg of lean body mass. In addition, as usual, existing deficits should be replaced by fluid containing an appropriate concentration of sodium and chloride to approximate extracellular fluid, and any ongoing abnormal losses should be replaced, milliliter for milliliter, as they occur, by fluid that approximates in concentration the lost fluid as outlined in Chapter 16. These volumes of fluid should contain 5 per cent glucose to supply an energy source to the cells.

Plasma levels of antidiuretic hormone (ADH) have been shown to be elevated in patients with status asthmaticus.[2] This elevation of ADH in asthma has been attributed to mild dehydration, stress, and beta-adrenergic drugs such as epinephrine and to decreased stimulation of the atrial volume receptors owing to decreased left atrial filling as a result of decreased pulmonary blood flow. The elevated ADH levels return to normal after the acute attack is over. This increase in ADH results in the production of a concentrated urine of low volume, even though excessive volumes of diluted fluids are given. This combination can produce water intoxication with hyponatremia, cerebral edema, and coma. Therefore, the production of small volumes of concentrated urine in an asthmatic patient should not be

considered, in itself, an indication of inadequate water administration or dehydration.

Excess fluid administration should, therefore, be avoided. Pulmonary edema can be produced by the combination of several factors.[5] The pleural pressure in patients with asthma has been recently found to be decreased.[5] This, coupled with the increased capillary pressure and decreased oncotic pressure that would be induced by overhydration, could lead to pulmonary edema, which might worsen respiratory distress. Patients with asthma should not be overhydrated and should be observed for signs of adequacy or excess of hydration by checking body weight, urine output, electrolytes, skin turgor, edema, breath sounds, venous distention, the size of the liver and spleen, and the clinical course of the condition as well as obtaining serial determinations of arterial blood gases and pH.

SALT REQUIREMENTS

Since most of the increased water requirements are due to insensible losses, the sodium and chloride requirements should be minimal, particularly since the increased steroid levels will reduce urinary Na^+ excretion. Therefore, only maintenance amounts of NaCl are necessary unless deficit is being replaced. Potassium losses in the urine may be increased by the steroids. These requirements can be met by the administration of an intravenous solution of 5 per cent glucose in water containing 40 mEq/l of NaCl and 20 mEq/l of potassium acetate. These required amounts of water and salt can be administered either orally or intravenously, with oral hydration favored in patients with mild disease and intravenous hydration mandatory for very sick patients.

INHALED WATER

If a patient is breathing room air through the nose, then the inspired air will be properly warmed and humidified, since the nose is well designed to do this. In hospitalized patients, this may not be the case, since they usually require oxygen administration to correct the hypoxia that accompanies even mild asthma in patients breathing room air. Oxygen coming from a compressed gas source will contain no water vapor, so it will be excessively drying. The hyperventilation of all but the most severely ill asthmatic patients will increase this drying effect still more. If the nose is bypassed by mouth-breathing, an oral or nasopharyngeal airway, or an endotracheal tube or tracheostomy, then the drying effect will be even more pronounced. This can turn what would otherwise be liquid airway secretions into a solid adhesive substance capable of obstructing the airway or totally plugging endotracheal tubes.

This extremely unpleasant development can be avoided by meticulous attention to humidification of the inhaled gases, which can be accomplished by the use of a heated humidifier or an efficient unheated or heated nebulizer. A humidifier puts molecules of water into the gas, whereas a nebulizer adds droplets of water. The disadvantages of the nebulizer are that the droplets may induce or worsen bronchospasm and may contain microorganisms and serve as a source of infection. Humidification may be a problem, since the amount of water a gas can hold increases with temperature. If gas at room temperature (25°C) with 100 per cent relative humidity is inhaled and warmed to body temperature at 36°C, it would then be at only 50 per cent relative humidity. If airway secretions are exposed to this gas, they will lose water to the gas and become inspissated. As water evaporates from a humidifier or nebulizer, the temperature of the remaining water actually drops to well below room temperature. Therefore, it is advisable to use a heater so that the inspired gases can be heated close to body temperature prior to inhalation.

Aerosols have an important role in asthma in the administration of drugs such as isoproterenol and other bronchodilators.[6, 7] These may be administered by self-contained canisters, by nebulizers with intermittent positive pressure breathing apparatus, or by spontaneous breathing. When necessary, the fluid used to dilute the medications can be sterile water or isotonic saline solution.

The administration of heated and humidified respiratory gases and the use of in-line nebulizers will decrease the amount of water lost in expiration. It is even possible to establish a positive water and salt balance in a patient by administering excessive amounts of fluids by aerosol. This extra source of water and salt should, therefore, be considered, and administration from other sources may need to be decreased accordingly. We are not able to give precise guidelines for this decrease, but we have not noted the development of clinical problems of hydration when we have administered fluids in the ranges specified in the preceding sections of this chapter.

OXYGEN

During an attack of asthma, the arterial PO_2 is lower than normal unless the patient is breathing oxygen. The main cause of the low PO_2 is ventilation perfusion inequality. If all the airways in patients with asthma sustained exactly the same degree of narrowing, hypoxia would not occur unless the less common complications of atelectasis and pneumonia (producing right-to-left shunting of blood) or general alveolar hypoventilation were present, since there would be no ventilation perfusion inequality. The patient would just have to breathe a little (or a lot) harder, and PO_2 (and PCO_2) would remain normal.

Unfortunately, asthma does not attack all airways symmetrically. Some are narrowed more than others, so that some alveoli get too little ventilation, some just enough ventilation, and some too much ventilation in proportion to blood flow to the respective alveoli. The blood perfusing poorly ventilated alveoli will not be completely oxygenated, although the blood perfusing those alveoli with just enough ventilation will be almost completely oxygenated. Those alveoli with excessive ventilation will not oxygenate the blood much better than will those with just enough ventilation, since the bulk of oxygen is carried in the hemoglobin, which will be almost fully saturated at the usual PO_2 found in normally ventilated alveoli. If the patient breathes harder, the PO_2 may be increased a little, but most of the air will go to alveoli already well ventilated and already oxygenating the blood well, so the PO_2 will stay low.

PCO_2 under the same circumstances may remain normal. This has been erroneously attributed to the faster rate of diffusion of CO_2 than of O_2. The speed of diffusion of O_2 is not the limiting factor. The reason that the PCO_2 may remain normal is that the overventilated alveoli can compensate for the underventilated alveoli with respect to CO_2 but not O_2, since extra CO_2 can be removed in the overventilated alveoli. This has to do with transportation and with the respective concentration gradients. For example, if a train is full of people, it is easier to get off (assuming you are near the door) than it is to get on. Extra oxygen cannot "get on," because the blood perfusing the hyperventilated alveoli is already full of oxygen, but extra carbon dioxide can easily "get off." In mild asthma, owing to hypoxia, anxiety, and reflex hyperventilation, the PCO_2 is usually actually low, in the range of 30 to 35 mm Hg.

Owing to ventilation perfusion inequality, even patients with a mild attack of asthma will have low arterial PO_2, in the range of 50 to 70 mm Hg, a level that is usually not low enough to produce cyanosis but that is close to the borderline. Patients can be made more comfortable if the attack does not respond quickly to therapy, by being treated with low ambient concentrations of oxygen of about 30 to 40 per cent. This will totally overcome hypoxia from a ventilation perfusion inequality, since even the poorly ventilated alveoli will now contain 50 to 100 per cent more oxygen at a higher partial pressure.

In a patient who has had chronically elevated carbon dioxide levels, the respiratory center may be responding only to the hypoxic drive. Giving such a patient oxygen may decrease ventilation further, producing more severe hypoventilation and perhaps death unless the level of oxygenation or ventilation is carefully controlled. Although this is a theoretic possibility in children with uncomplicated asthma, we have never seen such a patient. This fear should not, therefore, interdict the use of oxygen in the usual patient with asthma, although oxygen administration may be hazardous if the patient has been misdiagnosed or has other complicating or associated conditions such as cystic fibrosis or sleep apnea.[8] The presence of such longstanding complications as a cause of chronic hypercapnia may be made manifest by a positive base excess in the arterial blood, representing the metabolic compensation for the longstanding respiratory acidosis. In such patients, oxygen and other potential respiratory depressants should be used with caution.

With increasing severity of the asthma attack, the arterial PO_2 will drop further, owing to an increase in the ventilation perfusion inequality. If atelectasis or pneumonia develops, right-to-left shunting of blood will occur, which will cause the arterial PO_2 to drop even more, but this cause of hypoxia is not correctable by giving low (or even high) concentrations of oxygen. With right-to-left shunting, the arterial PCO_2 may remain unaffected for reasons of transportation, as previously outlined for ventilation perfusion inequality.

CARBON DIOXIDE

If the work of breathing increases to the point that alveolar hypoventilation and less work become preferable to the patient, the resultant rise in PCO_2 will be indirectly proportional to the decrease in alveolar ventilation, so that halving the alveolar ventilation will double arterial PCO_2.

The PO_2 falls about as much as the PCO_2 rises in arterial blood in a patient hypoventilating in room air. The hypoxia attributed to the hypoventilation can be corrected by giving oxygen, without directly affecting the PCO_2. In fact, if hypoventilation worsens, the PCO_2 can continue to rise to lethal levels without cyanosis developing and without obvious warnings. Paradoxically, as the PCO_2 rises above 60 to 70 mm Hg, it becomes a soporific and a respiratory depressant. As hypoventilation worsens, the wheezing may also stop. As a result, the patient may die, apparently suddenly, while sleeping quietly.

This possibility points up the importance of obtaining frequent arterial blood gases in seriously ill asthmatic patients. The level of arterial PCO_2, which can be used as a rough guide to therapy, should be directly proportional to the level of the physician's anxiety. If the PCO_2 is below 36 mm Hg, the physician's anxiety level should be 1+ and therapy should be the usual medical therapy. If the PCO_2 rises to "normal," around 40 mm Hg, anxiety should rise to 2+; medical therapy should be escalated and combinations of drugs at what may approach toxic levels should be used. The patient should have constant pediatric and nursing supervision, with a cardiac monitor for cardiac arrhythmias and tachycardia.

If the PCO_2 rises toward 50 mm Hg and is not rapidly responsive to medical therapy, 3+ anxiety is appropriate; help should be called for, if necessary, and the patient should be transferred, if possible, to an intensive care unit in case endotracheal intubation and respirator therapy become necessary. Appropriate preparations should be made for intubation and respirator therapy while maximal medical therapy continues. This includes large doses of steroids, oxygen, aerosol inhalation of isoproterenol or other bronchodilator by intermittent positive pressure breathing devices, intravenous aminophylline, intravenous isoproterenol, and intravenous fluids. It is sometimes not necessary to go on to intubation and respirator therapy, possibly because the patient is reassured (or frightened) by the large numbers of staff now present or by the passage of time, allowing the therapeutic measures to take effect. Intubation and respirator use are initiated at the 4+ level of anxiety if the PCO_2 continues to rise, if the patient seems to tire, if apneic episodes occur, if the PO_2 drops suddenly below 50 mm Hg, or if metabolic acidemia develops. Respirator therapy, when necessary, preferably with a volume-cycled ventilator, has become relatively routine and usually can quickly return blood gases toward normal.

pH

The arterial pH in mild asthma is usually elevated as a result of the hyperventilation-induced respiratory alkalosis. If the disease worsens, the PCO_2 will rise and the pH will then fall. If hypoxia or dehydration is also present, metabolic acidosis may develop, which, superimposed on the respiratory acidosis, will cause the pH to drop even further. Patients who are given oxygen to prevent hypoxia and sufficient fluids to prevent dehydration and circulatory insufficiency usually do not develop metabolic acidosis.

Rapid infusions of large dosages of sodium bicarbonate have been recommended by some to correct acidosis in status asthmaticus. Sodium bicarbonate infusions are not indicated for respiratory acidosis, since sodium bicarbonate will raise the PCO_2 even further and cross cell membranes rapidly, decreasing intracellular and intracerebral pH and making matters worse without much improving arterial pH. Theoretically, THAM (tris[hydroxymethyl]aminomethane) could be used, since it will lower PCO_2 while raising the pH, but it has not received much clinical favor and would not be necessary except in the most unusual circumstances.

If a severe metabolic acidemia develops (e.g., $-$ BE $>$ 15 mEq/l; pH $<$ 7.2), then something else has probably gone awry and time should be spent trying to discover and correct the underlying disturbance rather than reflexively pushing bicarbonate. With severe metabolic acidemia, nevertheless, a solution containing 150 mEq/l of $NaHCO_3$ with 5 per cent glucose and water may be infused at the rate appropriate for the requirement of the intravenous fluids. If cardiac arrest has occurred or seems imminent, one intravenous injection over several minutes of up to 3 mEq/kg of 0.5 molar $NaHCO_3$ may be given (but may not safely be repeated), followed by the isotonic sodium bicarbonate (150 mEq/l) solution. Arterial blood gases and pH should be carefully monitored so that the bicarbonate infusion can be stopped before metabolic alkalosis and alkalemia are produced. It should also be kept in mind that as the asthma improves, the kidneys, lungs, and tissues will eliminate acids and that the patient is not totally dependent on the infused bicarbonate for this purpose.

Less severe metabolic acidemia does not need specific therapy. With appropriate drug therapy of the asthma and provision of adequate fluids and oxygen, the acidosis will most likely be quickly and safely corrected by physiologic mechanisms.

REFERENCES

1. Deal EC Jr, McFadden ER Jr, Ingram RH Jr, et al: Airway responsiveness to cold air and hyperpnea in normal subjects and in those with hay fever and asthma. Am Rev Respir Dis 121:621, 1980.
2. Friedman AL, Segar WE: Antidiuretic hormone excess. J Pediatr 94:521, 1979.
3. Bard P: Medical Physiology. C.V. Mosby Co., St. Louis, 1956, p 580.
4. Davidson HD, Cayler GG: Oxygen cost of breathing in children. J Lab Clin Med 61:292:1963.

5. Stalcup SA, Mellins RB: Mechanical forces producing pulmonary edema in acute asthma. N Engl J Med 297:592, 1977.
6. Riley DJ, Liu RT, Edelman NH: Enhanced responses to aerosolized bronchodilator therapy in asthma using respiratory maneuvers. Chest 76:501, 1979.
7. Shim CS, Williams MH: Bronchodilator response to oral aminophylline and aerosol metaproterenol in asthma. Am Rev Respir Dis 123:64, 1981.
8. Kravath RE, Pollak CP, Borowiecki B: Hypoventilation during sleep in children who have lymphoid airway obstruction treated by ·nasopharyngeal tube and T and A. Pediatrics 59:865, 1977.

Chapter 31

CYSTIC FIBROSIS

Cystic fibrosis is the most common autosomal recessive disease among Caucasians, occurring at a rate of 1:2000. The underlying molecular defect remains unknown. The disease affects many parts of the body in a variety of ways that may seem unrelated, but its manifestations share a common pathogenetic mechanism, an unusual abnormality of the secretion of the exocrine glands. The disease has its major and most lethal impact on the respiratory system, in which tracheobronchial secretions, which seem to be poorly mobilized, plug the airways, with resulting bacterial infection and secondary damage to the airways and lungs, chronic pneumonia, bronchiolitis, bronchitis, and bronchiectasis. The reasons for this have been attributed to increased viscidity of mucus, abnormalities in the metabolism of calcium and other minerals, defects in ciliary transport, autonomic dysfunction, increased secretion of mucus, abnormalities of water transport, abnormal mucus glycoproteins, and abnormal electrolyte content of the mucus.[1-8]

LUNG, LIVER, AND PANCREAS

The electrolyte abnormalities of tracheobronchial mucus are shown in Table 31–1. Na^+ and Cl^- are lower in concentration in patients with cystic fibrosis than in normal controls, and K^+ and Ca^{2+} are higher. Therapy aimed at aiding in the removal of secretions by mist tents; inhalation of aerosols of water with propylene glycol and N-acetylcysteine; glyceryl guaiacolate; iodides; postural drainage; clapping; and bronchial lavage have not been as clearly useful as have vigorous antibiotic therapy and the encouragement of deep breathing and coughing.[1]

The repeated pulmonary infections with tissue destruction and airway obstruction produce hypoxia, initially through ventilation perfusion inequality, later through right-to-left shunting through atelectatic and infected areas of lung parenchyma, and later still through hypoventilation. Those components of the hypoxia that are due to the ventilation perfusion inequality and hypoventilation can be corrected by giving low concentrations of oxygen, with caution to avoid respiratory depression if the PCO_2 has been chronically elevated, but this will only minimally correct the component of the hypoxia due to right-to-left shunting.

With severe lung disease, chronic hypoventilation develops with respiratory acidosis and acidemia, so that metabolic compensation occurs, manifested by a base excess in arterial blood. Arterial pH will, therefore, show only a slight acidemia unless a superimposed acute illness suddenly raises PCO_2 even higher or hypoxia induces metabolic acidosis, in which case the pH may be very low.

The right-to-left shunting in the lungs, in addition to causing hypoxia, permits vasoactive substances that are usually inactivated by oxidation in the lungs to bypass this process and to enter the systemic circulation. It is possible that the focal biliary cirrhosis that occurs in cystic fibrosis may play a role in pathogenesis by liberating excess amounts of such a vasoactive substance from the diseased liver, which would further increase right-to-left shunting in the lung. The systemic effects of such a vasoactive substance are thought to be the development of hypertrophic pulmonary osteoarthropathy, with clubbing of the fingers and

Table 31–1. Electrolytes (in mmol/l) in Secretions of Patients with Cystic Fibrosis (CF) and Normal (Nl) Secretions[*]

Secretion	Na⁺ Nl	Na⁺ CF	K⁺ Nl	K⁺ CF	Cl⁻ Nl	Cl⁻ CF	Ca²⁺ Nl	Ca²⁺ CF
Sweat	22	103	9	15	18	97	0.44	0.47
Tears	140	137	26	23	134	133	2.5	4.8
Pancreatic juice (unstimulated)	107	125	11	10	94	90		
Tracheobronchial secretions	165	101	13.2	28	16.2	7.5	3.1	3.7
Saliva (parotid)	23.5	30.8	21.5	22.9	18.9	24.0	0.95	1.45
Saliva (submaxillary)	46.6	71.0	17.0	14.9	41.4	54.9	1.9	3.2

[*]Derived from data in Wood RE, Boat TF, Doershuk CF: Cystic fibrosis. In Murray JF (ed): Lung Disease, State of the Art, 1975–1976. American Lung Association, New York, 1977, p 275.

toes, hypertrophic bone changes, arthritis, and periostitis.[9]

The chronic hypoxia, hypercapnia, and acidosis can produce pulmonary hypertension, cor pulmonale, and heart failure.[10] The major factor in inducing the pulmonary hypertension is the hypoxia, which may worsen during sleep,[11, 12] with arterial blood PO_2 under 50 mm Hg being the critical level. If the PO_2 can be raised by administration of oxygen, antibiotics, and tracheal toilet, pulmonary hypertension may be reversed, at least temporarily, and heart failure corrected. Theophylline may be a potentially useful agent, since it increases the force of cardiac contractions, is a diuretic, and reduces pulmonary vascular resistance, but it requires further study in such patients.

The hepatic involvement in cystic fibrosis is probably due to inspissated biliary secretions. When the liver disease is severe, there may be insufficient production of serum albumin, with resulting hypoproteinemia and edema. Portal hypertension with enlargement of the spleen, hypersplenism, bleeding esophageal varices, and the development of ascites may also occur. These complications may be medically and surgically manageable to variable extents,[13] but the underlying liver disease has no specific therapy. While still relatively infrequent as a complication of cystic fibrosis, liver disease is likely to be seen more commonly as life expectancy increases as a result of more effective management of the pulmonary manifestations.

Pancreatic involvement also probably results from blockage of the duct from inspissation of exocrine secretions, which may produce maldigestion from pancreatic insufficiency. Endocrine secretion may

eventually also be impaired, with reduced secretion of both insulin and glucagon. This commonly results in impaired carbohydrate tolerance, with hyperglycemia and glycosuria, and occasionally results in frank diabetes mellitus, which is usually mild, but requires insulin for management.[14] Pancreatic juice (Table 31–1) has only a slightly elevated Na⁺ and decreased HCO_3^- in patients with cystic fibrosis.

Owing to the maldigestion and malabsorption, nutrients and fat-soluble vitamins are lost in the stools, which are characteristically large, bulky, soft, and foul-smelling. As a consequence of inspissation of intestinal contents, neonates may present with meconium ileus and older infants with its equivalent, and intussusception and rectal prolapse may also occur.[15] Vitamin D malabsorption, possibly combined with inadequate production of its active metabolites owing to hepatic dysfunction, may result, although uncommonly, in the development of rickets or osteopenia.[16] Vitamin K deficiency may result in bleeding, correctable by administration of the vitamin. Saliva has somewhat elevated levels of Na⁺, Cl⁻, and Ca²⁺ in patients with cystic fibrosis (Table 31–1), but this has no current role in diagnosis and pathogenesis.

Infants with cystic fibrosis may present after some months of relatively mild malabsorptive diarrhea with a chronic hypochloremic, hypokalemic metabolic alkalosis. Hyponatremia is also usually present. Several mechanisms may produce this, either singly or concurrently. First, potassium loss in the liquid stool may result in deficiency. Second, loss of NaCl in sweat may contribute to both chloride deficiency and hypovolemia. Hypovolemia may bring about increased aldosterone secretion, which augments potassium loss. If there is pulmonary disease, CO_2 retention also causes loss of potassium and chloride in the urine. Third, a low chloride concentration in plasma gives rise to potassium loss and alkalosis (Chapter 28).

Recent changes in infant feeding practices in the United States have increased the risk of this complication.[17] In 1977, manufacturers discontinued the practice of adding extra salt to infant foods (which had been added to make the food more tasty for the mother). At about the same time, cow's milk for infant feeding declined in use, replaced by commercial infant formulas and breast milk, which are lower in salt; thus, the amount of sodium in a 6-month-old infant's diet went from an average daily intake of 45 mEq of sodium down to 15 mEq. As a consequence of this reasonable change in national feeding practice, there has been an increase in the number of infants with cystic fibrosis who develop growth failure and anorexia with electrolyte depletion and metabolic alkalosis. This points up the need for alertness in diagnosis when such children are seen in the office, and the need for even more careful attention to salt losses in sweat in these modern infants, so that this may be prevented. It also should remind us of the often cryptic consequences of seemingly benign actions. Cystic fibrosis must be distinguished from congenital chloride diarrhea when these patients first present (Chapter 20).

SWEAT ANALYSIS

The electrolyte concentration of sweat plays a uniquely important role in the diagnosis of cystic fibrosis (Table 31–1). The sweat precursor initially secreted in the sweat gland of patients with cystic fibrosis is similar in salt concentration to extracellular fluid, as in normal individuals. As it passes up the sweat-gland duct, the normal degree of sodium and chloride reabsorption from the fluid does not occur, so that the sweat in patients with cystic fibrosis remains high in NaCl concentration. In sweat obtained by pilocarpine iontophoresis, normal concentrations of Na^+ range from 15.9 to 45.9 mEq/l, of Cl^- from 7.7 to 43.4 mEq/l, and of K^+ from 6.0 to 16.9 mEq/l. In patients with cystic fibrosis, sweat Na^+ concentrations range from 75.4 to 144.6 mEq/l, Cl^- from 78.6 to 148.2 mEq/l, and K^+ from 13.8 to 29.6 mEq/l.[18] Thus, there is essentially no overlap of values for Na^+ and Cl^- concentration in sweat between normal controls and individuals with cystic fibrosis.

Other diseases may produce an elevated NaCl concentration in sweat, such as untreated adrenal insufficiency, ectodermal dysplasia, nephrogenic diabetes insipidus, hypothyroidism, and malnutrition. Normal values for sweat NaCl concentration are higher in the first few days of life than later in childhood, and they double to the adult level during adolescence, but almost never to the level of patients with cystic fibrosis. Perhaps one or two per cent of patients with suspected cystic fibrosis will have a NaCl concentration in sweat at the borderline range, between 50 and 70 mEq/l. Diagnosis in these patients will depend on other factors, such as the NaCl content of nails, duodenal fluid assay, and the clinical picture over time.

Laboratory errors will usually be in the direction of a higher reported concentration of salt in sweat than actually exists, owing to evaporation of the sample. As a screening procedure, electrical conductivity of the collected sweat can be used, but this is not so reliable as a quantitative analysis of sweat collected on a weighed sample of filter paper for Na^+ and Cl^- concentration.

When sampling sweat that has not been absorbed on filter paper, care must be taken to mix the sample, since evaporation and condensation of the sweat may change the salt concentrations in various portions of the sample. This may be more of a problem with instruments that use electrical conductivity of sweat for analysis and with newer analytic instruments that require very small sample size and thus allow volumetric sampling of sweat collected by pilocarpine iontophoresis.

Given all these problems, the positive sweat test is still almost specifically diagnostic, but because of the serious prognostic implications, the diagnosis of cystic fibrosis should not be made until the test has been repeated in a reliable laboratory and until a history of either cystic fibrosis in the family or digestive or pulmonary insufficiency has been confirmed.

PATHOPHYSIOLOGY OF EXCESSIVE SWEATING

In hot weather, when large amounts of sweat are produced, patients with cystic fibrosis may lose excessive amounts of salt in their sweat. These patients lose proportionately more extracellular volume than do normal individuals, owing to the greater NaCl loss, and may develop heat prostration with hyperthermia, hyponatremia (if they drink unsalted water), and metabolic alkalosis.[19] This may be prevented by air conditioning, decreased exertion in the heat, and increased salt intake in hot weather. With severe exertion in extreme heat, a normal adult can secrete up to 2 l of sweat an hour and up to perhaps 13 l a day. If an adult patient with cystic fibrosis were to secrete this much sweat at a NaCl concentration of 140 mEq/l, it would total 140 mEq × 13 l, or 1820 mEq (1.82 moles) of NaCl, which equals, in turn, 106 gm (1.82 moles × 58.5, the molecular weight of NaCl). This is about five times the amount of salt required by normal adults at heavy work in the heat. The concentration of salt in the sweat of our hypothetical worker with cystic fibrosis is also about five times that in normal sweat. This amount of salt (almost one-quarter pound) should be taken as the extreme outer limit for the daily requirement for work in the heat, since actual requirements will almost always be less, since the salt concentration of the sweat of most patients with cystic fibrosis will probably be less than 140 mEq/l and sweating will unlikely be that extreme for that long.

For a 70-kg adult, 106 gm of NaCl is 1.51 gm per kilogram and 26 mEq/kg. If this amount were given quickly to anyone at one time, it would almost certainly be quickly lethal. The salt, in much lesser amounts, should be given as the losses occur, since salt will not be stored in the body and is harmful in overdose and since it is not possible to excrete a salt excess efficiently. Ingestion of salt tablets or powdered salt will likely lead to gastrointestinal distress, nausea, and vomiting. Eating salty foods and taking extra salt at meals may be encouraged, but excess salt ingestion should be avoided. Ingestion of fluids containing adequate concentrations of salt is probably the safest way to supplement salt. Most oral rehydration solutions used for treating diarrhea have too low a sodium and chloride concentration and too high a potassium concentration for this use (see Chapter 20). Commercially available chicken soup and beef broth contain concentrations of Na⁺ ranging from 114 to 251 mEq/l, with only 1.5 to 17 mEq/l of K⁺ and with osmolalities ranging from 293 to 507 mOsm/kg of H_2O.[20] Fruit juices, fruit-flavored drinks, beer, and carbonated beverages contain too little sodium to be useful. Chicken soup again finds a place in medical therapy and prevention(!) but should not be used as the sole source of fluid intake, lest hypernatremia develop.

REFERENCES

1. Wood RE, Boat TF, Doershuk CF: Cystic fibrosis. In Murray JF (ed): Lung Disease, State of the Art, 1975–1976. American Lung Association, New York, 1977, p 275.
2. Feigal RJ, Shapiro BL: Altered intracellular calcium in fibroblasts from patients with cystic fibrosis and heterozygotes. Pediatr Res 13:764, 1979.
3. Gibson LE, Matthews WJ Jr, Minihan PT, Patti JA: Relating mucus, calcium, and sweat in a new concept of cystic fibrosis. Pediatrics 48:695, 1971.
4. Johansen PG, Anderson CM, Hadorn B: Cystic fibrosis of the pancreas. Lancet, March 2, 1968, p 455.
5. Impero JE, Harrison GM, Nelson TE: Cystic fibrosis: isolation and physical properties of a salivary cystic fibrosis factor. Pediatr. Res 12:108, 1978.
6. Gillard BK, Feig SA, Harrison GM, Nelson TE: Cystic fibrosis: enzymatic detection of a ciliostatic factor. Pediatr Res 10:907, 1976.
7. Cherry JD, Roden VJ, Rejent AJ, Dorner RW: The inhibition of ciliary activity in tracheal organ cultures by sera from children with cystic fibrosis and control subjects. J Pediatr 79:937, 1971.
8. Hubbard VS, Barbero G, Chase HP: Selenium and cystic fibrosis. J Pediatr 96:421, 1980.
9. Kravath RE, Scarpelli EM, Bernstein J: Hepatogenic cyanosis: arteriovenous shunts in chronic active hepatitis. J Pediatr 78:238, 1971.
10. Stern RC, Borkat G, Hirschfeld SS, et al: Heart failure in cystic fibrosis. Am J Dis Child 134:267, 1980.
11. Francis PWJ, Muller NL, Gurwitz D, et al: Hemoglobin desaturation. Am J Dis Child 134:734, 1980.
12. Muller NL, Francis PW, Gurwitz D, et al: Mechanism of hemoglobin desaturation during rapid-eye-movement sleep in normal subjects and in

patients with cystic fibrosis. Am Rev Respir Dis 121:463, 1980.

13. Stern RC, Stevens DP, Boat TF, et al: Symptomatic hepatic disease in cystic fibrosis: incidence, course, and outcome of portal systemic shunting. Gastroenterology 70:645, 1976.

14. Lippe BM, Kaplan SA, Neufeld ND, et al: Insulin receptors in cystic fibrosis: increased receptor number and altered affinity. Pediatrics 65:1018, 1980.

15. di Sant'Agnese PA, Davis PB: Cystic fibrosis in adults. Am J Med 66:121, 1979.

16. Hahn TJ, Squires AE, Halstead LR, Strominger DB: Reduced serum 25-hydroxyvitamin D concentration and disordered mineral metabolism in patients with cystic fibrosis. J Pediatr 94:38, 1979.

17. Laughlin JJ, Brady MS, Eigen H: Changing feeding trends as a cause of electrolyte depletion in infants with cystic fibrosis. Pediatrics 68:203, 1981.

18. Shwachman H, Mahmoodian A, Neff RK: The sweat test: sodium and chloride values. J Pediatr 98:576, 1981.

19. Gottlieb RP: Metabolic alkalosis in cystic fibrosis. J Pediatr 79:930, 1971.

20. Wendland BE, Arbus GS, McCuaig CC, Malik AM: Oral fluid therapy: sodium and potassium content and osmolality of some commercial "clear" soups, juices and beverages. Can Med Assoc J 121:564, 1979.

Chapter 32

SPORTS AND EXERCISE

There is a surprising paucity of information on fluid and electrolyte problems in sports in the standard textbooks of pediatrics and in books and articles on sports medicine. Even books on marathon running give scant attention to water and salt requirements. This is probably because most individuals participating in sports are in good basic health with normal physiologic responses, so that drinking in response to thirst and the usual intake of salt and other minerals in the diet suffice to maintain homeostasis. Other responses to exercise, such as increasing respiration or cardiac output and the readjustments of circulation and renal blood flow, are autonomic and automatic and do not require the ministrations of a physician.

WATER

Nevertheless, there are several areas of interest and perhaps even usefulness to the physician. Sports activities obviously vary in their requirements for energy expenditure, as seen in Table 32–1.[1] This ranges, for a 70-kg adult or adolescent, from croquet at 135 cal per hour, to figure skating at 570 cal per hour, to running at 18.9 miles per hour, which, if one could do it, requires 9,480 cal per hour. For every 100 cal produced from carbohydrate, 20 l of oxygen are consumed and 20 l of carbon dioxide are produced. Water requirements parallel oxygen consumption and caloric expenditure. For every 100 cal expended, 100 ml of water is needed, including the water of oxidation from the carbohydrate, protein, or fat metabolized. Most of this increased water requirement is for insensible water loss through the skin and the lungs, with a small amount for urine, so that sodium and chloride requirements in the absence of sweating are minimal.

If sweating does occur, the water requirements are increased. The rate of sweating decreases with time, but rates of up to 2 l per hour are possible. Individual variability, temperature, humidity, degree of exertion, and level of training all exert an influence on the degree of sweating. With acclimatization to heat, larger volumes of sweat are produced with lower salt contents in the initial few weeks, but then sweat production falls as other measures of physiologic adaptation become active.

SALT

Water losses during exertion should be replaced as they occur, with major reliance on the thirst mechanism. Salt requirements in the absence of sweating are minimal, since most of the water lost does not contain salt. Since sweat may normally have a NaCl concentration of up to 70 mEq/l, substantial salt losses can occur with heavy sweating over a period of time. Even in marathon runners, however, it has not been shown to be necessary to replace the salt during a race, except in very hot weather, but water replacement is always necessary.[2] Salt as a powder or as tablets should not be given, since it may cause gastric distress, nausea, and vomiting and may easily lead to excessive use and overdosing. If salt solutions are used, they should be dilute, containing less than 50 mEq/l of salt. With extreme degrees of sweating and prolonged exertion, replacement of salt lost in sweat becomes mandatory, and it should be administered at a rate appropriate to the level of sweating.

217

Table 32–1. Energy Required by a 70-kg Person for Various Physical Activities*

ACTIVITY	TOTAL CALORIES PER HOUR
Sleeping	70
Mental work, seated	105
Standing	110
Croquet	135
Office work	145
Walking, 2 m.p.h.	170
Walking up stairs, 1 m.p.h.	180
Riding a bicycle, 5.5 m.p.h.	190
Bowling	215
Billiards	235
Dancing, moderate	250
Baseball (except pitching)	280
Rowing for pleasure	300
Dancing, vigorous	340
Table tennis	345
Baseball, pitching	390
Basketball	395
Bicycle riding, rapid	415
Swimming crawl stroke, 1 m.p.h.	420
Walking up 8.6% grade, 2.4 m.p.h.	430
Swimming breaststroke, 1.6 m.p.h.	490
Skiing, 3 m.p.h.	540
Figure skating	570
Walking up stairs, 2 m.p.h.	590
Rowing, 3.5 m.p.h.	660
Swimming crawl stroke, 1.6 m.p.h.	700
Parallel bar work	710
Horizontal running, 5.7 m.p.h.	720
Wrestling	790
Swimming backstroke, 1.6 m.p.h.	800
Horizontal running, 7 m.p.h.	870
Marathon running	990
Football	1000
Swimming sidestroke, 1.6 m.p.h.	1200
Horizontal running, 11.4 m.p.h.	1300
Swimming crawl stroke, 2.2 m.p.h.	1600
Swimming breaststroke, 2.2 m.p.h.	1850
Swimming backstroke, 2.2 m.p.h.	2000
Swimming sidestroke, 2.2 m.p.h.	3000
Horizontal running, 15.8 m.p.h.	3910
Horizontal running, 17.2 m.p.h.	4740
Horizontal running, 18.6 m.p.h.	7790
Horizontal running, 18.9 m.p.h.	9480

*Adapted from Morehouse LE, Miller AT: Physiology of Exercise. C. V. Mosby Co., St. Louis, 1976.

The caloric values are approximations that are based on oxygen consumption and include basal requirements.

A daily intake of 20 gm of salt per day should be adequate for exertion in a hot environment.[4] This is 341 mEq of NaCl and provides about 5 mEq/kg of body weight for a 70-kg adult. This provides enough salt for 10 l of sweat containing 34.1 mEq/l of NaCl. Six grams of salt per day for men working in a hot environment has proved inadequate. This dosage — 103 mEq, or about 1.5 mEq/kg of body weight — has been associated with increased temperature, pulse rate, nausea, vomiting, tachycardia, hypotension, and vertigo in 25 per cent of those taking this amount, ten times the incidence of those given 15 gm of salt per person. No advantage has been seen in increasing the salt intake to 30 gm per day.

The best drink during sports activities is pure cold water in large disposable cups. The favorite drink, following the activity, of marathon runners and other participants in sports requiring heavy physical exertion is beer, which is well suited to replace calories, water, and very mild salt deficits, since it contains approximately 3.6 per cent alcohol, 3.8 per cent carbohydrate, (0.42 cal/ml), 3 mEq/l of sodium and 6 mEq/l of potassium.[3]

EFFECTS OF EXERCISE

If water intake is inadequate, dehydration results, impairing metabolic function as well as further impairing the heat-dispersing mechanisms such as sweating and increased blood flow to the skin. At 5 per cent loss of body weight, performance becomes impaired.[5]

Even with ongoing water replacement during heavy exertion, significant weight loss and water loss still occur along with a decrease in plasma volume. Without replacement, the deficit may easily become excessive to the point at which physiologic adaptations may be impaired, as reflected by increasing heart rate and body temperature.

Efforts by wrestlers and boxers to make lower weight categories by forcing dehydration prior to weigh-in by the use of diuretics, sweating in a steam room or sauna, and exercise in a sweat suit, all accompanied by fluid restriction, are debilitating and should be discouraged, although some attempts at small amounts of weight loss are, realistically, probably inevitable. The resulting disturbance, particularly when diuretics are used, may persist into and beyond the athletic event, with the potential of adversely affecting performance and causing cardiac arrhythmia.

Exercise causes increased secretion of ADH, owing to both emotional stress and to water loss, and this results in the production of smaller amounts of concentrated urine.

As lactic acid accumulates in the blood and tissues owing to anaerobic metabolism, renal correction occurs with excretion of the acid, so that urine pH is low.

Constituents such as protein, red blood cells, casts, and sugar, which in other circumstance are considered abnormal, will be found in the urine of normal athletes following strenuous exercise with or without body contact. This has been called athletic pseudonephritis. After one week of rest these findings disappear. Hemoglobin may also be found in the urine of many athletes, and this has been found to be due primarily to running on a hard surface. The wearing of cushioned soles prevents damage to the blood cells in the soles of the feet and thereby alleviates the hemoglobinuria.[6]

During exercise, blood flow is diverted to the exercising muscles and away from the gastrointestinal tract so that digestive processes will not be efficient, although a light meal up to one-half hour before exercise has not been shown to be harmful.[6]

In addition to water, salt, and calories that must be replaced following exercise, there is an oxygen debt to be paid after extreme exercise for the restoration of oxygen stores in the myoglobin, blood, and tissues; for the restoration of creatine phosphate and ATP levels; for the metabolism of excess lactic acid; and for the repletion of glycogen.

In sustained exercise on land, PO_2 and PCO_2 do not change much beyond normal limits. On the other hand, moderate exercise may produce a fall in arterial blood pH to 7.25, and very severe exercise can produce a fall in pH to 6.8, which has been associated with a marked elevation of blood lactate.

Swimming and diving differ significantly from other sports in that breath-holding and hypoventilation frequently occur, so that hypoxia and hypercapnia are common. Breath-holding is of no particular medical consequence in the otherwise healthy individual, since there are strong physiologic mechanisms that will restore normal PCO_2 and PO_2 unless the individual has hyperventilated first, which can drive the arterial PCO_2 down quite a lot, from 40 mm Hg to 15 mm Hg, while raising the arterial PO_2 from 95 mm Hg to 120 mm Hg. Since the relationship between PCO_2 and blood content of CO_2 is linear, whereas that of oxygen follows the oxyhemoglobin dissociation curve, hyperventilation produces a large reduction in the amount of carbon dioxide and a relatively small increase in the amount of oxygen in the body. With breath-holding, the PO_2 will fall faster than the PCO_2 will rise. Since low PO_2 is a relatively weak respiratory stimulus, compared to a high PCO_2, it is possible to hold one's breath for a long period of time—so long, in fact, that one can lose consciousness and drown under water before developing the overwhelming desire to breathe that a higher PCO_2 would induce. Hyperventilation prior to swimming and diving should, therefore, be discouraged.

REFERENCES

1. Morehouse LE, Miller AT Jr: Physiology of Exercise. C. V. Mosby Co., St. Louis, 1976, pp. 136, 137.
2. Shephard RJ, Kavanagh T: Fluid and mineral needs of middle-aged and postcoronary distance runners. The Physician and Sportsmedicine, 6:90, 1978.
3. U.S. Government Agricultural Handbook #8, 1963.
4. Morehouse LE, Miller AT Jr: Physiology of Exercise. C.V. Mosby Co., St. Louis, 1976, Chapter 16.
5. Falls HB: Exercise Physiology. Academic Press, New York, 1968, Chapter 6.
6. Falls HB: Exercise Physiology. Academic Press, New York, 1968, Chapter 4.

Chapter 33

SPECIAL PROBLEMS OF THE FETUS AND NEONATE

This chapter will deal with some of the unique aspects of fluid and electrolyte balance in the neonatal period. This time of life is singled out for special emphasis because of the small size of the patients involved, their transition from fetal to neonatal life, and the dynamic nature of the evolving neonate. The margin for error is extremely small in the care of these patients. Several recent reviews of fluid, electrolyte, and mineral balance in the fetus and neonate provide the reader with multiple references on the topics discussed here.[1-4]

NORMAL FETAL AND NEONATAL PHYSIOLOGY

In the earliest stages of fetal life, water constitutes as much as 95 per cent of the total body weight of the developing embryo. By 32 weeks' gestation, total body water approximates 80 per cent of the body weight. At term, the normal fetus contains between 75 and 80 per cent of the total body weight as water. During development of the embryo, the proportion of the total body water represented in the extracellular space shifts, decreasing from approximately 60 per cent at the fifth month of gestation to only 45 per cent of the total body weight at term. The intracellular water, on the other hand, increases to approximately 33 per cent of the total body weight at birth. This is consistent with the hyperplasia and hypertrophy of cells in the developing fetus.

The fetus and mother are involved in major exchanges of water throughout pregnancy. There is a dynamic circulation among the fetus, the surrounding amniotic

fluid, and the mother. This three-compartment model for fluid and electrolyte exchange has been studied both in the non-human primate and, through isotope techniques, in the human. More than one liter of water per kilogram of fetal weight per hour is exchanged between the mother and fetus, with a small net positive balance to the fetus for growth. Isotope studies reveal that 40 per cent of the transfer of water from the amniotic fluid space back to the mother takes place through the fetus. Fetuses have been observed to swallow amniotic fluid at approximately 20 ml/hr at term and to micturate into the amniotic fluid between 20 and 30 ml/hr.

Maternal uterine blood flow ranges from 6 to 15 l per hour per kilogram of uterus and its contents, according to several species studies. Thus, a substantial portion of the plasma volume of the blood flowing through the uterine vessels is exchanged between mother and fetus. Hydrostatic and oncotic forces, which are responsible for the movement of fluid in and out of the intravascular space, are responsible for exchange between mother and fetus through the placental circulation as well. Multiple plasma electrolytes such as sodium, potassium, and chloride are exchanged as water moves in and out of the fetal compartment; thus, changes in the maternal milieu are rapidly reflected in fetal changes. In the early months of gestation, the amniotic fluid compartment reflects the fetal intravascular plasma concentrations of electrolytes. As the fetal kidneys mature, however, electrolyte concentration and osmolality increase in the amniotic fluid and no longer resemble concentrations found in fetal plasma.

The fetus will require large amounts of electrolytes and minerals for adequate growth and development. At term, the fetus contains approximately 25 to 30 gm of calcium, most of the accretion of which occurs in the last trimester. As early as the twentieth week of gestation, calcium balance studies have revealed an increase in calcium absorption in pregnant women. During the last trimester of pregnancy, total and ionized calcium levels in fetal plasma exceed those in the mother. The placenta plays an active role in transporting calcium ions from mother to fetus against a concentration gradient. It is postulated that this active transport occurs as a result of a calcium-stimulated ATPase found in placental membranes. Calcium is able to move bidirectionally across the placenta, but there is a net transfer rate from mother to fetus of six to ten times that required for fetal bone accretion.

The transition from fetal to neonatal life occurs with the clamping of the umbilical cord and the dramatic decrease in the influx of water, electrolytes, and minerals to the neonate. All neonates demonstrate an appreciable loss of body weight over the first few days of life. This is due largely to loss of extracellular fluid volume. Studies in animals have been interpreted as indicating that the excess fluid at birth not only serves during a period of less intake but may be regulated by hormonal mechanisms for more rapid excretion if exogenous fluid intake is maintained by intravenous infusion.[5]

Glomerular filtration rate in the kidney of the neonate is markedly decreased when compared with that of the adult. However, morphologic and physiologic studies have shown that there is an even more dramatic decrease in tubular reabsorptive or secretory capacity in the neonatal kidney. Thus, the neonatal kidney is functionally in a state of glomerular-tubular imbalance, with filtration capability surpassing reabsorptive capacity. By 35 weeks' gestation, the embryologic formation of the kidney is complete; however, the tubules have not grown to their ultimate relative length. The loops of Henle are very short, and their reabsorptive capacity is small, so that the ratio of glomerular surface area to tubular volume is very high.

Multiple factors in the neonate affect insensible water loss. Gestational age, respiratory rate, and temperature of the ambient environment as well as body temperature, activity, the use of exogenous heat sources such as radiant warmers and phototherapy lamps, and the use of heat shields to decrease evaporative heat loss through the skin all affect the amount of water lost from the skin and respiratory tract. Obligatory urine output in the neonate is affected by the amount of both solute and protein-generating urea in the diet. Although antidiuretic hormone and aldosterone are present in the neonate and can affect tubular function, the tubules themselves can only concentrate to a urine osmolality of approximately 800 mOsm/kg and dilute to approximately 30 mOsm/kg at term. For the term infant, insensible water loss represents approximately 35 ml/kg per day and obligatory urine loss is approximately 45 ml/kg per day; losses of sodium and potassium in these fluids are approximately 2 to 3 mEq/kg per day. Because the relationship between energy expenditure and body weight in neonates is linear, these fluid relationships can be expressed in relation to body weight.

Over the first 12 to 24 hours of life, all neonates exhibit a decrease in total and ionized calcium level in the plasma. This is not a result of increased losses or decreased amount of intake of calcium into the body; rather, it is a result of an inability to mobilize calcium from one compartment into the extracellular and intravascular space. The average neonate has approximately 150 to 200 ml of plasma and approximately 30,000 mg of calcium in his or her body. To maintain a normal plasma calcium level of greater than 8 mg/dl, the infant must maintain merely 12 to 16 mg of calcium in the intravascular space. This normal decrease in plasma ionized calcium in the neonate over the first two days of life stimulates homeostatic mechanisms within the vitamin D endocrine and parathyroid hormone systems in order to maintain normocalcemia.

NEONATAL DISORDERS

It is much more difficult to assess clinically the hydration state of a neonate than that of an older infant or child. The goal of fluid and electrolyte administration in the neonate is to prevent clinical and biochemical abnormalities and signs of dehydration without establishing a zero balance for water and electrolytes. Neonates weighing more than 1500 gm frequently lose up to 10 per cent of their body weight in the first few days of life. Much of this weight loss is water loss, and no attempt is made to replace it. Infants weighing less than 1500 gm frequently lose as much as 15 per cent of body weight in the first days of life.

Intravenous therapy in neonates attempts to replace insensible water losses and urinary losses and provide adequate water for growth and metabolism. Monitoring of the adequacy of fluid therapy is done primarily by measurement of the most important vital sign in the neonate — i.e., weight. Input and output, including accurate urine volumes, are obtained to assure that urinary output ranges from 1 to 4 ml/kg per hour. Urine osmolality between 75 and 300 mOsm/kg, which generally correlates with a urine specific gravity between 1.002 and 1.010, allows for normal hydration without undue stress on the neonatal tubules. Of course, urine specific gravity is of less value in the assessment of hydration status whenever there is glycosuria.

Reasonable fluid volumes to attain these goals in the full-term infant in the first days of life are 75 to 85 ml/kg per day, and they increase to approximately 150 ml/kg per day by the end of the first week of life. Sodium and potassium requirements are approximately 2 to 3 mEq/kg per day and should be provided in the intravenous solutions over the course of the entire 24-hour period beginning by the end of the first day of life. The anions are provided in a balanced ratio as described in the general sections on fluid and electrolyte therapy.

Neonatal Sodium Disturbances

Hypo- and hypernatremia are not infrequent occurrences during the neonatal period. Hyponatremia, defined as a serum sodium concentration of less than 130 mEq/l, is most frequently due to excessive hydration. Immaturity of renal glomerular and tubular function results in over-retention of fluid after excessive water intake. Excessive hydration frequently occurs in neonates who are hypoglycemic and require glucose infusions. Infusion rates to maintain adequate serum concentrations of glucose frequently result in greater water intake than is necessary.

Hyponatremia in the first hours of life may be due to maternal hyponatremia secondary to large volumes of water not containing adequate sodium in the maternal intravenous fluids during labor. Hyponatremia may also result from decreased sodium intake during the first weeks of life in those infants who have not received adequate sodium intravenously or who have been on low-sodium formulas or human milk. Abnormal losses of sodium secondary to surgical fistulae, diarrheal disease, or abnormal renal tubular function can result in hyponatremia. Lack of mineralocorticoid function either secondary to primary adrenal disease or due to pituitary-adrenal axis dysfunction can also present as hyponatremia usually associated with hyperkalemia. The "syndrome of excessive secretion of antidiuretic hormone" may occur in the neonate who has suffered any insult to the central nervous system secondary to hypoxia, hemorrhage, hypotension, or anesthesia and may be defined and treated, primarily by reduction of the maintenance water allowance, as discussed in Chapters 14 and 23.

Hypernatremia frequently occurs as a result of underhydration in the neonate. The thin skin and the ease of insensible water loss in the small premature infant, as well as the use of radiant heat and phototherapy light, can result in large water needs during the first days of life. Osmotic diuresis secondary to glycosuria can also cause excessive water loss and result in hypernatremia. True diabetes insipidus is a rare disorder in neonates, but it may occur. Excessive administration of sodium can result in hypernatremia. Flushes of intra-arterial or intravenous lines with sodium-containing solutions frequently are neglected in calculating the sodium intake of the small neonate. These flush solutions can provide a substantial proportion of salt and water intake in the neonate. The use of sodium bicarbonate infusions to correct acidemia can also result in large intakes of sodium in the neonatal period.

Correction of hypo- and hypernatremia can be accomplished in the neonate as in older infants and children. It should be emphasized that the need for slow correction of these abnormalities is crucial in the neonate, whose periventricular vessels are extremely fragile and prone to hemorrhage.

Prematurity

In the previous section we have described the increased insensible water losses in the premature neonate. The recommendation to begin 75 to 85 ml/kg per day in the first day of life and to increase to approximately 150 ml/kg per day by the end of the first week of life for full-term infants can be extended to premature infants weighing down to approximately 1500 gm. However, for premature infants weighing between 1000 and 1500 gm, increased insensible water losses mandate that 80 to 100 ml/kg for the first 24 hours be utilized and that by the third to fifth days of life as much as 175 ml/kg per day be administered to maintain normal hydration. In the very small premature infant, weighing less than 1000 gm, insensible water losses are so great that recommendations for appropriate fluid management can be made only in a general sense, and careful measurements of weight, heart rate, blood pressure, urine output, and specific gravity or osmolality must be determined every 8 to 12 hours in order to maintain adequate hydration.

Our recommendations for the very small neonate nursed in a radiant warmer are 100 to 125 ml/kg per day during the first 24 hours of life, increasing immediately to 150 ml/kg per day on the second day of life and to the range of 200 to 250 ml/kg per day by the third to fifth days of life. It is important to remember that, as these large volumes of water are utilized, the concentrations of glucose, sodium, potassium, and other electrolytes in the fluid must be decreased so that the total volume of these substances administered over a 24-hour period is not excessive. In the administration of intravenous solutions, determining the concentration of glucose on the basis of milligrams of glucose per kilogram per minute frequently helps in maintaining adequate levels of glucose in the plasma, preventing them from becoming excessive. The administration of excessive glucose can cause hyperglycemia and an osmotic diuresis.

Recent studies have suggested that overhydration of the very low birthweight infant may result in an increased incidence of patent ductus arteriosus and perhaps even accelerate the development of bronchopulmonary dysplasia. Thus, fluid needs in the premature infant must be very carefully assessed in order to maintain the delicate balance for appropriate hydration.

A frequent concomitant of prematurity is immature lung function, or respiratory distress syndrome. This disease of progressive atelectasis is caused by decreased formation of surface active phospholipids by the type II alveolar pneumocytes. The premature neonate with mild disease presents with respiratory distress as manifested by tachypnea, retractions, and increased work of breathing. Insensible water loss and caloric requirements increase in these sick neonates. Increase in the ambient oxygen requirement may be necessary to maintain appropriate partial pressures of oxygen in the blood. Nebulized or humidified oxygen must be utilized in order to decrease possible insensible water loss during breathing of dry gases, and warmed administration of gas is utilized in order to decrease cold stress and prevent the possible creation of temperature instability. If ventilatory assistance is required, humidified gases must be used to decrease insensible water loss from the respiratory tract. Humidification should be adequate but not excessive. Excessive water condensation on the endotracheal tube may result in a positive balance of water in the premature infant. This condensation can result in excessive water intake and hydration and electrolyte disturbances.

Premature infants with respiratory distress syndrome frequently manifest respiratory and metabolic acidemia and acidosis. Correction of respiratory acidosis is accomplished by ventilation of the patient, not administration of buffer. It is important to note that an ordinarily normal level of PCO_2, in the range of 40 to 45 mm Hg, is abnormal in the face of any metabolic acidosis. Appropriate respiratory compensation would force a decrease in PCO_2. Thus, neonates with mild acidosis and a "normal" PCO_2 are really manifesting abnormalities in ventilation. This is extremely important when correction of acidemia is considered. Only the metabolic components of acidosis can be or should be corrected by administration of base. When bicarbonate is utilized to buffer metabolic acidemia, the concentration of sodium and the osmolality of the infused solution are of critical importance. There is increasing evidence that rapid shifts of water due to rapid infusions of hypertonic bicarbonate in premature infants have resulted in an increased incidence of intraventricular hemorrhage.[6-8]

Metabolic acidemia in the neonate, as in other patients, should be corrected by the infusion of isotonic solutions of sodium bicarbonate — i.e., 150 mEq/l of sodium bicarbonate. This approach to correction of metabolic acidosis does result in increased fluid administration in the premature infant in order to correct acidemia. However, if the appropriate fluids are not provided exogenously, the hyperosmolar fluids administered will extract the necessary fluids from the extravascular and intracellular environment, resulting in serious cellular damage, particularly in the central nervous system.

A pathologic decrease of the plasma ionized calcium level occurs in approximately 35 to 50 per cent of premature neonates, depending upon weight, gestational age, and perinatal factors. Although many of these premature neonates remain without observable symptoms, we believe that this biochemical abnormality, defined as an ionized calcium level in the plasma of less than 3.0 mg/dl may result in central nervous system dysfunction that has yet to be defined. Neonates who become symptomatic from hypocalcemia may manifest seizures, apnea, neuromuscular irritability, vomiting, abdominal distension, poor feeding, cyanosis, and other nonspecific symptoms.

When the plasma ionized calcium level in the first days of life is less than 3.0 mg/dl or the total serum calcium level in the premature infant weighing less than 1500 gm is less than 6.5 mg/dl or in the larger premature infant less than 7.0 mg/dl, treatment of this early neonatal hypocalcemia can be accomplished by the intravenous infusion or oral administration of calcium salts. Intravenous calcium gluconate in a dose of 500 mg/kg per day can be added to the intravenous solution over 24 hours. Infants receiving intravenous calcium must have constant cardiac rate and rhythm monitoring because of the possibility of cardiac arrhythmias. Severe local damage can occur if calcium salts extravasate into the tissues.

Constant intravenous infusion of calcium salts with careful attention to the site of infusion results in a constant, normal plasma level of ionized calcium. Bolus infusions of calcium salts every four to six hours results in a normal level of calcium only during and shortly after the bolus infusion. For infants who are able to take formula at greater than 75 ml/kg per day and who are asymptomatic, calcium salts can be added to the formula to increase the ratio of calcium to phosphorus to 4:1 in the formula in order to decrease phosphorus absorption, enhance calcium absorption, and result in higher serum calcium levels. This supplementation to the formula is not calcium supplementation to the patient, but rather a treatment of the formula itself.

Attempts to utilize greater oral supplements of calcium than that proposed here results in severe gastrointestinal irritability and diarrhea. Recent preliminary studies have utilized, with some success, vitamin D metabolites, 25-hydroxycholecalciferol, and 1,25-dihydroxycholecalciferol in an attempt to prevent this disorder of prematurity.

Glomerular filtration rate and tubular reabsorption are quite minimal in the premature infant. Net acid excretion is also decreased in the premature infant; thus, a substantial proportion of normal premature neonates during the second week of life will exhibit metabolic acidosis sometimes associated with acidemia, which will result in poor weight gain and may result in lethargy and poor feeding behavior. This acidosis is secondary to an inability to handle the acid loads presented to the kidney by exogenous formulas that provide 3 to 4 gm/kg per day of protein to the premature neonate. Supplementation of these neonates with oral sodium bicarbonate (2 to 3 mEq/kg per day) in order to treat the metabolic acidosis frequently results in enhanced activity and growth. If oral sodium bicarbonate supplementation is not adequate, protein intake in the diet must be reduced in order to allow these infants to stabilize their acid-base status.

Infants of Diabetic Mothers

Infants born to diabetic mothers demonstrate a fetal embryopathy that results in an infant who is, on the average, 550 gm heavier and 1.5 cm longer at birth than normal infants with gestational ages between 36 and 38 weeks. Initially, many clinicians had the impression that these macrosomic infants were overhydrated. However, careful analysis demonstrates that the total body water in the infant of a diabetic is 70.2 per cent of body weight as compared to 78.2 per cent of the body weight in normal infants. Particularly, there is a significant reduction in extracellular water. Thus, infants of diabetic mothers, although large, require substantial administration of water and electrolytes in the early hours and days of life.

Frequently, these hyperinsulinemic neonates become hypoglycemic and require glucose supplementation. Excessive hydration may occur when large concentrations of glucose are needed for restoration of normoglycemia.

Approximately 20 to 30 per cent of infants born to diabetic mothers will demonstrate a pathologic decrease in ionized calcium level during the first four days of life. The approach to this problem in the infant of a diabetic should be similar to that in the premature neonate. Careful serial evaluation of serum calcium levels and the administration of intravenous or oral calcium salts when hypocalcemia is observed should result in the maintenance of normal biochemical homeostasis.

REFERENCES

1. Dreszer M: Fluid and electrolyte requirements in the newborn infant. Pediatr Clin North Am 24:577, 1977.
2. Roy, RN, Sinclair JC: Hydration of the low birth-weight infant. Clin Perinatol 2:393, 1975.
3. Fleischman AR: Fetal parathyroid gland and calcium metabolism. Clin Obstet Gynecol 23:791, 1980.
4. Fleischman AR, Rosen, JF, Nathenson G, Finberg L: Prevention and treatment of neonatal hypocalcemia. In DeLuca HF, Anast C (eds.): Pediatric Diseases Related to Calcium. Elsevier, New York, 1980. p. 345.
5. Coulter, DM, Avery ME: Paradoxical reduction in tissue hydration with weight gain in neonatal rabbit pups. Pediatr Res 14:1122, 1980.
6. Kravath RE, Aharon AS, Abal G, Finberg L: Clinically significant physiologic changes from rapidly administered hypertonic solutions: acute osmol poisoning. Pediatrics 46:267, 1970.
7. Simmons MA, Adcock EW, Bard H, Battaglia FC: Hypernatremia and intracranial hemorrhage in neonates. N Engl J Med 291:6, 1974.
8. Papile L, Burstein J, Burstein R, et al: Realtionship of intravenous sodium bicarbonate infusions and cerebral intraventricular hemorrhage. J. Pediatr 93:834, 1978.

Chapter 34

SPECIAL PROBLEMS OF SURGICAL PATIENTS, INCLUDING PARENTERAL NUTRITION

The act of surgery itself, apart from the underlying disorder for which it is performed, results in significant catabolism in all patients. Research has focused primarily on the adult surgical patient, and little is known about these catabolic effects on the neonate, infant, and child. However, it can be assumed that during the first week postoperatively, the surgical patient will be in a catabolic state of negative nitrogen balance. The surgical procedure itself, as well as this postoperative phase, will also be associated with major losses of electrolytes, minerals, and water. During the preoperative and intraoperative phases of stress, catecholamines, antidiuretic hormone, and glucocorticoids will be secreted in considerable amounts and the results of the secretion of these hormones will be evident in the first days postoperatively. The goal of the management of the surgical patient is not only to correct the abnormality that required surgical intervention, but also to allow the patient to maintain metabolic balance during the early postoperative phase and to reach a stage of anabolic restoration to allow normal growth and development. The challenge in the pediatric surgical patient is even greater than in the adult, because of the requirement that the patient not only heal but also maintain normal growth and development.

PREOPERATIVE, INTRAOPERATIVE, AND POSTOPERATIVE MANAGEMENT

Preoperative Management

The preventive management of the surgical patient is critical to the success of the surgical intervention and the postoperative restoration of normal function.

It has been observed that patients who have had surgery "converve" sodium postoperatively.[1] In fact, this sodium "conservation" is usually secondary to hypovolemia, which often has its genesis in preoperative dehydration, often of previously hydrated infants awaiting elective surgery. This occurs because the nothing-by-mouth order has been in effect too long, allowing rapid water turnover in infants and young children to result in hypovolemia.[2, 3] The remedy, of course, is to provide parenteral maintenance water preoperatively when time periods of more than three to four hours of oral fluid restriction are needed for infants.[2, 4]

The pediatrician must work in concert with the surgeon to fulfill the goals of the preoperative phase. Patients may frequently need to be resuscitated prior to surgical intervention. Maintenance of an adequate airway and cardiovascular integrity must be obtained. Preoperatively, the extracellular fluid volume must be restored. Assessment of adequacy of the intravascular space can be done by measurement of pulse, blood pressure, capillary filling in the skin, core temperature, and temperature of the extremities. Use of central venous pressure measurement is helpful when available. The emergent nature of the surgical intervention may preclude the correction of intracellular fluid composition or even a near-complete correction of the extracellular fluid composition. However, beginnings of such correction should be initiated in the preoperative phase, maintained throughout the operative course, and concluded in the postoperative phase.

Initial assessment in the preoperative management of the patient includes assessment of not only vital signs, but also accurate weight, plus electrolyte and blood gas analyses. In the neonate, measurement of serum glucose and calcium levels should also be done. Attempts should be made to correct any abnormalities encountered in this assessment. Frequently, surgical patients will maintain total body water but shift large amounts of protein and water into tissues or into potential spaces such as the peritoneal or pleural cavity. These so-called third-space losses are hard to quantitate. However, inadequate replacement of these losses will result in hypovolemia and shock. Infusion of colloid in the form of 5 per cent albumin, whole blood, or plasma-like products is required to maintain intravascular integrity in the face of significant protein losses and decreased oncotic pressure in the vascular space. This is a frequent concomitant of peritonitis, perforated viscus, congenital anomalies such as gastroschisis and omphalocele, intussusception, and crush injuries of any kind.

Peritonitis as a result of acute necrotizing enterocolitis in the premature neonate, intussusception in the older infant, chronic inflammatory bowel disease in the adolescent, or other causes will result in the transudation of protein from the intravascular space into the wall of the gastrointestinal tract as well as into the peritoneal cavity. This protein is accompanied by fluid that remains outside the vascular space because of the oncotic pressure of the protein and sometimes continued transudation or exudation. Loss of protein and fluid from the intravascular space can substantially deplete the intravascular volume and result in hypovolemic shock. Adequate resuscitation of the intravascular space includes the use of colloid and crystalloid in amounts adequate to maintain blood pressure and pulse within the normal range for age. Infection and necrotic bowel can result in significant build-up of metabolic acids. If acidemia is present, isotonic infusions of bicarbonate should be initiated in order to begin metabolic correction. It should be appreciated that in the face of necrotic bowel, only surgical extirpation will correct the acidosis.

Hirschsprung's disease (aganglionic megacolon), the most common cause of intestinal obstruction in the neonate, can result from the obstructive process in an acute enterocolitis. This complication is frequently fatal, owing to the massive losses of fluid, protein, and electrolytes from the vascular space into the lumen of the small intestines. Decompression of the obstructed bowel by colostomy to prevent this disorder is the treatment of choice. In the face of a severe enterocolitis with large fluid losses into the bowel, adequate fluid replacement is mandatory prior to surgery to ensure reasonable outcome.

In the severely ill patient, because intubation and artificial ventilation will begin anyway in the operating room, it is frequently helpful to intubate the patient in the preoperative phase of management. This allows complete control of ventilation and ensures that adequate carbon dioxide exchange will occur in the face of possible need for intravenous bicarbonate for correction of acidemia. Initial measurements of weight, hematocrit, vital signs, and total serum solids (assessed as an estimate of total serum proteins by the use of a drop of plasma on a refractometer) should be recorded for use in the postoperative management of the patient.

The preoperative phase of management of the surgical patient should be prolonged if it will result in enhancement of surgical outcome. Thus, preoperative management may be as short as minutes or as long as weeks in order to restore the metabolic and physiologic homeostasis of the patient and obtain an optimal operative risk. A good example of the positive use of a short delay in surgery is the case of gastric outlet obstruction.

Vomiting of gastric contents as a result of gastric outlet obstruction caused by duodenal atresia, a diaphragm or web, pyloric stenosis, intestinal bands, or malrotation results in chronic loss of gastric contents, primarily hydrogen and chloride ions. This results in a hypochloremic alkalosis. Chronic hypochloremic alkalosis will result in hypokalemia by renal compensation, conserving hydrogen ions at the expense of potassium loss. Preoperative management of patients with gastric outlet obstruction includes at least partial correction of the hypochloremic alkalosis by the infusion of chloride in the form of sodium chloride and potassium chloride. This will fully supply the body with chloride and potassium, and renal compensation will allow the correction of the alkalosis. Some authors have recommended the use of ammonium chloride for correction of alkalosis and hypochloremia, but we prefer the use of sodium and potassium salts. This metabolic correction preoperatively will greatly enhance surgical outcome.

Burns. When there has been thermal injury to the skin over more than 10 to 12 per cent of body surface, an edema of injury, or burn edema, accumulates at such sites. The total amount of burn edema may be estimated from the surface burned as a percentage of surface area. The estimating scheme given here is for second or third degree burns without charring.

When up to about 50 per cent of the body surface has been burned, the amount of edema formed is a linear function of the burn surface, with a slope approximately equal to the percentage of body weight that is extracellular fluid. Thus, for a burn of 30 per cent of the surface of a 12-month-old infant weighting 10 kg, the ECF (25 per cent of 10 kg = 2500 ml) times 0.3 (percentage of surface burned) equals 750 ml. When more than 50 per cent of the body surface has been burned, the linear relationship flattens out and little more edema is possible. Empiric data show that this edema accumulates over a 48-hour period, one half (375 ml in the example) in the first 12 hours, one quarter in the next 12 hours, and the final quarter in the second 24 hours. This fluid then is the deficit; the composition is that of ECF. Very little protein appears in this fluid unless plasma or blood transfusions are given. Over the next few days, however, plasma albumin levels fall because of increased catabolism and diminished anabolism.

When one should give plasma or albumin solution to burn patients is controversial; certainly it is not essential for survival during the immediate, or shock, phase. If it is given, a reasonable amount is one half of the first 12 hours' deficit. The deficit amount should be replaced as it occurs.

The ongoing insensible water losses are somewhat high, although variable, in burned patients. This factor is offset, however, by stimulus to high ADH production (pain, anxiety, and, in severe instances, hypovolemia). Therefore, urine output is scanty and concentrated. Overhydration is bad for the skin of these patients, so care must be taken to replace deficit and maintenance losses with a close tolerance. No rate of urine formation need be specified as long as there is some concentrated urine each hour.

The foregoing simplified scheme, while useful, must be tempered by many features of burns and therapy that are beyond the scope of this work. Burned patients often benefit after the initial hydration from parenteral nutrition, discussed later in this chapter.

Intraoperative Management

Preparation of the operating room for the pediatric patient is an important part of the surgical procedure. Heat loss during surgery is a major risk to the patient whose abdominal or pleural cavity is exposed. Therefore, room temperature should be increased depending upon the age and size of the patient and the risk of cold stress of the surgical procedure. Thermistor monitoring of patient temperature should be a routine part of all pediatric anesthesia. A warming mattress with manual controls should be placed on the operating table so that the anesthesiologist can maintain a warm environment beneath the patient. In the small infant and neonate, extremities may be wrapped to decrease heat loss. Fluids administered to the patient and blood and blood products can be warmed prior to infusion. All these procedures decrease the thermal stress and the risk of hypothermia.

Adequate monitoring of vital signs must be assured. The use of the Doppler blood pressure machine in recent years has allowed the noninvasive monitoring of blood pressure in infants and neonates. This has decreased the need for intra-arterial catheters and transducer-obtained blood pressure monitoring. However, intra-arterial catheters allow for the continual monitoring of blood gases during the operative procedure. Central venous pressure monitoring can be helpful in many major surgical procedures. Transcutaneous oxygen electrodes utilized in premature infants can allow the anesthesiologist to maintain the PO_2 in a range that will not induce retinal damage resulting in retrolental fibroplasia. Transcutaneous measurement of PCO_2 can be utilized to help the anesthesiologist maintain the PCO_2 in the normal range without the development of hyper- or hypocarbia. If transcutaneous monitoring is not available, blood gas analyses can be utilized to assist in monitoring these parameters.

Fluid volumes far in excess of maintenance fluid needs are required during surgical procedures in which body cavities are opened to the outside environment. Doubling of maintenance requirements when the abdomen is opened is a recommended first estimate for adequate fluid rate. Replacement of colloid, blood, and fluid losses must be carefully managed to maintain normal vital signs and cardiovascular integrity. Maintenance of adequate glucose levels during the stress of surgery is another important part of intraoperative management.

Whole blood and packed blood cells are provided with the anticoagulants of acid-citrate-dextrose or citrate-phosphate-dextrose. Both anticoagulants have large quantities of citrate that acutely chelate calcium. If large volumes of blood are utilized, the plasma ionized calcium level will be significantly decreased while the total calcium level may be maintained within the normal range. This is particularly important in patients undergoing open heart surgery in which large volumes of blood are utilized and in patients with liver disease or hepatic surgery in which citrate metabolism may be impaired.

Administration of exogenous calcium salts as calcium chloride or gluconate may be necessary in order to prevent acute hypocalcemia. Constant infusion in intravenous fluids is preferable to bolus infusion of calcium, because acute hypercalcemia can result in asystole and other cardiac arrhythmias. Blood-bank blood, particularly if more than three days old, has significantly elevated levels of potassium. Acute hyperkalemia may occur with large transfusions. Electrocardiographic monitoring should be maintained to assess potassium levels and arrhythmias.

Careful attention to all details in the maintenance of fluids, electrolytes, and glucose and calcium homeostasis during the surgical procedure, as well as temperature control, will greatly enhance the outcome.

Postoperative Management

The first phase in the postoperative management of the patient is the stabilization directly after the surgical procedure. Vital signs including weight should be obtained as soon as possible after the procedure. Goals in this phase are the maintenance of adequate cardiovascular integrity and intravascular fluid volume as well as the repair of any losses or the correction of any excesses that have resulted from the surgical procedure. The stress of surgery as well as the specific disorder for which the surgery was performed may have resulted in release of metabolic acids. Correction of acidemia is, therefore, often necessary. Postoperatively, besides the weight and vital signs, the patient should have serial monitoring of, specifically, serum electrolytes, calcium, and glucose levels, as well as blood gas analyses, hematocrit, and total serum solids.

Secretion of antidiuretic hormone (ADH) secondary to medications, stress, or anesthesia or specifically due to manipulation of the viscera or central nervous system can result in fluid retention at excessive levels in the postoperative period. Thus, after urinary output has been adequately assured, careful administration of fluids should be provided in an attempt to prevent excessive fluid accumulation. Ongoing losses such as those secondary to nasogastric suctioning or drainage through fistulae or dressings should be replaced every four to six hours or even more frequently, depending upon the volumes measured. The composition of replacement fluids should reflect an understanding of the electrolyte concentrations of the fluids being lost. Changes in weight in the acute postoperative period are virtually all due to losses or retention of fluid.

Following surgery several stimuli for ADH production may be operating independent of the osmolality. Hypovolemia may have been present at some point, although this should be corrected early in the postoperative period. Pain and anxiety are usually present. Drugs to control pain and anxiety (e.g., opiates) are often used. Each of these is a stimulus to ADH secretion. Therefore, the volume and rate of delivery of maintenance water must be monitored with care. Water intoxication, sometimes indicated symptomatically by a convulsion, is seen all too often following a routine surgical procedure in a child when the surgical team is accustomed to the fluid regimens in use for adult patients.

The recuperative powers of infants and children are far greater than those of adults. Thus, postoperative discomfort appears to most observers to be substantially less in children than in adults. Furthermore, peristaltic activity of the gastrointestinal tract appears to return earlier in young infants and children, and judicious attempts at feeding can be initiated relatively early in postoperative management. The extent of trauma and manipulation to the bowel and the length of the surgical procedure will determine the time at which gastrointestinal nutrition can be initiated.

A major goal of the early postoperative phase is to bring the patient out of a catabolic state and to begin anabolic healing, growth, and return to normal function. This requires adequate nutrition and supply of calories and protein. If adequate nutrition by the oral route cannot be supplied within four to five days of surgery, healing will be substantially impaired. We will discuss in the next section the use of parenteral nutrition to assist in the postoperative management of surgical patients.

Infection, either local or systemic, can be another cause of a prolonged catabolic postoperative phase and a patient's inability to become anabolic. Also, multiple surgical procedures within a few days of one another can result in an inability to enter the anabolic phase postoperatively.

TOTAL PARENTERAL NUTRITION

Total parenteral nutrition can be utilized to supply all of the necessary nutrients to patients who cannot be adequately nourished by the enteral route. Since the pioneering work of Dudrick in the late 1960s,[5] much has been learned in neonates, infants, children, and adolescents about the technique of intravenous nutrition to augment or fully replace enteral feedings.

There are three possible approaches to providing total nutrition by the intravenous route: first, hypertonic solutions of high concentrations of glucose can be infused through a central venous line; second, moderately hypertonic solutions of glucose can be infused through a peripheral line and supplemented to supply adequate calories by the use of intravenous fat; and third, moderately hypertonic solutions of glucose may be used through the peripheral route in

large volumes without the addition of intravenous fat. Each of these methods has been utilized with great success over the last ten years. We prefer to utilize total parenteral nutrition provided by the peripheral route with the supplementation of the intravenous solutions with a fat emulsion whenever possible.[6] This route is preferred because of the complications of the central venous lines, which will be discussed later in this section.

Indications for total parenteral nutrition include the medical problems of severe diarrhea and inflammatory bowel disease, in which the gastrointestinal tract mucosa has been denuded and is unable to absorb simple predigested nutrients.[7] The severe inanition of anorexia nervosa has also been treated by means of total parenteral nutrition. In surgical patients, intravenous nutrition can be used to restore metabolic homeostasis in the preoperative as well as the postoperative period until the gastrointestinal tract is adequate to be utilized for nutrition. Because of the need to facilitate the transition from the catabolic acute postoperative phase to the anabolic phase of postoperative management, it is generally appropriate to supply intravenous total nutrition if oral nutrition cannot be initiated within four to five days of a major surgical procedure.

Total parenteral nutrition solutions must provide an adequate source of protein in the form of protein hydrolysates, such as fibrin or casein, or crystalline amino acid solutions.[8] Amino acids should be provided at a concentration consistent with delivery of 2 to 4 gm/kg per day. The bulk of calories are provided by hypertonic solutions of glucose with or without the supplementation of fat emulsions. Intralipid, a 10 per cent soybean oil emulsion stabilized with 1.2 per cent egg phospholipid, supplies essential fatty acids and provides 1.1 cal/ml. This intravenous fat can be infused along with peripheral parenteral nutrition in an amount equal to 1 to 4 gm/kg per day.

Electrolytes, minerals, vitamins, and trace elements needed for growth and healing of tissues must also be provided in the intravenous solutions. Parenteral electrolyte requirements are similar to the usual oral maintenance needs. Mineral, vitamin, and trace element amounts provided intravenously are substantially lower than recommended oral intakes because of the variable absorption of these substances from the gastrointestinal tract.

Table 34–1 depicts a parenteral nutrition solution for use through a central venous line for patients up to approximately 30 months of age or 15 kg of body weight. This formula contains 25 per cent dextrose and 3.5 percent amino acids and provides 990 cal/l. Sodium, potassium, and chloride are provided as approximately 2 mEq/100 cal; about one fourth of the anion should be as organic base such as lactate or acetate. The trace element solution and folic acid are added only to the first liter daily in those patients requiring more than 1000 ml/day.

Peripheral total paenteral nutrition solutions are similarly constituted, except that the percentage of glucose is provided by 100 gm of dextrose per liter and equals 10 per cent. This peripheral parenteral nutrition solution is also utilized to begin total parenteral nutrition by the central route, thus allowing the patient to gradually become acclimatized to the high concentrations of glucose. The peripheral parenteral nutrition solution provides 480 cal/l and must be supplemented with fat emulsion to provide adequate calories.

Because of the use of the intravenous route rather than the gastrointestinal tract for nutrition, intravenous or intramuscular vitamin K should be provided after the completion of each two weeks of parenteral nutrition therapy. Vitamin B-12 should also be given every four weeks in order to supply the necessary requirements. Parenteral vitamin D also must be provided; we have found that the simple technique of injecting a dose of 100,000 to 600,000 units intramuscularly is adequate during a course of parenteral nutrition for six months in infants. The smaller doses are for infants weighing less than 3000 gm; for those weighing more than this, 600,000 units is used.

If central intravenous nutrition is utilized, placement of a nonreactive Silastic catheter in the superior vena cava via the facial or external jugular vein is the optimal approach. This catheter should be placed in an aseptic manner, preferably in the operating room. An x-ray should be obtained to assure appropriate placement of the catheter in the high-flow area near but not in the heart. Millipore filters are utilized to decrease the chances of bacterial invasion of the intravenous catheter. Compulsive care of the catheter and its site of entry into the skin is required to maintain an infection-free environment. Millipore filters are also utilized with the peripheral nutrition solu-

Table 34–1.   Central Total Parenteral Solution (1 Liter)

CONSTITUENT	AMOUNT	FORMULATION
Amino acids	35 gm	500 ml Aminosyn 7%
Dextrose	250 gm	500 ml dextrose U.S.P. 50%
Electrolytes		
Sodium	25 mEq	Sodium chloride concentrate
Chloride	25 mEq	
Potassium	25 mEq	Potassium phosphate
Phosphate	17 mmol	
Calcium	2.5 mEq	Calcium gluconate
Magnesium	2 mEq	Magnesium sulfate
Vitamins		
Vitamin C	50 mg	
Vitamin A	1000 units	
Vitamin D	100 units	
Thiamine HCl	5 mg	
Riboflavin	1 mg	Multiple-vitamin concentrate
Pyridoxine	1.5 mg	
Niacinamide	10.0 mg	
Panthenol	2.5 mg	
Vitamin E	0.5 unit	
Folic acid	0.5 mg	Folic acid
Trace Elements		
Zinc sulfate	0.8 mg	Zinc sulfate
Copper sulfate	0.4 mg	Cupric sulfate
Manganese sulfate	0.4 mg	Manganese sulfate

Table 34–2. Complications of Central Total Parenteral Nutrition

I. *Metabolic*
    Hypo- and hyperglycemia
    Acidosis
    Uremia
    Hyperammonemia
    Calcium and phosphorus abnormalities
    Trace metal deficiencies

II. *Organ Toxicity*
    Cholestatic jaundice
    Hepatopathy
    Hyperviscosity

III. *Infectious*
    Thrombophlebitis
    Sepsis
    Emboli

IV. *Technical*
    Thrombosis of the superior vena cava

V. *Ethical*
    When to stop?

tions. This allows any particles or bacteria to be filtered prior to entrance of the solution into the patient. It should be noted, however, that intralipid cannot go through the millipore filters and a Y connection must be provided distal to the filter in the peripheral intravenous line.

The possible complications of central total parenteral nutrition are enumerated in Table 34–2. Metabolic complications are rare when careful monitoring of the patient is done. Daily weights and serum evaluations of electrolytes, urea nitrogen, calcium, phosphorus, and magnesium, and multiple glucose determinations assure adequate monitoring of these substances. Weekly assessments of liver enzymes (SGPT), total and direct bilirubin, total protein, albumin, folate, vitamin B-12, prothrombin time, zinc, and complete blood count are necessary in order to prevent the metabolic complications listed in the table.

Hepatic damage and cholestatic jaundice resulting in hyperbilirubinemia of a direct variety as well as elevated serum transaminase levels and possibly hyperammonemia can be detected in patients on long-term total parenteral nutrition. Hyperviscosity and hyperlipidemia can result in

sludging in vessels in the lungs and other important organs. The central catheter is always a possible portal of entry for infectious agents of a bacterial or fungal nature. Peripheral catheters may be the site of thrombophlebitis, and both kinds of catheters may be the source of emboli. Central parenteral nutrition catheters have also been associated with thrombosis and the development of an obstruction to the superior vena cava. Because the solutions are caustic and hyperosmolar, extravasation of these fluids into the peripheral tissues when the intravenous solution accidentally infiltrates can result in severe sloughs.

Perhaps the most difficult complication of the central venous line occurs in the patients who are never able to maintain oral nutrition. The question of when to stop or when not to replace a line that is to be discontinued for another reason becomes an ethical question of major proportion.

Careful, comprehensive care of patients who require total parenteral nutrition, even for several years, can result in excellent long-term outcome.

REFERENCES

1. Moore FD, Ball MR: The Metabolic Response to Surgery. Charles C Thomas, Springfield, IL, 1952.
2. Calcagno PL, Rubin MI, Singh WS: The influence of surgery on renal function in infancy. I. The effect of surgery on the postoperative renal excretion of water: the influence of dehydration. Pediatrics 16:619, 1955.
3. Holliday MA, Segar WE: The maintenance need for water in parenteral fluid therapy. Pediatrics 19:823, 1957.
4. Rubin MI, Calcagno PL, Mukherji PK, Singh WS: The influence of surgery on renal function in infancy and childhood. II. The effect of surgery on the renal excretion of sodium. Pediatrics 22:923, 1958.
5. Dudrick SJ: Total intravenous feeding and growth in puppies. Fed Proc 25:481, 1966.
6. Coran AG: Total intravenous feeding of infants and children without the use of a central venous catheter. Ann Surg 179:445, 1974.
7. Avery GB, Villavicencio O, Lilly JR, Randolph JG: Intractable diarrhea of early infancy. Pediatrics 41:712, 1968.
8. Heird WC, Winters RW: Total parenteral nutrition — the state of the art. J Pediatr 86:2, 1975.

Appendix I
Definitional Glossary

acid

In Brönsted terminology, a molecule that donates a proton (hydrogen ion). The Lewis definition, which is useful in certain chemical applications, is "something that attaches itself to an unshared pair of electrons." Brönsted usage is customary in physiology.

acidemia

Sufficient excess of hydrogen ion in the blood to lower the pH below the physiologic range. A *metabolic acidemia* results from an increase in metabolic (or exogenous) hydrogen ions; a *respiratory acidemia* results from increased retention of CO_2. The two are not mutually exclusive.

acidosis

A change in hydrogen ion in the blood that reduces the bicarbonate ion concentration without changing the blood pH, because of simultaneous reduction in H_2CO_3 (CO_2) concentration. Either event may be the primary one, with the other compensating. The change in hydrogen ion is called *metabolic*; the change in PCO_2, *respiratory*.

alkalemia; alkalosis

See definitions of acidemia and acidosis, which are parallel terms. Addition of base (subtraction of acid) causes an increase in pH or an increase in both components of the buffer ratio $\dfrac{[HCO_3^-]}{[H_2CO_3]}$.

anion

The negatively charged portion of an electrolytically dissociated molecule.

anion gap (undetermined anion = R)

The anions (negatively charged particles) in plasma (serum or any biologic fluid) not determined in routine inorganic chemical analyses of plasma (or other fluid). The sum of the cations Na^+ and K^+ is usually about 20 mEq/l higher than the sum of Cl^- and HCO_3^-. In normal states, this group of anions includes $H_2PO_4^-$, HSO_4^-, and lactate. In disease states, ketoacids, drugs, and other substances may contribute to the "gap."

atomic weight

The relative weight of an atom compared to carbon-12, which is arbitrarily assigned the number 12. The unit is the dalton. The atomic weight expressed in grams is the *gram atomic weight*.

azotemia

An increase in nitrogenous compounds in the blood. The usual measurement is of urea in serum and is frequently expressed in terms of the nitrogen content. Hence, SUN or BUN is serum or blood urea nitrogen.

base

In Brönsted terminology, a proton acceptor (e.g., the hydroxyl ion). In Lewis terminology, a chemical species that possesses an unshared pair of electrons.

base deficit; base excess

Changes from normal in the buffer base of blood. Deficit is indicated by a minus sign (−), excess by a plus sign (+). A measure of the metabolic component of acidosis or alkalosis.

Bohr effect

The decrease in the affinity of hemoglobin for oxygen, with falling pH and rising PCO_2 reflected by a shift to the right on the oxyhemoglobin dissociation curve.

buffer base

The sum of all bases in 1 l of blood.

caloric expenditure

The energy released as heat over a designated time, expressed in Kcal (see *calorie*).

calorie (Calorie, Kcal)

The calorie is the amount of heat necessary to raise one gm of water at 15°C to 16°C. The Calorie, or Kcal, is the amount of heat required to raise 1 l of water from 15°C to 16°C, or 1000 calories. In this book, unless otherwise specified, the term calories (cal) means Kcal. One Kcal equals 4.187 kilojoules.

cation

A positively charged particle of a dissociated molecule.

chemical potential

The total quantity of chemical energy of a mass of substance that theoretically may be released. Defined precisely by Gibbs as follows: "If to any homogeneous mass we suppose an infinitesimal number of mols of any substance to be added, the mass remaining homogeneous (T and P unchanged), the increase of free energy, G, of the mass divided by the number of mols of the substance added is the chemical potential for that substance in the mass considered." Permitted to do so, substances move down a gradient of chemical potential. Going up such a gradient requires the expenditure of energy.

colloidal osmotic (oncotic) pressure

The pressure exerted by protein (or other colloids) in plasma across capillary membranes, that are (relatively) impermeable to the molecules.

dehydration

Loss of extracellular fluid (in physiology); loss of water (in simple English).

dielectric constant

A measure of the amount of electrical charge a substance can withstand. The dielectric constant of water is a measure of its ability to reduce the intensity of an external electric field. Water molecules have a strong permanent dipole moment that permits ions to move independently.

diffusion

The movement of a species of molecules through a system down a gradient until concentration in the system is everywhere equal.

Donnan factor	The number, experimentally determined, by which the concentration of a diffusible ion on one side of a semipermeable membrane is multiplied (or divided) to determine the concentration on the other side. For sodium and chloride in mammalian muscle, the Donnan factor is 0.95 to 0.96. (Multiply for sodium and divide for chloride in plasma to obtain interstitial fluid concentration.)
electrolyte	A substance that dissociates (ionizes) in water, making the solution capable of conducting electricity.
enthalpy	The sum of the internal energy of a system plus the product of pressure-volume work (PV) done on the system. Enthalpy (H) equals energy (E) plus PV.
entropy	The expression of disorder or degree of randomness of molecules in units of energy. Entropy always increases if a reaction is irreversible; it remains unchanged if the reaction is reversible (second law of thermodynamics).
equilibrium	A state in a closed chemical system in which all concentrations of reacting substances remain constant (i.e., forward reaction and reverse reaction have equal velocities).
equivalent weight	Atomic weight divided by valence.
extracellular fluid (ECF)	The water and solute outside cells. In the mammal this includes the plasma, the interstitial fluid, and other tissue fluids not in cells.
Fick's equation (law) of diffusion	The amount of a substance diffusing through a cross-section of area, A, is directly proportional to the concentration gradient across this section. In mathematical terms:

$$dQ/dt = DA \, (-dC/dx)$$

where Q = quantity
    t = time
    D = diffusion coefficient
    A = area
    C = concentration gradient
    x = distance

free energy (Gibbs)	Gibbs free energy (G) = enthalpy − absolute temperature × entropy. A thermodynamic function of state.
Gibbs-Donnan equilibrium	The expression of the concentrations of electrolyte reactants in a system involving a semipermeable membrane, at least one charged particle that is nondiffusible, and several other ions that are diffusible. For a general case involving, for example, Na^+, Cl^-, and P^- (nondiffusible):

$$\frac{[Na^+]_1}{[Na^+]_2} = \frac{[Cl^-]_2}{[Cl^-]_1}$$

Henderson-Hasselbalch equation	$$pH = pK' = \log \frac{[\text{conjugate base}]}{[\text{weak acid}]}$$

Where $K' =$ the apparent (measured) dissociation constant for a weak acid. For the bicarbonate system in blood:

$$pH = 6.1 + \log \frac{[HCO_3^-]}{[CO_2] \times \text{solubility factor}}$$

hypertonic	A term that describes solute concentration above that of normal body fluids.
hypotonic	A term that describes solute concentration below that of normal body fluids.
insensible water loss	Obligatory water loss from the interstices of skin and from the lungs, which is produced by heat expenditure.
interstitial fluid (IF)	Body fluid that bathes cells; a part of the extracellular fluid.
intracellular fluid (ICF)	The fluid of cells — water and solute.
ion	The charged dissociated particle of a molecule in solution.
isotonic	Describes solute concentration identical to that of body fluids.
joule	A unit of heat. 1 Kcal = 4.187 kilojoules.
milliequivalent (mEq)	Concentration unit equaling one thousandth of an equivalent; usually expressed as milligram atomic wt/valence.
milliosmol (mOsm)	The unit of concentration of particles in solution, independent of size of particles.

Concentration (in mOsm) = amount of solute (in mmol) $\times$ number of particles (n) in solution after dissociation.

For glucose, $n = 1$; for NaCl, $n = 2$; and for $MgCl_2$, $n = 3$.

molal	One gram mole of a substance per kilogram of solvent (water).
molar	One gram mole of substance per liter of solution.
mole fraction	The number of moles of a substance in solution divided by the sum of all the moles of solute in the solution. The solvent is one component.
molecular weight	The sum of atomic weights in a molecule measured in daltons. *Gram molecular weight* is this weight expressed in grams.
Nernst equation	Mathematical expression of the potential difference across a membrane separating two solutions. For example:

$$\pi = \frac{RT}{ZF} \ln \frac{[Na]_1}{[Na]_2} = 58 \log \frac{[Na]_1}{[Na]_2}$$

where $\pi =$ potential in millivolts
  $R =$ gas constant
  $T =$ absolute temperature (here, 18°C)
  $Z =$ valence
  $F =$ Faraday's constant

"normal" saline; "physiologic" saline	A solution containing 9 gm of NaCl (154 mEq) per liter (0.9%), which is neither "normal" in the chemical sense nor "physiologic," because sodium and chloride ions are not equally present in body fluids. The solution is approximately isotnic (300 mOsm/l). The expression "half normal saline" for a 0.45% solution of NaCl is a barbarism!
normal (N) solution	A solution containing in each liter an amount of solute equal to the gram molecular weight of the solute divided by its hydrogen equivalent (i.e., one *gram equivalent weight* of solute). "Normal" saline is *not* a normal solution.
oncotic	A term used for the colloid osmotic pressure of plasma.
osmolality; milliosmolality	The number of osmols (milliosmols) per kilogram of water (solvent), measured by an osmometer on the basis of either freezing point or vapor pressure. This measure, not osmolarity, is the chemically significant concentration.
osmolarity; milliosmolarity	The number of osmols (milliosmols) per liter of solution. Not measured by any instruments currently available. This concentration may be achieved precisely by diluting a known amount of solute to a measured volume or by calculation from measured osmolality.
osmosis	The movement of a solvent through a membrane to equalize the concentration of the solvent on both sides.

osmotic pressure
  (gas law) equation

Mathematically:

$$\pi V = \frac{gm}{M} RT$$

where π = osmotic pressure (in mmHg)
   V = volume in liters
   gm = grams of solute
   M = molecular weight
   R = gas constant
   T = absolute temperature (°Kelvin)

PCO_2	The partial pressure of carbon dioxide (CO_2), measured in millimeters of mercury (mm Hg) or, if corrected for altitude above sea level, in torr.
pH	A measure of hydrogen ion concentration. In a system with a glass electrode, a measure of activity.

$$pH = \frac{1}{\log [H^+]}$$

The normal pH of blood is 7.4; the $[H^+]$ is 40 nmol/l.

pK, pK′	Experimentally determined constants for the Henderson-Hasselbalch equation relating to the degree of dissociation of $[H^+]$ at a given temperature. The normal pK′ of carbonic acid–bicarbonate in plasma is 6.10.
PO_2	The partial pressure of oxygen (O_2) measured in millimeters of mercury (mm Hg) or, if corrected for altitude above sea level, in torr.

Poiseuille flow

The steady laminar flow of a fluid through a narrow horizontal cylinder.

$$u = (\tfrac{1}{4}V) (pg) (a^2 - r^2)$$

where u = fluid velocity along cylinder's axis at distance r from the axis
V = dynamic viscosity
pg = pressure gradient
a = radius of cylinder
r = distance from axis of cylinder

renal clearance

The amount of plasma "cleared" of a given substance by the kidney per unit of time, measured in milliliters per minute. Creatinine and inulin clearances approximate glomerular filtration. PAH clearance approximates renal blood flow.

$$\frac{\text{Clearance}}{(\text{ml/min})} = \frac{UV}{P}$$

where U = concentration of substance in urine
P = concentration of substance in plasma
V = urine volume/time in minutes

saline

Salt (NaCl) solution. See also *normal saline*.

secretion

An active (energy-dependent) process of moving substances across a surface (membrane).

semipermeable
   membrane

A membrane that permits passage of some particles (ions, molecules) but not others in the solutions separated by the membrane.

serum

Plasma minus fibrin and other clotting factors.

solubility

The concentration of a substance in a solvent when the undiluted solute is in equilibrium with the solution.

solubility product (K_s)

A mass action expression of a dissociated salt in solution. For compound BA:
$$[B^+] [A^-] = K_s$$

solute

A substance dissolved in a solvent.

solution

Solutes in a solvent.

solvent

A substance (usually liquid) in which other substances dissolve.

steady state

A term describing a group of reactants in an open system in which the reactants maintain constant concentration because input equals output for each.

sweat

An aqueous secretion of the sweat glands.

thermodynamics, laws of

I. When mechanical work is transformed into heat or heat into work, the amount of work is always equivalent to the amount of heat (conservation of energy).

II. It is impossible by any continuous self-sustaining process for heat to be transferred from a colder to a hotter body (energy runs "downhill");

or

given the opportunity, a system will spontaneously go in the direction that increases the disorder, or randomness, of its molecules (maximal entropy).

torr

A unit of pressure equal to 1 mm Hg at the earth's gravity at sea level. In honor of the Italian scientist Torricelli.

total body water (TBW)

The sum of all body water compartments. In health, about 70 per cent of the lean body mass.

valence

The property of an atom describing the number of hydrogen atoms with which it combines (negative valence) or which it displaces (positive valence). The number of unitary electrical charges of an atom.

water of oxidation

The water produced by the oxidation of food. For example, in the following reaction, 6 H_2O is the water of oxidation:

$$C_6H_{12}O_6 + 6\ O_2 \longrightarrow 6\ CO_2 + 6\ H_2O$$

Normally, about 12 ml of water is produced for each 100 cal expended.

Appendix II
Time Line

This time line provides a pediatric perspective of contributions to the understanding of problems of fluid and electrolyte physiology and to the application of that understanding to therapy. The years are listed chronologically, and the name of an individual is given before the contribution in order to honor those to whom credit is usually given. This system is, of course, subject to error because of personal ignorance or bias.

Up to the twentieth century, initially scientists and later clinicians in general medicine dominate the time line because pediatrics had not yet become a distinct branch of medicine. From 1925 on, only a pediatric pathway is followed in this chronology, highlighting major specific contributions to child medicine. Many of these were seminal advances in adult medicine as well.

3400–500 B.C.E.*
  Comments on diarrheal disease may be found in the earliest Egyptian, Sumerian, Hebraic, Greek, Indian, and Chinese writings. In the documents available to us, these comments comprise descriptions and treatment regimens and, therefore, are not strictly contributions to understanding in the current sense.

460–370 B.C.E. Hippocrates
  Introduced method of making systematic clinical observations and rational deductions from them. Contributed many writings on diarrhea.

400–100 B.C.E.
  Talmudic scholars wrote on medicine and diarrhea but did not add new insights to those of previous times.

100 B.C.E.–1600 C.E.
  Advances in descriptive medicine but not, so far as we are aware, in physiology as it bears on water and mineral metabolism.

Circa 1600 C.E. Sanctorius (Santorio Santorio, 1561–1636)
  Experimentally demonstrated insensible water loss by the use of a weighing chair.

1616 Thomas Harvey
  Lectured on the circulation.

---

*B.C.E. and C.E.—"before the common era" and "after the common era"; equivalent to B.C. and A.D.

1666   Richard Lower
Performed first transfusion of blood in lower mammals.

1667   Jean Baptiste Denys
Performed first blood transfusion in humans.

1748   Jean Nollet
Discovered the diffusion of liquid through a membrane.

1827–32   René Dutrochet
Described (but did not name) osmosis, deducing the important elements. Coined terms *endosmose and exosmose* to indicate bidirectional flow of fluids.

1831   W. B. O'Shaughnessy
Analyzed the chemical changes in the serum caused by cholera, then prevalent in London, and described a theoretic approach to intravenous therapy.

1832   Thomas Latta
Utilizing O'Shaughnessy's data, treated 16 patients intravenously with sodium chloride and sodium bicarbonate salts in water. Eight survived. Similar reports were published by T. Weatherhill and S. Miller the same year. These reports were largely ignored by clinicians in succeeding years. Even after the rediscovery of parenteral therapy by Arnaldo Cantani in Naples (1892), acceptance lagged for two more decades until 1910, when A. W. Sellards published his work on the treatment of diarrhea in the Philippines. In 1921, L. Rogers added studies from India.

1844   J. L. M. Poiseuille
Found that foodstuffs move from the stomach to the blood by osmosis and diffusion.

1850   Carl Schmidt
Published detailed studies of the chemical anatomy of blood and serum in normal controls and in patients with cholera. Recognized dehydration with normal sodium concentration and with low or high sodium concentration. Virtually no clinical application followed during his lifetime.

1854–61   Thomas Graham
Introduced the term "osmosis," recognizing the phenomenon as a passage of water. Divided solutes into colloids and crystalloids.

1855   A. Fick
Formulated the general law of diffusion.

1859   Claude Bernard
Conceptualized the "milieu interieur" in terms of its function and role in physiology.

1874   A. Kussmaul
Described air hunger in diabetic dehydration and acidemia.

1876–78   J. W. Gibbs
Developed thermodynamics and physical chemistry to their modern level by rigorous mathematical treatment. First formulated Gibbs-Donnan theory.

1877   W. F. P. Pfeffer
Introduced the concept and the term "osmotic pressure."

1887   J. H. van't Hoff
Correlated osmotic pressure in biologic systems with physical and chemical properties of solution and with gas laws. Investigated and conceptualized semipermeable membranes. (Was awarded Nobel Prize in 1901.)

1891–1901 W. Ostwald
  Recognized "colligative properties" of solutions.
1896 E. H. Starling
  Developed theory of oncotic versus hydrostatic forces in the circulation.
1903 S. Arrhenius
  Introduced the concept of electrolytic dissociation and investigated the behavior of ions in solution (Was awarded Nobel Prize in 1903.)
1909 S. P. L. Sörensen
  Developed hydrogen electrode; suggested the symbol pH.
1909–13 L. J. Henderson
  Developed mass action equation for equilibrium of hydrogen ion in biologic systems.
1910 A. W. Sellards
  Demonstrated empirically the value of bicarbonate in intravenous fluids.
1911 F. G. Donnan
  Obtained experimental data on Gibbs's theory, leading to Gibbs-Donnan equilibrium formulation.
1915 L. E. Holt, A. Courtney, and H. L. Fales
  Performed electrolyte analyses of the stools of infants.
1915–16 A. K. Hasselbalch
  Conceptualized "compensated acidosis"; devised the logarithmic form of Henderson's equation.
1916 J. Howland and W. M. Marriot
  Investigated acidosis in diarrhea.
1917 O. M. Schloss and R. E. Stetson
  Investigated acidosis in diarrhea.
1918 D. D. Van Slyke
  Made a series of contributions on the measurement of CO_2 and hydrogen ion in blood. Classified acid-base disorders in collaboration with J. P. Peters.
1919 Lewis H. Weed
  Studied CSF changes after intravenous infusion of hypertonic solutions in animals.
1919 W. M. Marriot
  Investigated effects of dehydration on circulation.
1926 G. P. Powers
  Developed comprehensive plan of treatment of infantile diarrhea.
1932 A. F. Hartmann and M. J. E. Senn
  Investigated use of lactate in intravenous fluids.
1933–50 A. Butler
  Studied parenteral fluid therapy.
1933–55 J. L. Gamble
  Made many contributions to the understanding of the chemical anatomy of body fluids and to electrolyte physiology in general.
1935–60 D. C. Darrow
  Made many contributions to electrolyte physiology and to the clinical management of dehydration. Established the role of potassium in therapy in 1946 with C. Govan (and later with R. E. Cooke).
1946 S. Rapoport and K. Dodd
  Described "postacidotic syndrome," later better understood as hypernatremia.

1946 H. E. Harrison and D. C. Darrow
  After consultation with each other, simultaneously introduced scientifically designed oral hydration solutions for prevention of dehydration and for postparenteral maintenance therapy.
1951 H. Wirz, B. Hargitay, and W. Kuhn
  Introduced countercurrent hypothesis for renal concentration of urine solutes.
1952 W. B. Weil and W. M. Wallace; L. Finberg and H. E. Harrison
  Described hypernatremic dehydration in infants.
1950–81
  When trying to sort out the weight of contributions made during the period of one's own career, perspective becomes perilously clouded by proximity.

The direct contributors to pediatric knowledge are more easily identified than those who contributed more general and basic knowledge. In addition to those already mentioned, they include P. Astrup, D. B. Cheek, R. E. Cooke, P. Dodge, G. B. Forbes, B. Friis-Hansen, S. Hellerstein, M. Holliday, E. Kerpel-Fronius, P. Kildeborg, J. Metcoff, E. L. Pratt, W. E. Segar, O. Siggaard-Andersen, J. Sotos, R. Torres-Pinedo, C. D. West, and R. W. Winters.

Indeed, many others working in fields other than pediatrics — such as physiology, biochemistry, internal medicine, and surgery — have contributed much that has been utilized at the bedside and in the clinic and additional important work that has not yet been implemented in clinical settings. From a pediatric perspective, the following investigators stand out among the many such contributors:

A. I. Arieff
R. W. Berliner
D. A. K. Black
C. C. J. Carpenter
F. P. Chinard
E. J. Conway
J. J. Danielli
T. W. Danowski
H. Davson
H. E. deWardener
I. S. Edelman
J. R. Elkington
W. O. Fenn
M. Field
J. S. Fordtran
G. G. Giebish

C. W. Gottschalk
A. B. Hastings
R. M. Hays
J. P. Kassirer
C. R. Kleeman
V. Koefoed-Johnson
A. Leaf
G. N. Ling
R. H. Maffly
J. F. Manery
M. H. Maxwell
R. A. McCance
F. B. Moore
R. A. Philips
R. F. Pitts
R. Podolsky

F. C. Rector
A. Relman
B. M. Schmidt-Nielsen
S. G. Schultz
W. B. Schwartz
D. Seldin
N. B. Shock
H. Smith
A. K. Solomon
H. B. Steinbach
M. B. Strauss
H. Ussing
M. Walser
L. G. Welt
E. M. Widdowson
K. Zierler

The list is necessarily incomplete, and we apologize to those whose names were left off. We think it better to identify most despite the risk of inadvertent offense to a few.

Index

Page numbers in *italics* indicate illustrations; t indicates table.

Acetaminophen, poisoning with, 201t
Acetylsalicylic acid, poisoning with, 201
Acid(s), and bases and electrolytes, 41t
  definition of, 233
Acid-base balance, combined disturbances of,
    treatment of, 101
  renal regulation of, 53, *54*
  respiratory alterations in, *101*
Acidemia, 90
  definition of, 50, 233
  in asthma, 210
  in premature infants, 224
Acidosis, compensatory, 50
  definition of, 50, 233
  dilution, 52
  metabolic, 93–97
    changes in, 101t
    clinical signs of, 94
    mechanisms of, 94t
    therapy for, 95
    with respiratory acidosis, 99
    with respiratory alkalosis, 99
  primary, 50
  respiratory, 90–93
    changes in, 101t
    clinical signs of, 90
    therapy for, 93
    with metabolic acidosis, 99
Addison disease, 173
Adrenal gland, disorders of, electrolyte disturbances
  in, 171–185
Adrenal hemorrhage, 173
Adrenal hyperfunction, 174–176
Adrenal hyperplasia, congenital, 176–183
  results of cortisol therapy in, *179*
Adrenal hypoplasia, congenital, 172
  treatment of, 180t
Adrenal insufficiency, acute, 183
  clinical and biochemical features of, 177t
  in infancy and childhood, 171–172
    causes of, 172t
    clinical manifestations of, 171t
  preparation for surgery in, 181, 182t
Adrenocorticotropic hormone (ACTH), disorders of,
  172
  hereditary adrenocortical unresponsiveness to, 173
  in congenital adrenal hyperplasia, levels of, *181*
Aerosols, in asthma, 208
Albumin, laboratory analysis of, 140
  loss of, edema in, 109

Aldosterone, in regulation of plasma potassium, 59,
  59
  selective deficiency of, 173
Alkalemia, definition of, 50, 233
Alkaline phosphatase, in bone mineralization, 69
Alkalosis, compensatory, 50
  contraction, 52
  definition of, 50, 233
  metabolic, 97–99
    clinical signs of, 98
    mechanisms of, 98
    therapy for, 99
    with respiratory acidosis, 99
    with respiratory alkalosis, 99
  primary, 50
  respiratory, 97
    clinical signs of, 97
    therapy for, 97
Anion gap, definition of, 233
Antidiuretic hormone (ADH), and abnormal water
  loss, 20
  and thirst, 20–21
  in postoperative patient, 229
  in status asthmaticus, 207
  syndrome of inappropriate secretion of (SIADH),
    113, 199
  synthesis of, 20
Anuria, in acute glomerular nephritis, 163–164
  in hypernatremic dehydration, treatment of, 131
Arrhenius S., 243
Arterial puncture, 141
Aspirin poisoning, 201
Asthma, 206–211
  arterial pH in, 210
  carbon dioxide in, 209
  inhaled water in, 207
  oxygen in, 208
  salt requirements in, 207
  water requirements in, 206
Atomic weight, definition of, 233
Azotemia, definition of, 234

Bacterial infections, invasive, as cause of diarrhea,
  149
Bacterial toxin infections, as cause of diarrhea, 150
Bartter syndrome, 199
  hyperaldosteronism in, 176

Base(s), and acids and electrolytes, 41t
  definition of, 234
  excess, determination of, 45–46
Bernard, Claude, 242
Bicarbonate, increase of, in respiratory acidosis, 91
  measurement of, 46
Bicarbonate ion, laboratory analysis of, 137–138
Blood, and water regulation, 32
  arterial, obtaining specimens of, 141
  venous, obtaining specimens of, 142
Blood-brain barrier, *167*
  and Starling hypothesis, *27, 28*
Blood gases, hydrogen ion, and pH, 35–55
  laboratory analysis of, 138–139
Blood urea nitrogen (BUN). See *Serum urea nitrogen
  (SUN)*.
Body fluid(s), composition and chemical anatomy of,
  11–16
  distribution in body of, *11*
  ionic profiles of, *10, 14*
  methods of analysis of, 12
Body fluid spaces, maintenance of, 9–10
Body water compartments, as percentage of body
  weight, *15*
Bohr effect, definition of, 234
Bone, mineralization of, 68
  role in storage of sodium, 58
Bone matrix, 68
Brain, osmotic solutes in, 168
Brain trauma, and hypoxia, 168–169
Bromate salts, poisoning with, 201t
Buffer base, definition of, 234
Buffering, in acid-base imbalance, 51
Burns, evaluation of patient in, 228
Butler, A., 243

Calcitonin, in regulation of calcium, 65
Calcitriol, 63
  in regulation of calcium, 64–65
Calcium, absorption of, 63
  body content of, 62
  homeostasis of, in dehydration, assessment of, 120
  in metabolism and regulation, 62–66
  in premature infants, 224
  ionized, 62
  laboratory analysis of, 139
  loss of, in hypernatremic dehydration, 86
  physiologic role of, 62
  regulatory hormones and, 64–65
  renal regulation of, 63
  requirement and intake of, 63
Caloric expenditure, basal, 18t
Calorie, as unit of energy, 17
  definition of, 234
Campylobacter fetus, as cause of diarrhea, 149
Capillaries, and Starling hypothesis, *25, 26*
  brain, and Starling hypothesis, *27, 28*
  circulatory role of, 25–27
  glomerular, 30
  of lung, and Starling hypothesis, *27, 29*
Carbon dioxide (CO_2). See also PCO_2.
  in asthma, 209
  in blood, 36
  laboratory analysis of, 137–138. See also PCO_2.
  partial pressure of, in lung, 36
    measurement of, 43
  role in acid-base metabolism, 35
  total, measurement of, 44

Carbon dioxide (CO_2) electrode, *43*
Carbon tetrachloride, poisoning with, 201t
Carbonic acid, measurement of, 48–49
Cardiac failure. See *Heart failure*.
Cardiac output, 23
Catheterization, arterial, 141
  venous, 142
Central nervous system (CNS), anatomy and
  physiology of, 167–170
  hemorrhage in, in hypernatremic dehydration, 83,
  84
Cerebrospinal fluid (CSF), electrolytes in, 168
  pressure changes in, effect of glucose infusion on,
  130
  in hypernatremia, 83, 85
Cerebrospinal fluid (CSF)-brain barrier, *167*
Chemical potential, definition of, 234
Chloride, and sodium, laboratory analysis of, 137
  in metabolism and regulation, 59–60
Cholera, as cause of diarrhea, 150
Cholesterol desmolase deficiency, 178
  clinical and biochemical features of, 177t
Circulatory system, and regulation, 23–34
Cirrhosis, 193–194
Colloidal osmotic pressure, definition of, 234
Compensation, metabolic, of acid-base imbalance, 50
Copper sulfate, in total parenteral solutions, 231t
Creatinine, laboratory analysis of, 139
Cushing disease, 174–175
Cyanosis, 39
Cystic fibrosis, 212–216
  electrolytes in secretions in, 213t
  lung, liver, and pancreas in, 212–214
  sweat analysis in, 214

Darrow, D. C., 243
Dehydration, assessment of, 117–120
  clinical evaluation of, 115–120
  clinical history of patient in, 115
  definition of, 234
  diabetic, 196
  examination of patient in, 116
  hypernatremic, 78–89
    epidemiology of, 79
    etiology of, 80
    historical background of, 79
    mild, case history of, 132–133
    moderate, case history of, 131–132
    pathophysiology of, 81–86
    symptoms of, 80–81
    therapeutic management of, 129–135
    therapeutic regimen for, 130t
    with shock, case history of, 133–134
  hyponatremic, 77, 112
    case history of, 125–126
    severe, case history of, 127–128
    therapy for, 121–128
  hypotonic, 77
    effect on blood of, 32
  in gastrointestinal fluid loss, therapy of, 121–128
  in malnutrition, treatment of, 161
  isonatremic, 75–77, *75*
    and hyponatremic, emergency treatment of, 122
      repletion phase in treatment of, 123
    mild, case history of, 126
    therapy for, 121–128
  isotonic, 75–77
    and hyponatremic, 73–77

Dehydration (*Continued*)
  isotonic, treatment schedule for first 24 hours in, 123t
    with enteritis, case history of, 123–125
    with enteritis and vomiting, case history of, 155
  laboratory studies in, 117
  pathogenesis of, 76
  volume assessment in, 117
  water distribution in, 82
Denys, Jean Baptiste, 242
Diabetes insipidus, 198
  nephrogenic, 198–199
Diabetes mellitus, 195–197
Diabetic mothers, infants of, 224–225
Diarrhea, congenital chloride, 151
  dehydration from, 74–75
  drug therapy for, 154
  etiology, epidemiology, and pathogenesis of, 147–151
  general principles of therapy for, 154–155
  in malnutrition, 160
  intractable, of infancy, 151
  mild, in breast-fed infant, case history of, 156
  noninfectious secondary, 151
  noninfectious secretory, 151
  therapy of, 152–156
    case histories in, 155–156
  water losses due to, 19
Diarrheal diseases, of infancy, 147–157
Dielectric constant, definition of, 234
Diet, infant, in heart failure, 190t, 191
Diffusion, 7
  definition of, 234
  facilitated, 9
Digitalis, in heart failure, 188
Diuretics, in heart failure, 188, 188t
  mode of action of, 110–111
Donnan, F. G., 243
Donnan factor, 8
  definition of, 235
Dutrochet, René, 242
Dysentery, bacillary, 149

Edema, definition of, 108
  effect on fluid movement of, 27
  hypervolemic, 109
  hypoproteinemic, 109
  in abnormal water loss, 20
  in cirrhosis, 193
  in heart failure, 108
    relief of, 191
  in hyponatremia, 113
  in portal obstruction, 109
  pathophysiology of, 108–110
Electrolyte(s), and acids and bases, 41t
  and water, in metabolic disorders, 198–200
  content and distribution of, in malnutrition, 159–160
  definition of, 235
  dietary, in heart failure, 189
  in cystic fibrosis, 213t
    analysis of, 214
  in solutions, 143
  in stool water, concentrations of, 75t
  in total parenteral solutions, 231t
  physiology of, and growth and development, 3
    early history of, 2

Electrolyte(s) (*Continued*)
  urinary, during diuresis, 188t
Electrolyte disturbances, in adrenal gland disorders, 171–185
  in poisonings, 201–205
Electrolyte imbalance, in malnutrition, 161
Electrolyte-glucose mixtures, for diarrhea, 153
Energy, requirements in physical activities, 218t
Energy metabolism, 17
Entamoeba histolytica, as cause of diarrhea, 151
Enteric disease, isotonic constriction in, 75
Enteritis, as cause of diarrhea, 149
Enthalpy, definition of, 235
Entropy, definition of, 235
Equilibrium, definition of, 235
  Gibbs-Donnan, 8
Escherichia coli, as cause of diarrhea, 149
  enterotoxigenic, as cause of diarrhea, 150
Evolution, and comparative physiology, 1–2
Exercise, and sports, 217–219
  energy requirements in, 218t
  effects of, 218
Extracellular fluids (ECF), chloride in, 59–60
  definition of, 235
  in beginnings of life, 1
  measurement of, 13
  organic molecules in, effects on physiology of, 71–72
  osmols in, 82, 83
    in hypernatremia, 83
Extracellular water, as percentage of body weight, 15, 16t

Fanconi syndrome, 199
Fetus, normal physiology of, 220–221
Fetus and neonate, special problems of, 220–225
Fibrosis, cystic, 212–216. See also *Cystic fibrosis*.
Fick, A., 242
Fick principle, in cardiac output, 23
Fick's equation of diffusion, definition of, 235
Fluid(s), administration of, 143
  extracellular (ECF). See *Extracellular fluid*.
  interstitial and intracellular, ionic profiles of, 10
Fluid deficit, in dehydration, assessment of, 117
Fluid loss, gastrointestinal, therapy of dehydration in, 121–128
Fluid therapy, early history of, 2–3

Galactosemia, 200
Gamble, J. L., 243
Gastrointestinal tract, physiological aspects of, 25
Giardia lamblia, as cause of diarrhea, 151
Gibbs, J. W., 242
Gibbs-Donnan equilibrium, 8
  definition of, 235
Gibbs free energy, definition of, 235
Globulin, laboratory analysis of, 140
Glomerular membrane, 30
Glossary, definitional, 233–239
Glucocorticoids, characteristics of, 180t
  enzymatic deficiencies of, 174
Gluconeogenesis, in diabetes mellitus, 195
Glucose, 72
  changes in level of, in hypernatremia, 86
  in diabetes mellitus, 195

Glucose (*Continued*)
  in treatment of diarrhea, 152
  laboratory analysis of, 140
  solutions of, 143
Glucose-electrolyte solutions, for malnutrition, 161
Graham, Thomas, 242
Growth and development, and changes in electrolyte
  physiology, 3

Harrison, H. E., 244
Hartmann, A. F., 243
Harvey, Thomas, 241
Hasselbalch, A. K., 243
Heart, physiologic and metabolic aspects of, 23–25
Heart failure, 25, 186–192
  edema in, 108
  therapy for, 187–191
Heat loss, body, 17
Hemoglobin, oxygen concentrations in, 38
Hemoglobin concentration, mean corpuscular
  (MCHC), and osmolality, 32, 33
Hemorrhage, CNS, in hypernatremic dehydration,
  83, *84*
Henderson, L. J., 243
Henderson-Hasselbalch equation, 40
  definition of, 236
Hippocrates, 241
Historical highlights, 241–244
Howland, J., 243
Humidification, in asthma, 208
Hydration, water distribution before and after, 82
Hydration problems, in renal disorders, therapy for,
  163–166
Hydrogen ion, control of levels of, 52–54
Hydrogen ion concentration, and pH, measurement
  of, 41
  relationship to pH of, 42
Hydrogen ion disturbance, in dehydration, assessment of, 119
  pathophysiology of, 90–107
Hydrogen ion metabolism, changes in, in hypernatremia, 86
11-Hydroxylase deficiency, 179
  clinical and biochemical features of, 177t
  treatment of, 179
17α-Hydroxylase deficiency, 178
  clinical and biochemical features of, 177t
21α-Hydroxylase deficiency, 178
  clinical and biochemical features of, 177t
  treatment of, 179
3β-Hydroxysteroid dehydrogenase (3β-HSD)
  deficiency, 178
  clinical and biochemical features in, 177t
Hyperaldosteronism, 175–176
  causes of, 175t
Hypercalcemia, 66
Hypercapnia, 40
Hypercortisolism, 174–175
Hypermagnesemia, 68
Hypernatremia, definition of, 78
  histologic appearance of, 87
  in dehydration, 78–89
  neonatal, 222
  pathology of, 86–87
Hyperosmolality, effect on blood of, 32
Hyperparathyroidism, in hypercalcemia, 66
Hypervolemia, edema in, 109

Hypoaldosteronism, selective, 173
Hypocalcemia, 65–66
Hypomagnesemia, 68
Hyponatremia, dehydration in, 112
  emergency treatment of, 122
  dilutional, 113
  edema in, 113
  in infection, 113–114
  in malnutrition, 114
  in SIADH, 113
  neonatal, 222
  pathophysiology of, 112–114
Hypophosphatemia, 67
  in diabetes mellitus, 197
Hypoproteinemia, edema in, 109
Hypoxia, and brain trauma, 168–169
  physiological aspects of, 40

Idiogenic osmols, 81–82
Immunodeficiency disease, as cause of diarrhea, 151
Infant formula, content of, 190t
Infection, hyponatremia in, 113–114
Interstitial fluid, composition of, 15
  volume of, 15
Intracellular fluid (ICF), composition of, 15
  measurement of, 14
Intracellular water, as percentage of body weight, *15*,
  16t
Ion(s), and equilibria, 7–8
  skeletal, in dehydration, assessment of, 120
Ion losses, intracellular, in dehydration, assessment
  of, 119
Ion mixture 25–25, for hypernatremic dehydration,
  154t
Ion mixture 75–15 (rehydration), 153t
Ion mixture 49–20, in treatment of diarrhea, 152t
Irritants, noninfectious, as cause of diarrhea, 151
Isotonic constriction, in enteric disease, 75

Kidney, action of diuretics in, 110–111
  excretion of potassium in, 58
  excretion of sodium in, 57
  physiological aspects of, 27–32
  role in water metabolism, 19
Kidney disease, edema in, 109
  hydration problems in, therapy for, 163–166
Kussmaul, A., 242
Kwashiorkor, 158–162

Laboratory analyses, interpretation of, 136–140
Latta, Thomas, 242
Law of mass action, 44
Lead, poisoning with, 201t
Lean body mass (LBM), in infant, body fluids in, *11*
Liddle syndrome, 200
Liver, in cystic fibrosis, 212
Liver disease, edema in, 109
Liver failure, problems in, 193–194
Lower, Richard, 242
Lung, capillaries of, and Starling hypothesis, 27, *29*
  in cystic fibrosis, 212

Magnesium, absorption of, 68
  in metabolism and regulation, 68
  laboratory analysis of, 139
Malnutrition, 158–162
  effects of disease in, 160–161
  effects of treatment in, 161–162
  electrolyte content and distribution in, 159–160
  hyponatremia in, 114
  protein-calorie, 158
  water content, distribution, and turnover in, 158–159
Manganese sulfate, in total parenteral solutions, 231t
Marasmus, 158–162
Marriot, W. M., 243
Membranes, permeability of, 7
Meninges, infections of, 169
Meningitis, bacterial, 169
  tuberculous, 169–170
Mercury, poisoning with, 201t
Metabolic disorders, water and electrolytes in, 198–200
Milk, in infant feeding, electrolyte content of, 190t
Mineralocorticoids, characteristics of, 180t
  enzymatic deficiencies of, *174*

Neonatal disorders, 221–225
Neonate, normal physiology of, 220–221
Nephritis, acute glomerular, and acute renal failure, 163–164
Nephron, permeability of, 31t
  physiological aspects of, *30*, 31
  sites of diuretic action in, *110*
Nephrotic syndrome, 164–165
Nernst equation, definition of, 236
Nitrogen, partial pressure of, 35
  in lung, 36
  serum urea (SUN), laboratory analysis of, 139
Nollet, Jean, 242
Nutrition, total parenteral, 230–232
    complications of, 232t
    solutions in, 231, 231t

Oliguria, in acute glomerular nephritis, 163–164
  in chronic renal failure, 165
Oncotic pressure, 9
Ondine's curse, 199
Orthohydroxybenzoate poisoning, 201
O'Shaughnessy, W. B., 242
Osmol production, idiogenic, 81, 82, 83
Osmolality, and hemoglobin concentration, 32, *33*
  definition of, 237
  in dehydration, assessment of, 118
Osmosis, 8
Osmotic pressure equation, definition of, 237
Ostwald, W., 243
Oxygen, in asthma, 208
  in blood, 36
  in heart failure, 187
  partial pressure of, 35
    in lung, 36
    measurement of, 44
  role in acid-base metabolism, 35
Oxyhemoglobin dissociation curve, 38, *39*

Pancreas, in cystic fibrosis, 212
Paralysis, periodic, 200
Parasitic diseases, as cause of diarrhea, 151
Parathyroid hormone (PTH), in hypocalcemia, 66t
  in regulation of calcium, 64
Parenteral nutrition, total, 230–232
Parvoviruses, as cause of diarrhea, 149
PCO_2, in asthma, 208
  in exercise, 219
  in premature infants, 223
  laboratory analysis of, 138
Permeability, and transport, 8–9
  of membranes, 7
Pfeffer, W. F. P., 242
pH, and hydrogen ion concentration, measurement of, 41
  arterial, in asthma, 210
  in acid-base balance, 40–41
  laboratory analysis of, 138
  regulation of, 52–54
  relationship to hydrogen ion concentration, 42
Phosphate, in metabolism, 67
Phosphorus, in metabolism and regulation, 66–68
  laboratory analysis of, 139
  normal levels, at various ages, 139t
  renal regulation of, 67
  requirement and intake of, 67
Physiology, comparative, and evolution, 1–2
  electrolyte, and growth and development, 3
    early history of, 2–3
Plasma, composition of, 14
  volume of, 12
    measurement of, 14
Plasma proteins, 71–72
PO_2, in asthma, 208
  in exercise, 219
P_AO_2, in alveolar air equation, 36, *37*
Poiseuille, J. L. M., 242
Poiseuille flow, definition of, 238
Poiseuille-Hagan equation, 24
Poisonings, electrolyte problems in, 201–205
Poisons, common, effects on fluid and electrolyte metabolism, 201t
Portal obstruction, edema in, 109
Potassium, body content of, 58
  excretion and regulation of, 58
  in diabetes mellitus, 195
  in metabolism and regulation, 58–59
  laboratory analysis of, 138
  plasma, control of, 59
  requirements and intake of, 58
Powers, G. P., 243
Prematurity, special problems of, 223–224
Pressure, oncotic, 9
Proteins, plasma, 71–72
    in oncotic pressure, 9
  total serum, laboratory analysis of, 140
Pseudohyperaldosteronism, 200
Pseudohypoaldosteronism, 174, 199–200

Rapoport, S., 243
Rehydration, in malnutrition, 161
  in treatment of diarrhea, 152
Rehydration Solution, Oral (ORS), 153t
Renal clearance, definition of, 238
Renal disorders, hydration problems in, therapy for, 163–166

Renal failure, acute, and acute glomerular nephritis, 163–164
  chronic, 165–166
  edema in, 109
Renal tubule, bicarbonate-carbonic acid-carbon dioxide equilibrium system in, 52
Renin, in regulation of plasma potassium, 59
Renin-angiotensin-aldosterone system, in regulation of sodium, 58
Rotaviruses, as cause of diarrhea, 148

Salicylate, plasma concentrations of, and degree of intoxication, *202*
Salicylate (orthohydroxybenzoate) poisoning, 201–205
  acute, 203
  chronic, 204
Saline, normal, definition of, 237
Saline solution, hypertonic, changes produced by, *144*
Salmonella, as cause of diarrhea, 149
Salt, in cystic fibrosis, 215
  requirements in asthma, 207
  requirements in exercise, 217
Salt poisoning, case history of, 134–135
  in hypernatremic dehydration, treatment of, 131
Sanctorius, 241
Schloss, O. M., 243
Schmidt, Carl, 242
Secretions, gastrointestinal, composition and volume of, *74*
Sellards, A. W., 243
Serum urea nitrogen (SUN), laboratory analysis of, 139
Sex hormones, enzymatic deficiencies of, *174*
Shigella, as cause of diarrhea, 149
Shock, in hypernatremic dehydration, treatment of, 131
  with hypernatremic dehydration, case history of, 133–134
Siggaard-Andersen alignment nomogram, in acid-base metabolism, 46, *47*
  in complicated acid-base disturbances, *102, 105, 106*
  in respiratory acidosis, 92
Skeleton, role in sodium storage, 58
Sodium, and chloride, laboratory analysis of, 137
  body content of, 56
  disturbances of, neonatal, 222
  effect on distribution of body fluids, 12
  excess, in dehydration, 78–89
  excretion of, 57
  in dehydration, assessment of levels of, 119
  in metabolism and regulation, 56–58
  in treatment of diarrhea, 153
  regulation of, 57–58
  requirements and intake of, 56
  restriction of, in heart failure, 191
Sodium deprivation, 113
Sodium loss, in dehydration, 77
Sodium phosphate, poisoning with, 201t, 205
Sodium/potassium ATPase, in active transport system, 10
"Sodium pump," 10
Solutions, administration of, 143
  and techniques, 141–145
  commercially prepared, 143

Solutions (*Continued*)
  hypertonic saline, changes produced by, *144*
  thermodynamics of, 6
Solvent drag, 10
Sorenson, S. P. L., 243
Sports, and exercise, 217–219
Staphylococcus aureus, as cause of diarrhea, 150
Starling, E. H., 243
Starling hypothesis, and blood-brain barrier, 27, 28
  in lung capillary, 27, *29*
  of capillary action, 25, *26*
Status asthmaticus, antidiuretic hormone in, 207
Steroid therapy, withdrawal of, in adrenal insufficiency, 182
Surgical patients, intraoperative management of, 228
  postoperative management of, 229
  preoperative management of, 226
  special problems of, 226–232
Sweat, analysis of, in cystic fibrosis, 214
Sweating, excessive, in cystic fibrosis, pathophysiology of, 215
  water losses from, 19

Taurine, as idiogenic osmol, 81–83
Theophylline, in heart failure, 189
Thermodynamics, laws of, 238
  of solutions, 6
Thirst, and antidiuretic hormone (ADH), 20–21
Thirst center, absence of, 199
Total body water (TBW), as percentage of body weight, *15*, 16t
  measurement of, 13
Transport, active, 9
  coupled, 10
Tuberculous meningitis, chloride of CSF in, 114
Tumors, as cause of diarrhea, 151

Undernutrition, 158–162
Urea, 72
  in urine, role of, 32
Urine, water loss in, 18

Van Slyke, D. D., 243
van't Hoff, J. H., 242
van't Hoff's law, 8
Vibrio cholerae, as cause of diarrhea, 150
Viral infections, as cause of diarrhea, 148
Vitamins, in total parenteral solutions, 231t
Vomiting, water losses due to, 20

Water, and electrolytes, in metabolic disorders, 198–200
  as percent of body, 11
  body, in malnutrition, 158–159
  inhaled, in asthma, 207
  molecular physics of, 6
  of oxidation, definition of, 239
  requirements in asthma, 206
  requirements in exercise, 217
  restriction of, in heart failure, 191

Water (*Continued*)
 structure and properties of, 5–7
 thermodynamics of, 6
 transcellular, 12
Water intoxication, *130*
Water losses, abnormal, 19–20
 in urine, 18
 insensible, 18
 obligatory, 18–19
Water metabolism regulation, 17–22
Water vapor, in air, partial pressure of, 35

Weed, Lewis H., 243
Weil, W. B., 244
Wirz, H., 244

Yersinia enterocolitica, as cause of diarrhea, 149

Zinc sulfate, in total parenteral solutions, 231t